Foundations
of
NURSING
THEORY

Notes on Nursing Theories

SERIES EDITORS

Chris Metzger McQuiston
Doctoral Candidate, Wayne State University

Adele A. Webb
College of Nursing, University of Akron

Notes on Nursing Theories is a series of monographs designed to provide the reader with a concise description of conceptual frameworks and theories in nursing. Each monograph includes a biographical sketch of the theorist, origin of the theory, assumptions, concepts, propositions, examples for application to practice and research, a glossary of terms, and a bibliography of classic works, critiques, and research.

All monographs are available for individual purchase.

Foundations of
NURSING THEORY

Contributions of 12 Key Theorists

Edited by
Chris Metzger McQuiston
Adele A. Webb

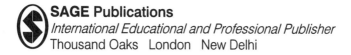
SAGE Publications
International Educational and Professional Publisher
Thousand Oaks   London   New Delhi

For information address:

SAGE Publications, Inc.
2455 Teller Road
Thousand Oaks, California 91320

SAGE Publications Ltd.
6 Bonhill Street
London EC2A 4PU
United Kingdom

SAGE Publications India Pvt. Ltd.
M-32 Market
Greater Kailash I
New Delhi 110 048 India

Printed in the United States of America

Library of Congress Cataloging-in-Publication Data

Main entry under title:

Foundations of nursing theory: Contributions of 12 key theorists /
    edited by Chris Metzger McQuiston, Adele A. Webb.
        p. cm.
    Includes bibliographical references and index.
    ISBN 0-8039-7136-2 (cl). — ISBN 0-8039-7137-0 (pb.)
    1. Nursing—Philosophy. 2. Nursing models. I. McQuiston, Chris
Metzger. II. Webb, Adele A.
    [DNLM: 1. Nursing Theory.   WY 86 F771 1995]
RT84-5F68 1995
610.73′01—dc 20
DNLM/DLC
for Library of Congress   94-37205

            97 98 99 10 9 8 7 6 5 4 3

Production Editor: Astrid Virding
Copy Editor: Joyce Kuhn   Typesetter: Christina Hill

Contents

Foreword

Given birth by Florence Nightingale, the rich body of theoretical works now available in nursing represents a coming of age. Viewed together, the writings of nurse theorists spanning more than 100 years, show a pattern of evolution and a resulting maturity that provides a solid foundation for nursing practice; a foundation worthy of modern challenges. Knowledge of this volume of theoretical work has the potential of enabling nurses to develop a critical self-consciousness regarding the underpinnings and ramifications of their practice. Such an understanding, developed among a broad base of nurses, coupled with reflection on current nursing practice, creates the possibility for further enrichment and expansion of the theory development movement. *Foundations of Nursing Theory* represents the authors' efforts to make these ideas more accessible to the nursing community. These ideas are the rightful inheritance of every contemporary nurse. We seek to provide you access to this wealth.

Foundations of Nursing Theory is an organized collection of 12 monographs which include: Nightingale's visionary understanding of the affects of the environment on patient's well-being, Betty Neuman's systems approach with prevention as an intervention, Parse's simultaneity paradigm, Patterson and Zderad's humanistic nursing, Leininger's cultural care and universality, Orlando's nurse-patient process. We have also included: Peplau's interpersonal focus, Margaret Newman's expanding consciousness, Orem's self-care agency and self-care, Rogers's human energy fields, Roy's patients as bio-psycho-social beings, and King's goal attainment. In each part the author discusses the origin of the theorist's ideas, the presumptions she used in developing the theory, and implications of these assumptions. Each nurse theorists' conceptual model represents a different view of nursing. Some of the views are complimentary such as Margaret Newman and Martha Rogers. Clear threads are traceable from Peplau to Orlando. Others such as Leininger chart completely new and separate ground.

Foundations of Nursing Theory offers glimpses of different paradigms, or world views. This sampling should allow you to more easily examine various theories, better enabling you to reflect on your view of nursing care. *Foundations of Nursing Theory* was designed to support your creative thinking around serious nursing questions. How could nursing theory relate to and guide your research? What are its implications for your real world practice? Only in answering these basic questions do the nursing theories presented here have value.

The **Notes on Nursing Theories** series was originally designed to make theory more accessible to students. The premise behind the books is that a clear, basic understanding of these sometimes complex and difficult theories would lead students to access and appreciate the original works. It was further hoped that an appreciation for nursing theory would perpetuate its use in practice and research, and further theory development.

Foundations of Nursing Theory is not an inclusive collection of nursing theory, nor was it meant to be. Instead it is a collection chosen because of historical significance or diversity in thinking which mirrors the diverse views of nurses.

Chris Metzger McQuiston
Adele Webb

PART I

Martha Rogers
The Science of Unitary Human Beings

LOUETTE R. JOHNSON LUTJENS

Biographical Sketch of a Scientist in Nursing: Martha E. Rogers, ScD, RN, FAAN

Born: May 12, 1914, Dallas, TX

Diploma: Knoxville General Hospital School of Nursing, TN, 1936

BS: Public Health Nursing, George Peabody College, TN, 1937

MA: Teachers College, Columbia University, NY, 1945

MPH: Johns Hopkins University, Baltimore, MD, 1952

ScD: Johns Hopkins University, Baltimore, MD, 1954

Fellow: American Academy of Nursing

Position: Professor Emerita, Division of Nursing, New York University; consultant, speaker

Foreword

Conceptual models are representations of the universe; therefore, one's perception of reality relates to the particular model used. Rogers's Science of Unitary Human Beings is a particular lens with which to view the universe, whereby a reality is created that requires specific beliefs about the relationships of human beings and their environments. The broad generalizations of the Science of Unitary Human Beings enable nurses to peer into the wholeness of the universe and to be creative and imaginative in their participation in the emerging science of wholeness.

The Science of Unitary Human Beings presents a framework for the construction of theories to understand the pattern of the wholeness of reality. The broad generalizations and theories guide perceptions in the way people think and what they look for in phenomena and their relationships. Through such a process, nursing science advances through the generation of *nursing* knowledge. This knowledge of the wholeness of human beings is necessary to help people participate knowingly in unfolding their potentials.

This section is a tribute to Martha E. Rogers. It whets one's appetite to go to her original writings to comprehend the details of her prophetic vision, especially how it participated in the shaping of the science of nursing. The author accomplishes this through a succinct presentation that synthesizes the major ideas in Rogers's writings.

The author swiftly leads the reader along a path of enlightenment of Rogers's science through concise writing. This intellectual journey includes the current thinking of Rogers, where effective use of figures and tables highlights major structural characteristics. The importance of this journey is recognized through demonstrating that nursing is concerned with the *to know* rather than just the *to do*, signifying that a scientific body of knowledge is required.

A specific example illustrates the use of the Science of Unitary Human Beings in a clinical situation, where the enigma of health is clarified from a Rogerian perspective. Rogers's futuristic perspectives are synthesized to illustrate how health and human potentials need to be viewed differently.

The unfolding of Rogers's science does not end but continues in her theories. The author shows briefly that the thoughts and paths of other nurse theorists have as their wellspring Rogers's Science of Unitary Human Beings.

This section is a testament that nurses in the future will resonate with the rhythms of Rogers's vision. Rogerian scholars will have the joy of being the "hundredth monkey" in the advancement of nursing science within a science of wholeness.

JOHN R. PHILLIPS, RN, PHD
Associate Professor,
Division of Nursing
School of Education, Health,
Nursing, and Arts Professions
New York University

Preface

Dr. Martha E. Rogers presented an evolutionary model of humans in *An Introduction to the Theoretical Basis of Nursing* (1970). Her view of nursing as a science of unitary human beings pioneered a radical shift in thinking within the profession.

The Science of Unitary Human Beings challenges traditional ways of thinking about the world and about nursing. This new worldview, characterized by energy fields, continuous mutual change in humans and their environment, no causality, and a reality unbounded by space and time, is called an abstract system by Rogers. This abstract system is science and not to be confused with the more commonly used terms of conceptual model or theory (Rogers, personal communication, November 11, 1990). The terms used in the Science of Unitary Human Beings are unique to the abstract system. The two common reactions of students to this abstract system are either one of immediate bonding with Rogers's way of thinking or one of disregard because her science is viewed as too abstract to be useful in nursing practice. Most would agree that the ideas put forth by Martha Rogers are exciting.

There are many nurse scholars who conduct research and practice based on Rogers's abstract system. They have formed the Society of Rogerian Scholars, which holds conferences and publishes the *Rogerian Nursing Science Newsletter*. Also, many doctoral students at New York University (where Rogers is Professor Emerita) and other universities in the United States and other countries use the Science of Unitary Human Beings for their dissertation research. This science also serves as the basis for programs in nursing education and practice and administrative decision making in nursing service.

Martha Rogers, as one of the foremost thinkers in nursing today, serves as an inspiration to faculty as well as students. She continues to develop her science based on research and new thinking. The evolutionary nature of her abstract system is apropos to a view of humans as forever changing and evolving. The ongoing development of the Science of Unitary Human Beings challenges students of nursing theory to keep current. Examples of the continuing development of this science are described throughout Part I.

In her early writings, Rogers used the term *man;* thus quotes from her writings prior to 1983 use the term *man* rather than *human beings.* The change in words was an update to reflect sensitivity to the goal of gender-free language.

This section presents a current, succinct description of Rogers's abstract system. The objective of this description is a basic understanding of a nontraditional worldview and the role of the nurse based on that worldview. Serving as a summary of the abstract system, this section supplements original sources, most recently a chapter in Barrett's (1990) book. Moreover, the latest thinking of Dr. Rogers, which was gleaned from conversations between Dr. Rogers and the author in November 1990, is incorporated herein.

This section is intended primarily for undergraduate students who are studying several conceptual models, theories, and the Science of Unitary Human Beings with their differing terms, language, and specific definitions of common concepts. It also could be used as a review by nurse faculty and graduate students.

Although several theories have been generated from this abstract system, they are not addressed herein. The abstract nature and/or scope of these theories demand individual attention.

A bibliography is provided to direct readers to appropriate sources for in-depth information on the Rogers abstract system, theories derived from this science, nursing practice based on this abstract system, applications to practice and education, and analysis and critique of the abstract system. It is hoped that this description of Rogers's Science of Unitary Human Beings will entice readers to make use of the references provided in the bibliography.

I would like to acknowledge the careful and thoughtful critique by Dr. Barbara Girardin of California State University, San Diego, California. Special thanks also to Dr. Martha Rogers for her review and comments on an earlier draft. She is indeed inspirational.

—LOUETTE R. JOHNSON LUTJENS

1

Evolution of
the Abstract System

The evolution of the Science of Unitary Human Beings began 30 years ago with the early writings of Dr. Martha E. Rogers. The development of her abstract system was strongly influenced by an early grounding in the liberal arts and an educational background in science at the University of Tennessee (1931-1933) that began two years before she entered nursing school. Her interest in space began with a fascination for air travel as a small child.

In the 1960s, Rogers advocated nursing science as unique and essential in realizing nursing's contribution to human science. For Rogers, the uniqueness of nursing as a science is its long-established concern and interest in people and their world. The Science of Unitary Human Beings was not derived from other sciences, but, rather, originated as a synthesis (not a summation) of facts and ideas from multiple sources of knowledge; a new product. The uniqueness is in the phenomena central to its concern: people and their environment. As defined in this abstract system, the uniqueness of nursing is its focus on unitary human beings and their world.

An abstract system of mutuality generates no causality (acausality). A Rogerian view of acausality emerges from an infinite universe of open systems. Cause and effect are contradictions of open systems. Similar findings with regard to acausality have been reported in the physical world. Specifically, these findings include Heisenberg's principle of uncertainty, quantum theory, and Einstein's theory of relativity, to name but a few. Thus any words implying linear or causal relationships (e.g., cause, effect, adaptation, sequence, influence) are inconsistent with a Rogerian viewpoint. In earlier writings, Rogers used such terms as *continuum* and *unidirectional.* These linear words have been deleted in later writings to correct earlier misinterpretations.

The Science of Unitary Human Beings provides a world view of a universe that is beyond our current understanding or familiarity. It includes possibilities for the future and recognizes change as basic to existence. The aim of the Science of Unitary Human Beings is to advance nursing as a learned profession, both the science and art of nursing (Rogers, 1990). As a learned profession, the art and science of nursing could be empowered to provide compassionate service to humankind now and "spacekind" in the future. The purpose of nurses is "to promote health and well-being for all persons and groups wherever they are" (Rogers, personal communication, November 11, 1990). (A Rogerian view of health is discussed later.)

Rogers identifies and uses the word *nursing* as a noun, a learned profession. This new view differs from the traditional use of nursing as a verb or action word. Rogers's abstract system of Science of Unitary Human Beings, which was formally proposed in 1970, established her as a vanguard of a new view and vision of nursing. Her futuristic perspective is unrivaled.

Assumptions

Assumptions are givens—statements assumed to be true without proof. In *An Introduction to the Theoretical Basis of Nursing,* Rogers (1970) put forth five assumptions that underlie her science of nursing. However, it must be recognized that this book was published 25 years ago and that the Science of Unitary Human Beings has developed substantially over the past 25 years based on research and new thinking. Therefore, the 1970 book contains terms and language that have been replaced with terminology consistent with emerging knowledge and the development of Rogerian science (Rogers, personal communication, November 11, 1990). However, *An Introduction to the Theoretical Basis of Nursing* is considered a seminal text of historical significance. It put forth a new world view of nursing as a discipline by declaring it a science.

2

Building Blocks
of the Abstract System

As Rogers worked on the development of her abstract system, it became necessary that she become more specific. Energy fields, openness, pandimensionality, and pattern have been identified as building blocks of her abstract system (Table 2.1). These building blocks, which correspond to contemporary knowledge, have been used to develop a language of specificity for the Science of Unitary Human Beings. This science was developed to address nursing's long-held concern with persons and their environment, specifically their health.

At the time of the initial development of the Science of Unitary Human Beings, systems theory was among the many schools of thought that had a bearing on general thinking, the major features of that model being the system (unitary human being) and its environment in a mutual process that is active and dynamic. Rogers refers to a universe of open systems, and her view of systems proposes a mutual process of change in human beings and environment that is continuous. Human beings and their environments are defined as energy fields.

TABLE 2.1 The Building Blocks of the Abstract System

Energy Fields
Openness
Pandimensionality
Pattern

Energy Fields

Energy fields are "the fundamental units of the living and the non-living" (Rogers, 1990, p. 7). This is a notion that is different for those who learned that the cell was the fundamental unit of living systems, such as human beings. Field is the concept that unites humans and their environments. Energy signifies the dynamism of the human and environmental fields. Fields are infinite, in continuous motion, and always changing mutually; in essence, they are without boundaries.

Person. According to Rogers, people and their environments are the phenomena central to the focus of nursing. Human beings are wholes, not merely collections of body parts (heart, lungs) or body systems (cardiovascular, neurological). Wholeness is irreducible.

The notion of wholeness is becoming more commonplace. Recently, an exhibition of Monet serial paintings was held at art institutes across the United States. Guided tours were available on audiotapes. At one point the narrator advised patrons to stand back from the individual paintings and look at the series as a whole. This would provide a perspective of the series collection as a whole that was different than the sum of the individual paintings. Rogers's human energy fields, viewed as a whole, provide a perspective that is also irreducible and indivisible, manifesting characteristics specific to the whole. A Rogerian would not discuss or study a part of a human being since doing so would be a contradiction of wholeness.

Human beings have "the capacity for abstraction and imagery, language and thought, sensation and emotion" (Rogers, 1970, p. 73). They have the ability to perceive the universe and wonder about it. Unique human energy fields are differentiated by pattern just as fingerprints or voice prints are unique to individuals.

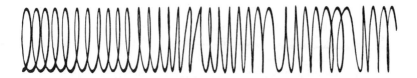

Figure 2.1. Rogers used a Slinky to illustrate the openness and rhythmical nature of the life process.
NOTE: Slinky,® James Industries Inc., Hollidayburg, PA. Used by permission.

Environment. The environmental field is also a whole with its own identity and is also irreducible, indivisible, and differentiated by pattern. Human and environmental energy fields are integral with one another. The mutual process of the energy fields is observed in manifestations of pattern. Martha Rogers uses the analogy of an overlay to help others understand the integrality of the fields (Rogers, personal communication, November 11, 1990). When a transparent image is laid over another image the two images are united and thus integral.

Openness

The integrality of human and environmental energy fields is possible because both are open systems. Openness between human beings and their environment is continuous—that is, they are *always* open. Energy is in continuous movement. In *An Introduction to the Theoretical Basis of Nursing*, Rogers used a Slinky as a symbol of openness and the rhythmical nature of the life process (Figure 2.1). She used the Slinky initially as an aid to thinking. Although she no longer sees a need to use a Slinky to illustrate her point (Rogers, 1990), it is a useful symbol for students learning the Science of Unitary Human Beings.

Human and environmental energy fields evolve and continuously change at the same time. Through the continuous process of humans and their environment, people are different today than they were yesterday. Therefore, human beings can *never* go back. One never walks the same stream twice. The person is different and so is the stream (Rogers, Doyle, Racolin, & Walsh, 1990). Human beings do not adapt to their environment; they are integral with their environment. For that reason, the environment cannot cause something to happen to humans. "Causality is a contradiction of open systems" (Rogers, 1988, p. 100). Rogers asserted (personal communication, November 11, 1990) that adaptation, causality, equilibrium, homeostasis, and similar terms have been outmoded since the 1950s because they are unsupported in a universe of open systems.

Pandimensionality

Human beings are unique energy fields that cannot be divided or reduced. The human field is integral with its unique environmental field, which also cannot be divided or reduced. Both fields have infinite dimensions. Because we live in a three-dimensional reality, we understand it, but that does not mean that there are no other realities. We have limited our thinking to the traditional three-dimensional world view. In earlier writings, Rogers used the term *four-dimensionality* to define a reality without spatial or temporal attributes. As her abstract system continued to develop, it became increasingly clear that four-dimensionality was not consistent with the definition that had emerged, and multidimensionality (Rogers, 1990) was substituted for four-dimensionality for a brief time. These two terms are now viewed as misnomers and have been replaced by *pandimensionality*, which better corresponds with the definition of a nonlinear domain without spatial and temporal attributes. The term refers to a reality that is different than a three-dimensional world view. Pandimensionality is a new reality, a way of perceiving that is a new and different way to view the world. Paranormal events, such as déjà vu, clairvoyance, and other phenomena, can be explained with Rogers's view of pandimensional reality, unique human energy fields united with their unique environment in an infinite domain.

Pattern

Human energy fields can be differentiated from their environmental energy fields by pattern. Pattern is an abstraction that cannot be seen; however, manifestations of a pattern can be observed. The pattern is in the form of a single wave. Field patterns demonstrate increasing variation and continual change. Therefore, the field patterns are unpredictable, dynamic, creative, and continuously innovative.

Manifestions of pattern unite humans and environments in the variations in their patterns. They represent expressions of the unique relationship of individual human beings and their environment. Manifestations of patterns can be observed in a manner similar to looking into a kaleidoscope to see continually changing patterns brought about by unique relationships among bits of colored glass and reflecting surfaces. As the instrument is rotated, similar to the passage of time, there is constant change, continuous variations in form, revealing new, creative, and innovative manifestations of pattern. Some of the changes are subtle, but the observed patterns are *never* the same. There is order to the display, but it contains variations, differences, and a uniqueness with each rotation of the kaleidoscope.

In humans, patterns are abstractions that display themselves as nonrepeating rhythms in human behavior, such as sleep and waking and perceptions of time and motion. In Rogers's earlier writings, the manifestations of field patterning were called correlates. Pattern manifestation signifies mutual process of human and environmental energy fields. This process occurs continually in infinite dimensions. Manifestations of the diversity in field patterning can be seen in, for example, perceptions of time. One person may experience a day as very long, while another may talk about how the day just flew by. It is not uncommon for a person to think that it takes longer to get someplace than to come home from that place though the distance is the same. It should be clear that the evidence or manifestation of human field patterns is specific to the whole person, not just to one of the parts. For example, as Rogers's abstract system clarifies nursing, it would be inappropriate to treat only a part of the whole person, such as the cardiovascular system of a patient. However, you could facilitate comfort during chest pain with guided imagery and observe the change in the duration of chest pain. Rogers views human bodies as manifestations of field. This view of humans and the purpose of nurses is distinct to Rogers's abstract system.

Nursing is also concerned with groups. Two or more people constitute a group, which is its own energy field, integral with its own unique environmental field. Nurses must decide whether they are going to focus on a group energy field, such as family, community, or mother/baby dyad, or an individual energy field, such as family member, community member, mother, or baby (Rogers, 1990). Group energy fields, like human energy fields, are irreducible and indivisible. Therefore, information about group members does not provide information about the group or vice versa. In other words, one cannot generalize from a part (individual group member) to a whole (group). The focus of nursing on human beings and their world as wholes as defined by the Science of Unitary Human Beings is unique to nursing.

3

Nursing

Nursing is a learned profession—that is, it is a science and an art (Rogers, 1990). "Nursing is the study of unitary, irreducible, indivisible human and environmental [energy] fields" (p. 6). It is an organized body of abstract knowledge about people and their world. The art of nursing involves the imaginative and creative use of nursing knowledge (science). The purpose of nurses is to promote health and well-being for all persons and groups wherever they are using the art and science of nursing. Rogers emphasizes that health (versus sickness) services should be community based. Sickness services are traditional to health care settings. Thus Rogers challenges nurses to consider the nursing needs of all people, including future generations of spacekind, as life continues to evolve from earth to space and beyond. The Science of Unitary Human Beings provides a different world view that encompasses a practice of nursing for the present time and for the imagined and yet-to-be imagined future. Rogers envisions a nursing practice of noninvasive modalities, such as therapeutic touch (Krieger, 1979; Quinn, 1989), humor, guided imagery (Butcher & Parker, 1988), use of color, light (Girardin, 1990), music, and meditation focusing on the health potential of the person.

4

Principles of Homeodynamics

The Science of Unitary Human Beings has generated three principles of homeodynamics that provide a foundation for nursing practice: integrality, resonancy and helicy (Table 4.1). These principles provide "fundamental guides to the practice of nursing" (Rogers, 1990, p. 8). The four building blocks (energy field, openness, pandimensionality, pattern) previously described are evident in the principles of Rogers's science and propose a view of change as evolutionary. All of the principles of homeodynamics are characterized by continuous change.

Integrality

The principle of integrality states that human and environmental fields are a continuous and mutual process. The two fields are open systems integral with one another. Use of such terms as simultaneous, changing together, and exchange, to name a few, would be incongruent with the principle of integrality because they imply separateness rather than unity.

The continuous mutual flow of energy of human beings and their environments creates constant changes in the life process. Human beings and their environments are continually being identified by different manifestations (Rogers, 1970). As the mountain climber ascends to higher altitudes, continuous changes occur from the dy-

TABLE 4.1 Principles of Homeodynamics

| Integrality |
| Resonancy |
| Helicy |

namic mutual process of the human and the environment. Thus the change in altitude does not *cause* changes in the climber, nor does the climber *adapt* to the altitude. The principle of integrality firmly rejects the idea of causality.

Resonancy

The principle of resonancy asserts that manifestations of patterns characterizing human and environmental energy fields are continuously changing from lower frequency, longer waves to higher frequency, shorter waves. The life process in human beings is a symphony of rhythmical vibrations that gives intensity to the life process. The life process becomes increasingly diverse. There are more variations, greater differences. Each turn of the spiral in the Slinky (see Figure 2.1) symbolizes the rhythmical nature of life. Human beings experience their environment by resonating patterns.

Helicy

The principle of helicy tells us that human and environmental field patterns are continuous, innovative, unpredictable, and increasing in diversity. In 1990, Rogers substituted the word *unpredictable* for *probabilistic*. The deletion of probability in favor of unpredictability was associated with the emergence of chaos theory discussed in the recent works of such authors as Mallove, and Peterson, as well as others. The change to unpredictability "strengthens consistency and supports the nature of change proposed in the principles of homeodynamics" (Rogers, 1990, p. 7).

The life process is evolutionary in that constant change is taking place that draws upon the past. Through continuous change, new, nonrepeating rhythmical patterns continue to emerge, becoming more diverse, possessing more variation, and becoming unpredictable. This is *becoming.*

Nursing practice chiefly involves assessment and identification of the manifestations of patterns that emerge from the mutual person and environmental energy field process and deliberative patterning through a nurse and person mutual process. The nurse's energy field and the person's energy field together participate in patterning toward optimum health potential. Unique and constantly changing human and environmental field patterns require nursing interventions that are different for each person. Through its practice, nursing seeks to promote harmony of human and environmental energy fields, to strengthen coherence and integrity of human fields, and to participate in direct and redirect patterning of human and environmental energy fields toward the goal of optimum health potential (Rogers, 1970). An excellent example of nursing practice with a focus on patterning can be found in Madrid (1990).

5

Clinical Example

Madrid (1990) recounts a clinical experience with a young man hospitalized for gastrointestinal bleeding secondary to Acquired Immune Deficiency Syndrome (AIDS), providing a view of the transformation of this man, manifesting patterns of energy depletion, pain, and restlessness to patterns of peace, enjoyment, and interest in self and his environment. The transformation occurs through the process of mutual (person and nurse) patterning of the self and environment using Rogerian practice modalities.

Madrid used imagination and imagery to achieve a picture of what this man's life was like before he became ill. These techniques enabled her to experience a richer perception of him as a unitary human being that transcended his present ill health. She promoted comfort through deep breathing, relaxation exercises, and therapeutic touch. Music was used to achieve a sense of peace, and guided imagery was utilized to capture enjoyable moments from the past. Also, her *presence* as a nurse was used as a therapeutic modality to promote comfort. Throughout this experience, Madrid used Rogerian practice methodology of pattern manifestation appraisal and deliberative mutual patterning involving the nurse and the sick person's energy fields in mutual process.

6

Health

Rogers does not give an explicit definition of health. She considers it an ambiguous term that is used in many different ways. She states that both health and sickness are expressions of the life process and are determined by individuals and cultures; therefore, they are value-laden words. Contemporary major American health problems are iatrogenesis (induced by physicians), nosocomial (induced by hospitals) infections, and nosophobia (fear of disease) according to Rogers (1990, p. 5). Behaviors of low value to an individual or culture may be labeled *sick*, whereas behaviors of high value may be labeled *health*. Some values change over time. At one time homosexuality was generally considered a sick behavior, a behavioral disease, in the United States. Persons exhibiting such behavior were hospitalized in psychiatric units, and great effort was extended to change their homosexual behavior to heterosexual behavior. Rogers seems to prefer the term *human betterment* over health because the former is less ambiguous. Having a diagnosis, a label, is sometimes enough to cripple action (e.g., cardiac cripples). Also, Rogers does not use the term *patient*. She considers the term too restrictive. The word patient does not encompass the majority of people, and people are nursing's concern (Rogers, personal communication, November 11, 1990).

From a futuristic perspective, Rogers explains that what is disease or sickness today may not be pathological in the future (Rogers, 1990). Current physiological parameters of a normal hemoglobin or pulmonary vital capacity may not hold for future generations. Loss of calcium has been observed in astronauts; perhaps, spacekind will not need the amount of calcium required by humankind. Rogers believes a new species will emerge: spacekind. "Homo spacialis" will evolve and transcend homo sapiens. The normal parameters for the great-grandchildren of the young adults of today that will be residing in a space station in the year 2050 may be entirely different from those of their great-grandparents residing on earth. Humankind will change and evolve continuously and mutually with its environments to spacekind and beyond.

Future health services are predicted to be community based, with an orientation to health, as contrasted with what now might better be called hospital or sickness orientation. Health promotion rather than cure of disease will be the focus. The practice of nursing will be identified through noninvasive modalities with a purpose of promoting human betterment.

7

Related Theories

A science generates many theories. Among the theories proposed by Rogers, three have received the most attention in the literature: accelerating change, paranormal phenomena, and rhythmical manifestations of change.

The theory of accelerating change holds that change is speeding up and that there is greater diversity of human and environmental fields. This theory provides an explanation for the hyperactivity observed more frequently in children today.

The theory of paranormal phenomena provides an explanation for precognition, déjà vu, clairvoyance, and telepathy. In a pandimensional world, there are no limits imposed by space and time. Human and environmental fields are integral. Therefore, the present is relative to the person.

"The theory of rhythmical [manifestations] of change focuses on human and environmental field rhythms" (Fawcett, 1989, p. 278). This theory deals with manifestations of human and environmental field patterns, such as sleep/wake patterns (Floyd, 1983) and perceptions of time passing (Fitzpatrick, Donovan, & Johnston, 1980), to name but a few manifestations.

The Science of Unitary Human Beings was foundational for the development of some theories of nursing. These theories are in varying stages of development. One example is Margaret Newman's Model of Health as an Expansion of Consciousness (1986). The focus of her theory is the nature of health. The three definitions of health proposed by Newman (expanding consciousness, disease-nondisease fusion, person and environment) have pattern as a common element. Additionally, the concepts of consciousness, movement, time, and space with which Newman views health reflect the influence of Rogers.

Rosemarie Rizzo Parse's Man-Living-Health model (1981) is considered Rogerian science that has been modified to include existential phenomenological thought. The focus of Parse's theory is the meaning underlying the behavior of human beings as they relate with the environment.

Rogerian scholars conduct basic and applied research using the Science of Unitary Human Beings. Basic research is theoretical research that extends the base of knowledge for the sake of knowledge itself. An example is Barrett's theory of power (Barrett, 1990), which was derived from Rogers's principle of helicy: "Power is defined as the capacity to participate knowingly in the nature of change characterizing the continuous patterning of the human and environmental fields as manifest by awareness, choices, freedom to act intentionally, and involvement in creating change" (p. 108). The concepts of awareness, choices, freedom to act intentionally, and involvement in creating change were used as empirical indicators of power to test the hypothesis that power was related to human field motion (Barrett, 1990). Barrett developed an instrument, the Barrett Power as Knowing Participation in Change Test, to measure field patterns of power.

Another example of applied research using the Science of Unitary Human Beings is Ference's research in human field motion. A theory of motion was derived from the principle of resonancy. This theory "proposes that as a human field engages in ever-higher levels of human field motion, the pattern evolves toward greater . . . diversity and differentiation" (Ference, 1989, p. 123). The Ference Human Field Motion Tool was developed to measure evaluation of change. Ference (1989) found in her research that human field motion expanded with greater physical motion. Other researchers have found that human field motion also expands with meditation, risk-taking, and higher levels of participation in change (Ference, 1989).

Applied research seeks to find solutions to practical problems. An example of applied research using Rogerian science is Andersen's LIGHT model (Andersen & Smereck, 1989). This is a prescriptive model synthesized from Aristotle's theory of ethics and the Science of Unitary Human Beings. The Personalized Nursing LIGHT model has two tracks. One track, personalized care, consists of all actions taken by a nurse on behalf of persons with the intent of improving their well-being. The other track, personalized action, consists of all actions taken by the person to achieve well-being. "Both tracks are described with the acronym LIGHT" (Andersen & Smereck, 1989, p. 122). The Personalized Nursing LIGHT Model "has been implemented successfully with patients confined to a psychiatric institution, with persons treated in a mental health nursing clinic, and with persons who are intravenous drug abusers in urban community outreach programs in three states" (Andersen & Smereck, 1989, p. 120).

Martha Rogers continues to have a profound influence on nursing as a profession and as a science. Rogerian scholars believe the Science of Unitary Human Beings is *the* nursing science. They constitute probably the best organized band of theory scholars of any of the nurse theorists. These scholars are developing an ever widening program of research to clarify, expand and extend understanding of the Science of Unitary Human Beings. Even those who do not promote Rogers's abstract system recognize that Martha E. Rogers has challenged traditional ways of thinking and encouraged futuristic thinking. More important, she has identified what is unique to nursing.

Glossary

Building Blocks

Energy field
"The fundamental unit of the living and the non-living. Field is a unifying concept. Energy signifies the dynamic nature of the field; a field is in continuous motion and is infinite" (Rogers, 1990, p. 7).

Environmental field (environment)
"An irreducible, indivisible, pandimensional energy field identified by pattern and integral with the human field" (Rogers, 1990, p. 7).

Four-dimensionality
Retitled pandimensionality (Rogers, personal communication, November 11, 1990).

Human field
See *unitary human beings.*

Pandimensionality
"A nonlinear domain without spatial or temporal attributes . . . provides for an infinite domain without limit" (Rogers, 1990, p. 7). Formerly titled four-dimensionality and multidimensionality.

Pattern
"The distinguishing characteristic of an energy field perceived as a single wave" (Rogers, 1990, p. 7).

27

Unitary human beings (human field)

"An irreducible, indivisible, pandimensional energy field identified by pattern and manifesting characteristics that are specific to the whole and which cannot be predicted from knowledge of the parts" (Rogers, 1990, p. 7).

Principles of Homeodynamics

"Provide fundamental guides to the practice of nursing" (Rogers, 1990, p. 8).

Helicy

"Continuous, innovative, unpredictable, increasing diversity of human and environmental field patterns" (Rogers, 1990, p. 8).

Integrality

"Continuous mutual human field and environmental field process" (Rogers, 1990, p. 8). Formerly titled complementarity.

Resonancy

"Continuous change from lower to higher frequency wave patterns in human and environmental fields" (Rogers, 1990, p. 8).

Related Terms

Health

"Unitary human health signifies an irreducible human field manifestation" (Rogers, 1990, p. 10); human betterment (Rogers, 1990, p. 10); an expression "of the process of life" (Rogers, 1970, p. 85); a value defined by individuals and cultures.

Nursing

"Learned profession"; "a science and an art" (Rogers, 1990, p. 5); a basic science (Rogers, personal communication, November 11, 1990); "study of unitary, irreducible, indivisible human and environmental fields: people and their world (Rogers, 1990, p. 6).

> *Art of nursing:* "Creative use of the science of nursing for human betterment" (Rogers, 1990, p. 6); imaginative and creative use of nursing knowledge (Rogers, 1990, p. 387).

Purpose of nurses: "Promote health and well being for all persons and groups wherever they are" (Rogers, personal communication, November, 11, 1990).

Uniqueness of nursing: The "focus on unitary human beings and their world" (Rogers, 1990, p. 6).

Science
"An organized body of abstract knowledge" (Rogers, personal communication, November 11, 1990); "a synthesis of facts and ideas; a new product" (Rogers, 1990, p. 6).

References

Andersen, M., & Smereck, G. A. D. (1989). Personalized nursing LIGHT model. *Nursing Science Quarterly, 2,* 120-130.

Barrett, E. A. M. (1990). Health patterning with clients in a private practice environment. In E. A. M. Barrett (Ed.), *Visions of Rogers' science-based nursing* (Pub. No. 15-2285, pp. 105-115). New York: National League for Nursing.

Butcher, H. R., & Parker, N. I. (1988). Guided imagery within Rogers' science of unitary human beings: An experimental study. *Nursing Science Quarterly, 1,* 103-110.

Fawcett, J. (1989). *Analysis and evaluation of conceptual models of nursing* (2nd ed., pp. 263-305). Philadelphia: F. A. Davis.

Ference, H. M. (1989). Nursing science theories and administration. In B. Henry, C. Arndt, M. Di Vincenti, & A. Marriner-Tomey, *Dimensions of nursing administration: Theory, research, education, practice* (pp. 121-131). Boston: Blackwell Scientific.

Fitzpatrick, J. J., Donovan, M. J., & Johnston, R. L. (1980). Experience of time during the crisis of cancer. *Cancer Nursing, 3,* 191-194.

Floyd, J. (1983). Research using Rogers' conceptual system: Development of a testable theorem. *Advances in Nursing Science, 5*(2), 37-48.

Girardin, B. (1990). *The relationship of light wave frequency and sleepwakefulness frequency in well, full-term Hispanic neonates.* Unpublished doctoral dissertation, Wayne State University, Detroit.

Krieger, D. (1979). *Therapeutic touch: How to use your hands to help and heal.* Englewood Cliffs, NJ: Prentice Hall.

Madrid, M. (1990). The participating process of human field patterning in an acute-care environment. In E. A. M. Barrett (Ed.), *Visions of Rogers' science-based nursing* (Pub. No. 15-2285, pp. 93-104). New York: National League for Nursing.

Newman, M. (1986). *Health as expanding consciousness.* St. Louis: C. V. Mosby.

Parse, R. R. (1981). *Man-living-health: A theory of nursing.* New York: John Wiley.

Quinn, J. F. (1989). Therapeutic touch as energy exchange: Replication and extension. *Nursing Science Quarterly, 2,* 79-87.

Rogers, M. E. (1970). *An introduction to the theoretical basis of nursing.* Philadelphia: F. A. Davis.

Rogers, M. E. (1988). Nursing science and art: A prospective. *Nursing Science Quarterly, 1,* 99-102.

Rogers, M. E. (1990). Nursing: Science of unitary, irreducible, human beings: Update 1990. In E. A. M. Barrett (Ed.), *Visions of Rogers' science-based nursing* (Pub. No. 15-2285, pp. 5-11). New York: National League for Nursing.

Rogers, M. E., Doyle, M. B., Racolin, A., & Walsh, P. C. (1990). A conversation with Martha Rogers on nursing in space. In E. A. M. Barrett (Ed.), *Visions of Rogers' science-based nursing* (Pub. No. 15-2285, pp. 375-386). New York: National League for Nursing.

Bibliography

Biography of Dr. Martha E. Rogers

Gioiella, E. (1989). Professionalizing nursing: A Rogers legacy. *Nursing Science Quarterly, 2*, 61-62.

Hektor, L. M. (1989). Martha E. Rogers: A life history. *Nursing Science Quarterly, 2*, 63-73.

Parse, R. R. (1989). Martha E. Rogers: A birthday celebration. *Nursing Science Quarterly, 2*, 55.

The Abstract System

Barrett, E. A. M. (1990). Health patterning with clients in a private practice environment. In E. A. M. Barrett (Ed.), *Visions of Rogers' science-based nursing* (Publication No. 15-2285, pp. 105-115). New York: National League for Nursing.

Chinn, P. L., & Kramer, M. K. (1991). *Theory and nursing: A systematic approach* (3rd ed., pp. 182-183). St. Louis: C. V. Mosby.

Daily, J. S., Maupin, J. S., Satterly, M. C., Schnell, D. L., & Wallace, T. L. (1989). Martha E. Rogers: Unitary human beings. In A. Marriner-Tomey (Ed.), *Nursing theorists and their work* (2nd ed., pp. 402-412). St. Louis: C. V. Mosby.

Falco, S. M., & Lobo, M. L. (1990). Martha E. Rogers. In J. B. George (Ed.), *Nursing theories: The base for professional nursing practice* (pp. 211-230). Norwalk, CT: Appleton & Lange.

Leddy, S., & Pepper, J. M. (1989). *Conceptual bases of professional nursing* (2nd ed., pp. 188-190). Philadelphia: J. B. Lippincott.

Malinkski, V. (Ed.). (1986). *Explorations on Martha Rogers' Science of Unitary Human Beings*. Norwalk, CT: Appleton & Lange.

Newman, M. (1986). *Health as expanding consciousness.* St. Louis: C. V. Mosby.

Parse, R. R. (1981). *Man-living-health: A theory of nursing.* New York: John Wiley.

Rogers, M. E. (1970). *The theoretical basis of nursing.* Philadelphia: F. A. Davis.

Rogers, M. E. (1988). Nursing science and art: A prospective. *Nursing Science Quarterly, 1,* 99-102.

Rogers, M. E. (1989). Nursing: A science of unitary human beings. In J. P. Riehl-Sisca (Ed.), *Conceptual models for nursing practice* (3rd ed., pp. 181-188). Norwalk, CT: Appleton & Lange.

Rogers, M. E. (1990). Nursing: Science of unitary, irreducible, human beings: Update 1990. In E. A. M. Barrett (Ed.), *Visions of Rogers' science-based nursing* (Publication No. 15-2285, pp. 5-11). New York: National League for Nursing.

Rogers, M. E., Doyle, M. B., Racolin, A., & Walsh, P. C. (1990). A conversation with Martha Rogers on nursing in space. In E. A. M. Barrett (Ed.), *Visions of Rogers' science-based nursing* (Publication No. 15-2285, pp. 375-386). New York: National League for Nursing.

Reeder, F. (1984). Philosophic issues in the Rogerian science of unitary human beings. *Advances in Nursing Science, 6,* 14-23.

Sarter, B. (1988a). *The stream of becoming: A study of Martha Rogers's theory* (Publication No. 15-2205). New York: National League for Nursing.

Sarter, B. (1988b). Philosophical sources of nursing theory. *Nursing Science Quarterly, 1,* 52-59.

Sarter, B. (1989). Some critical philosophical issues in the science of unitary human beings. *Nursing Science Quarterly, 2,* 74-78.

Smith, M. J. (1989). Four dimensionality: Where to go with it. *Nursing Science Quarterly, 2,* 56.

Analysis and Evaluation of the Science of Unitary Human Beings

Cerilli, K., & Burd, S. (1989). An analysis of Martha Rogers' nursing as a science of unitary human beings. In J. P. Riehl-Sisca (Ed.), *Conceptual models for nursing practice* (3rd ed., pp. 189-194). Norwalk, CT: Appleton & Lange.

Fawcett, J. (1989). Rogers' science of unitary human beings. *Analysis and evaluation of conceptual models of nursing* (2nd ed., pp. 263-305). Philadelphia: F. A. Davis.

Quillin, S. I. M., & Runk, J. A. (1989). Martha Rogers' unitary person model. In J. J. Fitzpatrick & A. L. Whall (Eds.), *Conceptual model of nursing* (2nd ed., pp. 285-300). Norwalk, CT: Appleton & Lange.

Whall, A. L. (1987). A critique of Rogers's framework. In R. R. Parse (Ed.), *Major paradigms, theories and critiques* (pp. 147-158). Philadelphia: W. B. Saunders.

Extensions of the Science of Unitary Human Beings to Groups

Alligood, M. R. (1989). Rogers' theory and nursing administration: A perspective on health and environment. In B. Henry, C. Arndt, M. Di Vincenti, & A. Marriner-Tomey (Eds.), *Dimensions of nursing administration: Theory, research, education, practice* (pp. 105-111). Boston: Blackwell Scientific.

Ference, H. M. (1989). Nursing science theories and administration. In B. Henry, C. Arndt, M. Di Vincenti, & A. Marriner-Tomey (Eds.), *Dimensions of nursing administration: Theory, research, education, practice* (pp. 121-131). Boston: Blackwell Scientific.

Gueldner, S. H. (1989). Applying Rogers's model to nursing administration: Emphasis on client and nursing. In B. Henry, C. Arndt, M. Di Vincenti, & A. Marriner-Tomey (Eds.), *Dimensions of nursing administration: Theory, research, education, practice* (pp. 113-119). Boston: Blackwell Scientific.

Hanchett, E. S. (1989). *Nursing frameworks and community as client: Bridging the gap.* Norwalk, CT: Appleton & Lange.

Hanchett, E. S. (1990). Nursing models and community as client. *Nursing Science Quarterly, 3,* 67-72.

Research and Applications to Practice

Alligood, M. R. (1991). Testing Rogers' theory of accelerating change: The relationships among creativity, actualization, and empathy in persons 18 to 92 years of age. *Western Journal of Nursing Research, 13*(1), 84-96.

Andersen, M. D., & Smereck, G. A. D. (1989). Personalized nursing LIGHT model. *Nursing Science Quarterly, 2,* 120-130.

Barrett, E. A. M. (1988). Using Rogers' science of unitary human beings in nursing practice. *Nursing Science Quarterly, 1,* 50-51.

Barrett, E. A. M. (Ed.). (1990a). *Visions of Rogers's science-based nursing: Unit 2. Practice.* (Publication No. 15-2285). New York: National League for Nursing.

Barrett, E. A. M. (Ed.). (1990b). *Visions of Rogers's science-based nursing: Unit 3. Research* (Publication No. 15-2285). New York: National League for Nursing.

Benedict, S. C., & Burge, J. M. (1990). The relationship between human field motion and preferred visible wavelengths. *Nursing Science Quarterly, 3,* 67-72.

Butcher, H. K., & Parker, N. I. (1988). Guided imagery within Rogers; science of unitary human beings: An experimental study. *Nursing Science Quarterly, 1,* 103-110.

Compton, M. A. (1989). A Rogerian view of drug abuse: Implications for nursing. *Nursing Science Quarterly, 2,* 98-105.

DeFeo, D. J. (1990). Change: A central concern of nursing. *Nursing Science Quarterly, 3,* 88-94.

Floyd, J. (1983). Research using Rogers' conceptual system: Development of a testable theorem. *Advances in Nursing Science, 5*(2), 37-48.

Girardin, B. (1990). *The relationship of light wave frequency and sleepwakefulness frequency in well, full-term Hispanic neonates.* Unpublished doctoral dissertation, Wayne State University, Detroit.

Heggie, J. R., Schoenmehl, P. A., Chang, M. K., & Grieco, C. (1989). Selection and implementation of Dr. Martha Rogers' nursing conceptual model in an acute care setting. *Clinical Nurse Specialist, 3,* 143-147.

Heidt, P. R. (1990). Openness: A qualitative analysis of nurses' and patients' experiences of therapeutic touch. *Image, 22,* 180-186.

Krieger, D. (1979). *The therapeutic touch: How to use your hands to help or heal.* Englewood Cliffs, NJ: Prentice Hall.

Madrid, M., & Winstead-Fry, P. (1986). Rogers's conceptual model. In P. Winstead-Fry (Ed.), *Case studies in nursing theory* (pp. 73-102). New York: National League for Nursing.

Mason, T., & Patterson, R. (1990). A critical review of the use of Rogers' model within a special hospital: A single case study. *Journal of Advanced Nursing, 15,* 130-141.

Phillips, J. R. (1989). Science of unitary human beings: Changing research perspectives. *Nursing Science Quarterly, 2,* 57-60.

Quinn, J. F. (1989). Therapeutic touch as energy exchange: Replication and extension. *Nursing Science Quarterly, 2*(2), 79-87.

Schodt, C. M. (1989). Parental fetal attachment and couvade: A study of patterns of human-environment integrality. *Nursing Science Quarterly, 2,* 88-97.

Smith, M. C. (1988). Testing propositions derived from Rogers' conceptual system. *Nursing Science Quarterly, 1,* 60-67.

Smith, M. C. (1990). Pattern in nursing practice. *Nursing Science Quarterly, 3,* 57-59.

Wynd, C. A. (1990). Analysis of a power theory for health promotion activities. *Applied Nursing Research, 3,* 118-120.

Applications to Education

Barrett, E. A. M. (Ed.). (1990). *Visions of Rogers' science-based nursing: Unit 4. Education* (Publication No. 15-2285). New York: National League for Nursing.

Rogers, M. E. (1985a). Nursing education: Preparation for the future. In *Patterns in education: The unfolding of nursing* (pp. 11-14). New York: National League for Nursing.

Rogers, M. E. (1985b). The nature and characteristics of professional education for nursing. *Journal of Professional Nursing, 1,* 381-383.

PART II

Imogene King

A Conceptual Framework for Nursing

CHRISTINA L. SIELOFF

Biographical Sketch of the Nurse Theorist: Imogene M. King, EdD, RN

BSN: St. Louis University, St. Louis, Missouri
MSN: St. Louis University
PhD: Education, Teachers College, Columbia University,
New York
Past Professor of Nursing: University of South Florida,
Tampa
Professor Emeritus: University of South Florida
Member: American Nurses' Association/Florida Nurses'
Association/District IV
Board Member: Operation PAR, Inc.
President: Florida Nurses' Foundation

Foreword

Nursing science has come of age. The multiple publications of conceptual systems and theories in nursing have demonstrated advance in the scientific movement in nursing. This section by Christina Sieloff presents my conceptual system from which a theory of goal attainment was derived. The author is well qualified to do this. She has demonstrated very clearly the difference between a conceptual system and a theory derived from it and has displayed a thorough understanding of theory construction and testing in research. In addition, she has shown an understanding of the theory and the use of my nursing process of interactions that lead to transactions and then to goal attainment.

In the past few years, several nurses have published ways in which they have used knowledge of the concepts of the theory and my nursing process in caring for patients. These publications have shown that the theory is useful in caring for patients in critical care units, in oncology units, in psychiatric units, in community health, and in gerontological nursing situations. One group of nurses in Canada published the way they organized all of the nursing diagnoses under the concepts of this theory. Two nurses in Canada published their ideas about how they planned and implemented change in a hospital and used my conceptual system.

Some of the criteria used by accrediting agencies such as the Joint Commission of Accreditation for Healthcare Organizations, indicate an expectation that nurses understand the theoretical basis for their practice. Use of a conceptual system and theory such as mine helps nurses meet this criterion. Several nursing departments in medical centers and community hospitals have used this theory to implement theory-based practice. This section increases the focus on nursing science.

IMOGENE M. KING, EDD, RN
Professor Emeritus
University of South Florida
Tampa, Florida

Preface

Nurses routinely set goals for, and frequently with, clients. And yet, how often is that process examined from a nursing theory perspective? Dr. Imogene M. King began writing about nursing theory in 1964 and published her first book in 1971. She developed a conceptual framework for nursing and within this framework developed a theory for nursing that focused on the process of mutual goal setting by nurse and client. By developing a systems approach that focused on a holistic view of human beings, Dr. King (1981)

1. identified concepts of relevance to nursing,
2. developed and tested the Theory of Goal Attainment, and
3. developed the Goal Oriented Nursing Record (1981).

The purpose of this book is to provide a descriptive overview of King's framework and theory. A brief biography of Dr. King is presented. The origin of her conceptual framework is discussed and the framework described. Concepts from the proposed metaparadigm for nursing are then examined. The Theory of Goal Attainment is presented and the assumptions and hypotheses discussed. Application of the theory to practice and research is examined. The bibliography includes publications both by and about Dr. King.

—CHRISTINA L. SIELOFF

8

Origin of the Conceptual Framework

Imogene King began developing her conceptual framework in 1961 in order to cultivate a master's program in Nursing at Loyola University in Chicago (Ackermann et al., 1986). As a beginning step, she examined society and identified several trends in health care, many of which are still applicable today: (a) a knowledge explosion, (b) increasing technological advances, (c) changes in the composition of the population, and (d) mobility of employees. The environment was becoming increasingly complex.

Because nurses were, and are, key persons in health care systems, King developed several questions about nursing:

1. What is the nursing act?
2. What is the nursing process?
3. What is the goal of nursing?
4. Who are nurses, and how are they educated for practice?
5. How and where is nursing practiced?
6. Who needs nursing in this society? (King, 1975a, p. 37)

King reviewed the literature in psychology, sociology, and nursing as she searched for the answers to her questions. She identified words that consistently appeared in the nursing literature. Following an analysis of these words, three initial concepts were identified: interpersonal relations, perception, and organization. In addition, one concept was identified as a major component of the other words—energy.

After reviewing the literature, King discussed her findings at conferences and with colleagues. Through this process of critical thinking, using inductive and deductive processes, she began developing her framework (King, 1975a).

Conceptual Framework

King's work resulted in the development of a conceptual framework and the Theory of Goal Attainment. Her conceptual framework will be discussed first, followed by a review of her theory.

A conceptual framework differs from a theory in several ways:

1. A conceptual framework is usually more abstract than a theory and cannot be directly applied to practice situations. A theory may be used to guide practice.
2. A conceptual framework presents a broad view of an area of interest, for example, human interactions. In contrast, a theory presents a narrower view—for example, the goal attainment aspect of nurse-client interactions.
3. Although both a conceptual framework and a theory contain concepts, the linkages between concepts in a theory are more clearly delineated than in a conceptual framework. (Meleis, 1985)

Systems Framework

King used a systems framework as the basis for developing her conceptual framework. General systems theory was developed in the early 1930s by a group of individuals to counteract logical positivism and to offer another approach in the search for scientific knowledge (King, 1990). Logical positivism focused on mechanistic relationships—dividing wholes into parts and determining the relationships of these parts. General systems theory is concerned with wholes rather than parts (Bertalanffy, 1968). In examining wholes, one does not examine the total of the parts of a system, for the whole is different from this total—a view consistent with nursing's perspective of an individual.

Elements of any system include structure, function, resources, and goals. In attempting to provide a "structure for nursing as a discipline and as a profession" (King, 1989a, p. 151), King developed a systems framework. According to her theory, the structure of a system may be reflected by a person interacting with an environment. Nursing functions include viewing, recognizing, observing and measuring, synthesizing and interpreting, and analyzing. However, these functions are conducted not in a stepwise manner, but simultaneously within the context of the nursing process. Resources involved are of two types: human and material. The goal of the system is health.

King used this systems framework to determine that health concerns related to nursing can be grouped into "three dynamic interacting systems: (a) personal systems, (b) interpersonal systems, and (c) social systems" (King, 1989a, p. 151). Figure 8.1 illustrates this relationship. In addition, following a review of the literature, King identified concepts that are relevant to nursing and nursing practice:

- Authority
- Body image
- Communication
- Decision making
- Growth and development
- Interaction
- Organization
- Perception
- Power
- Role
- Self
- Space
- Status
- Stress
- Time
- Transaction

The three "systems, along with identified concepts, provide a way of organizing one's knowledge, skills, and values" (King, 1989a, p. 152).

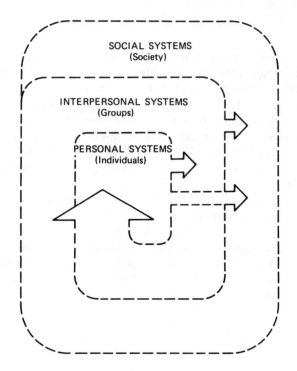

Figure 8.1. A conceptual framework for nursing: Dynamic interacting systems.
SOURCE: King (1971, p. 20).

Personal Systems

King conceptualized a personal system as an individual, using information that would assist nurses in understanding individuals. Understanding an individual as a whole is critical before a nurse can understand groups and communities. The concepts of body image, growth and development, perception, self, space, and time are particularly relevant to the personal system.

The personal system focuses on individual human beings. Therefore, it is fitting to discuss King's view of this concept. The concept of a human being is synonymous with that of a personal system within the conceptual framework.

Although King did not define the personal system specifically, she identified several characteristics of a human being. A human being is a complex, open living system that "copes with a wide range of events, persons and things over time" (King, 1975b, p. 6). This human being has the following fundamental health needs: "(a) usable health information at a time when he/she needs it and is able to use it, (b) preventive care, and (c) care when ill" (King, 1971, p. 83).

Human beings are rational and feeling and react to their expectations, other individuals, events, and objects. They react on the basis of their "perceptions, expectations, and needs" (King, 1981, p. 20). They react as a whole, individuals being viewed as an entity, a living system.

Human beings are time-oriented and have an awareness of the past, present, and their future goals. By choosing among alternatives, human beings make decisions. They select goals upon which to focus, and then identify the means to attain them. In addition, a human being, "depending upon habits, abilities, age and situation, has functions to be performed; age, the place in the family, and roles being critical variables" (King, 1975b, p. 6).

Interpersonal Systems

Interpersonal systems focus on groups of individuals, including dyads, triads, or small or large groups. A group's complexity and variability increase concurrent with its size. Concepts more important to interpersonal systems include communication, interaction, roles, stress, and transaction. The interpersonal system is the system in which the nursing process primarily occurs (King, 1981). King (1975a) defined the nursing process as a "series of acts that connote action, reaction, interaction, and transaction between nurse and health client" (p. 37).

Social Systems

A social system is defined by King (1981) as "an organized boundary system of social roles, behaviors and practices developed to maintain values and the mechanisms to regulate the practices and rules" (p. 115). Individuals within a social system share common goals and interests. The social system exists in order to address the specific concerns of these individuals and the subgroups they form within the social system (Gulitz & King, 1988). Families, religions, educational systems, work places, and health care settings are examples of social systems.

All social systems have certain common characteristics. Among these are age gradation, authority, behavior patterns, roles, social interactions, status, structure, and values. However, King (1981) identified the following concepts from the conceptual framework as particularly relevant to a social system: authority, decision making, organization, power, and status.

An individual "functions in social systems through interpersonal relationships in terms of . . . perceptions which influence . . . life and health" (Daubenmire & King, 1973, p. 512). Therefore, it is important for nurses to know about the impact of social systems on individual's and groups' behaviors.

When nursing within a social system, practice focuses on the health needs and wants of a social system. Utilizing the nursing process, a nurse works with individuals and groups within the social system to address the health needs of clients and the wants of the social system. Therefore, "the establishment of mutually set goals, the planning of programs, and the evaluation of outcomes need to focus on the goals of the social system being served" (Gulitz & King, 1988, p. 130).

Assumptions

An assumption is "a statement of principle that is accepted as true on the basis of logic or reason" (Woods & Catanzaro, 1988, p. 552). The following are the original assumptions upon which King's (1971) conceptual framework was based:

(a) Nurses, in the performance of their roles and responsibilities, assist individuals and groups in society to attain, maintain, and restore health.

(b) In the process of functioning in social institutions, nurses assist individuals to meet their basic needs at some point in time in the life cycle when they cannot do this for themselves.

(c) An understanding of basic human needs in the physical, social, emotional, and intellectual realm of the life process from conception to old age, within the context of social systems of the culture in which nurses live and work, is essential and basic content for learning the practice of nursing. (Fawcett, 1984, pp. 88-89)

King states that the 1981 version of her conceptual framework is based on the following assumption: "The focus of nursing is human beings interacting with their environment leading to a state of health for individuals, which is an ability to function in social roles" (Fawcett, 1984, p. 89).

Concepts

Although the concepts of King's (1981) conceptual framework are placed in specific systems, they "are so interrelated in the interactions of human beings with their environment that the placement within each of the three systems is an arbitrary decision" (King, 1989a, p. 151). Thus each concept is applicable to each of the three dynamic interacting systems (personal, interpersonal, and social) and may be discussed, examined, and used within each system. In this section, the concepts have been presented in alphabetical order so that the reader can more easily locate them. These concepts are authority, body image, communication, decision making, growth and development, interaction, organization, perception, power, role, self, space, status, stress, time, and transaction.

The concepts of King's conceptual framework are presented in a consistent format, which includes the following:

- Title of a concept
- Characteristics of, and information regarding, a concept
- An example of the concept

Definitions of the concepts are included in the glossary. Each concept may include one or more of the following types of definitions: (a) conceptual, (b) theoretical from the Theory of Goal Attainment, or (c) operational.

Authority

Authority is the ability "to make decisions that guide the actions of self and others" (King, 1981, p. 122). It may be either formal or functional and is the "legitimate power given to a person by virtue of role and position in a social system" (King, 1981, p. 122). Authority resides in (a) a position that enables an individual to dispense rewards and sanctions, (b) expertise that results from special knowledge and skills, and (c) the leader of a group (King, 1981).

Authority is universal. It is present in every culture and "provides order, guidance, and responsibility for actions" (King, 1981, p. 123). There is a reciprocal relationship between an individual exercising authority and an individual accepting authority. In addition, authority varies with the situation in which it occurs.

In order to function effectively in an organization, nurses need to understand authority. A department of nursing within a health-care organization should have the authority to make nursing-related decisions. To have this authority, nurses within a department need to understand their organizational position and the authority and power related to that position (King, 1981).

Example: A client requested that the bed bath be done later in the morning rather than directly after breakfast. Because the primary nurse was responsible for the completion of the client's care, he had the authority to rearrange the order of that care to meet the client's request.

Body Image

Everyone has a body image, although cultural factors affect the perception of a body image. An individual's body image is personal, subjective, and unique. It cannot be duplicated by another individual. Body image develops over one's life span as input is received regarding the image one, and others, perceive about the body. Thus body image is dynamic; it changes over time as additional input is received from others and as an individual becomes aware of bodily changes.

Disturbances in one's body image may result from trauma, loss of body parts, or actual or perceived threats to one's person. It is important for a nurse to be aware of a client's perception of body image because the nurse and client work together to develop goals and means to achieve these goals. If a client perceives that a body image may limit the ability to achieve a goal, whether or not this is true, a nurse needs to recognize this perception as real and work with the client in order to provide additional feedback.

An individual's body image is not the only image that affects an individual. The image that family members and friends hold of an individual also influences the individual's perception of body image. Hence it is important to include a client's family and friends when addressing goals that involve a client's body image. Touch contributes to an individual's development of a "healthy body image" (King, 1981, p. 72). Because nurses frequently touch clients while delivering nursing care, it is important that nurses recognize the impact of a client's perception of touch on body image.

Example: A client recently was informed that she has diabetes. Even though there was no overt physical change in her body image, she expressed that she felt ugly and marred. She believed that her body image had been negatively altered.

Communication

Communication occurs through both verbal and nonverbal exchanges. Verbal exchanges can include both spoken and written communications. Nonverbal communication is also extremely important because it provides "accurate information about another person's attitudes and feelings" (King, 1981, p. 71). When the client is unable to verbally communicate, nonverbal communication is a key factor in determining whether or not mutual goal setting occurs. Examples of nonverbal communication include appearance, distance, facial expressions, posture and touch (King, 1981). While communicating, it in important to listen, be silent, and observe how an individual communicates nonverbally.

The interpretation of communication depends upon the situation in which it occurs. Once communication takes place, it cannot be recalled. The impact of communication remains even if subsequent communications attempt to change or eliminate it.

Communication involves the perceptions of both a sender and a receiver. Through communication, transactions may be made between the two individuals (see the discussion on transactions). Each individual's communication is different. No one can say the exact same words in the exact same way with the exact same results.

Communication involves an "interchange of thoughts and opinions among individuals and is a means whereby social interaction and learning take place" (King, 1981, p. 62). Open systems (human beings) continuously communicate through interactions with the environment (King, 1981). This communication may be intrapersonal and primarily nonverbal, or interpersonal (between individuals) and both verbal and nonverbal.

The following factors can influence the "patterns of communication" between individuals: the situation in which the individuals are communicating; the roles, expectations, and goals of each individual, and the barriers to communication (King, 1981).

For communication to be most effective, an environment must exist in which a nurse and a client respect and wish to understand each other. This environment provides motivation for the understanding and utilization of information (King, 1981).

Information "is crucial in the care, cure and recovery" (King, 1981, p. 78) of clients. Thus communication facilitates the delivery of nursing care because it "establishes a mutuality between care givers and recipients of care" (King, 1981, p. 146). Nurses have the primary responsibility to maintain open communication with the client in order to mutually set goals (King, 1981).

Communication also occurs in nurses' interactions with other nurses, providers, and family members. Hence it is important that nurses have a knowledge of communication and communication skills (King, 1981).

Example: A nurse observes a comatose client's nonverbal responses to a range of motion exercises. In response to nonverbal communication interpreted negatively by the nurse (e.g. grimaces, frowns), the nurse moves through the exercises more slowly. The nurse and the client have communicated.

Decision Making

Decision making is a personal process that involves subjective behaviors; it is individual. Decision making is also situational because it is affected by the time of the decision, the information available, and the individuals participating (King, 1981). Because each decision results in the need for additional decision-making behaviors, the decision-making process is continuous. Decision making occurs to achieve a goal.

There are three components to every decision: (a) the process, (b) the decision maker, and (c) the resulting decision. Situational variables impact the decision-making process by influencing clients' decisions regarding goal prioritization and the means to achieve these goals (King, 1981). Variables related to a nurse and a client occur as a result of their "knowledge, background of experience, goals, values, and perceptions of the situation" (King, 1981, p. 134).

Participation in decision making leads to decreased resistance to decision implementation, and learning occurs. Decision makers are viewed as having authority and power. Decision making affects the quality of care delivered throughout a health care setting (King, 1981). Hence decision making is a key factor in both the delivery of nursing care and in the administrative functions of a department.

Example: After identifying the possible goals available, the nurse and client began to prioritize them. After ranking the goals, they selected one goal. They engaged in decision making.

Growth and Development

Growth and development is a "function of (a) genetic endowment, (b) meaningful and satisfying experiences, and (c) an environment conducive to helping individuals [and groups] move toward maturity" (King, 1981, p. 31). Growth and development also include behavioral, cellular, and molecular changes.

Age is an important variable in determining an individual's growth and development. The age of a system defines "the stage of each [system's] developmental tasks" (King, 1981, p. 148).

Groups can also experience growth and development, moving from a potential to an actualization of their abilities and goals. Through knowledge of social systems and related concepts, a nurse can assess a group's level of growth and development.

Knowledge of growth and development patterns is useful if nurses are to help clients through stressful periods. Familiarity with the normal patterns of growth and development enables a nurse to identify disruptions in these patterns and to assist clients in establishing goals to alleviate those disruptions.

Example: When completing an admission assessment with a 12-year-old girl, the nurse assessed the child's developmental and chronological age. The nurse assessed the child's level of growth and development.

Interaction

All human beings and groups interact with values influencing each interaction. When individuals and groups interact, they respond to each other through mutuality—"interdependence in the situation in which both achieve goals" (King, 1981, p. 84). Verbal and nonverbal communication are present in every interaction.

The process of an interaction moves forward; it is unidirectional. Occurring within a time-space context, an interaction is a continuous process. Once an interaction occurs, it cannot be repeated.

Certain factors are to be considered when viewing interactions. These factors include (a) the situation, (b) the context of the interaction, (c) the closeness of the participants, and (d) the interdependency of each person. Inferences are made as a result of an interaction, and their accuracy results from verification with the other person.

> In nursing, the primary purpose of interactions is to assist an individual to cope with a health problem or concern about health. . . . Nurses and [clients] respond through interactions to the humanness of each other, to the presence of each other, and to the reciprocally contingent relationship. Interactions help nurses and [clients] clarify the shared environment. (King, 1981, pp. 85-86)

Purposeful interactions require that nurse and client openly share information and agree on the means to achieve goals. By being open to cues given during an interaction, each participant is more able to process information. Purposeful, goal-oriented interactions in nursing situations also enhance the effectiveness of care and create positive outcomes for those involved (King, 1981).

King (1981) presented the following assumptions about nurse-client interactions:

1. Perceptions of nurse and of client influence the interaction process.
2. Goals, needs, and values of nurse and client influence the interaction process.
3. Individuals have a right to knowledge about themselves.
4. Individuals have a right to participate in decisions that influence their life, their health, and community services.
5. Health professionals have a responsibility to share information that helps individuals make informed decisions about their health care.
6. Individuals have a right to accept or reject health care.
7. Goals of health professionals and goals of recipients of health care may be incongruent. (King, 1981, pp. 143-144)

Example: A client turned on her call light. The nurse responded by entering the client's room and asking if he could help her. The client responded that she had questions about her discharge plans. The nurse began to answer the client's questions. The nurse and client interacted.

Organization

An organization ensures an arrangement of positions and actions. It has structure. Within this structure, an organization is associated with roles, positions, and actions to be executed; an organization demonstrates function (King, 1981).

All organizations have goals, and resources are used for goal achievement. Successful decision making is crucial for an organization to exist and to be productive (King, 1981).

Organizations arrange individuals in a variety of ways that are designed to attain organizational goals (King, 1981). The focus of an organization is to achieve goals. The system view of an organization "emphasizes the design of communication, information flow and decisions" (King, 1981, p. 118). An organization, as a system, connects questions and answers.

Components of an organization include the following:

1. Human values, behavior patterns, needs, goals, and expectations
2. A natural environment in which material and human resources are essential for achieving goals
3. Employers and employees or parents and children, who form groups that collectively interact to achieve goals
4. Technology that facilitates goal achievement (King, 1981, p. 116)

A knowledge of the concept of organization is essential for nurses working within social systems. To function professionally and to achieve quality care standards, nurses must exert influence on an organization (King, 1981).

King (1989b, p. 42) proposed the following criteria for the analysis of an organization:

- Philosophy of the organization
- Goals of the organization
- Structure of the organization

- Functions of the organization
- Resources available to accomplish the goals
- Constraints in the organization
- Clarity of the lines of communication and responsibility
- Who makes the decisions

King (1981, p. 121) suggests the following techniques for successful functioning within an organization once the nurse has analyzed the organization:

1. Assess the organization, using objective criteria, to determine if your professional and personal goals mesh with the organizational goals.
2. Agree with the written philosophy and its implementation.
3. Agree with the goals of the organization.
4. Know who makes decisions that affect care.
5. Identify the lines of formal and informal communication and the power.
6. Assess the kind of management that prevails.

Example: A hospital is an organization with a formal structure (organizational plan) and specific functions assigned to designated individuals and groups. Using available resources, individuals and groups focus on achieving goals.

Perception

Every human being perceives, and each person's perceptions are different from those of others. Perception involves the individual taking action at the present time (King, 1981).

Perception is a basic concept (King, 1981). Perception occurs through the use of both "sensory (functioning sense organs) and intellectual (brain processes) tools" (King, 1981, p. 20). Perception is related to an individual's or group's education, experiences, goals, needs, physiology, self-concept, socioeconomic status, temporal-spatial relationships, and values (King, 1981).

The perceptual process for open systems (human beings) involves the following elements: "(a) import of energy from the environment organized by information, (b) the transformation of energy, (c) processing of information, (d) storing of information, and (e) export of information in overt behavior" (King, 1981, p. 146).

Perception "gives meaning to one's experience, represents one's image of reality and influences one's behavior, and is the basis for developing a concept of self" (King, 1981, pp. 24-25). Perception enables a human being to know (a) self, (b) others, and (c) "objects in the environment" (King, 1981, p. 19). Reflective of this importance of perception, it is important to note that perception may be distorted by stress and sensory overload or deprivation (King, 1981).

In addition, perceptual congruence is an important element in nurse-client interactions and is the "first step in mutual goal setting" (King, 1981, p. 24). Nurses need to recognize factors that influence perceptions to avoid making inferences on the basis of limited behavioral cues (King, 1981). Hence, by understanding perceptions, nurses can better understand their selves and their clients (King, 1989a).

Example: A client developed an understanding of her upcoming surgery from talking with the physician, the anesthetist and the recovery room nurse. The client's primary nurse identified that this understanding was not accurate because the client believed that she would be able to get out of bed immediately after surgery. The client's perception of what she was told was different from the information that had been provided.

Power

Power is universal and related to a situation, not a person. Because power is situational, and situations change, power also changes. Directed toward the achievement of a goal, the exercise of power within a relationship depends on the acceptance of power. The existence of power "implies a dependency relationship" (King, 1981, p. 126).

The concepts of authority, influence, and status are related to power. Authority is the "legitimate power given to a person by virtue of role and position in a social system in a formal organization" (King, 1981, p. 123). "Influence is an instance of power in which outcomes are not predetermined" (King, 1981, p. 126). Status can be interpreted as personal power (King, personal communication, 1990).

Power is a characteristic of a social system and is equivalent to energy "in the physical world" (King, 1981, p. 126). Uses of power within a social system include budget control, decision making, information control, and reward/sanction control (King, 1981). Power "protects relationships among people to maintain order and to achieve goals" (King, 1981, p. 128) and is "essential in an organization for the maintenance of balance and harmony" (King, 1981, p. 126). Power involves a method of obtaining needed resources that facilitate the production of organizational efficiency (King, 1981).

According to King (1981, p. 127), power (a) enhances group cohesiveness and (b) is a function of human interactions and decision making.

"Each person," wrote King (1981), "has the potential power . . . which is determined by individual resources and the environmental forces encountered" (pp. 127-128). Power results from one's role and position, but it is limited by the amount of resources available and the existence of goals. Without goals, power cannot exist (King, 1981). With power, one can exercise "some control over the process of change in an organization" (King, 1981, p. 127).

Example: A nurse asked a unit clerk to rearrange the multiple tests scheduled for a client in order to provide the client with rest periods. The nurse used his power to rearrange the client's scheduled tests.

Roles

Roles are "learned from functioning in a variety of social systems within society" (King, 1981, p. 92). Roles are complex and situational. Individuals or groups may exchange roles depending on the situation.

The concept of roles requires individuals to communicate and to "interact in purposeful ways to achieve goals" (King, 1981, p. 91). The role of a nurse can be defined as an "interaction between one or more individuals who come to a nursing situation in which nurses perform functions of professional nursing based on knowledge, skills, and values identified as nursing" (King, 1981, p. 93).

Nurses have both expressive roles, which focus on maintaining balance in a system, and instrumental roles, which focus on actions that assist a system in achieving goals. For nurses to function professionally, they must define their role. If employer expectations differ from professional expectations, role conflict will result. Role conflict may then reduce the effectiveness of nursing care and produce stress. Therefore, a knowledge of the concept of roles is important for professional nurses (King, 1981).

Example: During the week, a nurse functioned as a primary nurse with a caseload of 5 patients. During weekends, the nurse assumed additional managerial responsibilities for the unit. She assumed the role of charge nurse.

Self

The self is an open system. As an individual has new experiences, the self changes to incorporate information from these experiences. An individual or a group "directs activities toward fulfillment of self" (King, 1981, p. 27); the self is goal directed.

"Knowledge of self is a key to understanding human behavior," wrote King (1981, p. 26). Both a nurse and a client have a self. For a nurse to assist a client, the nurse must understand the client's self-perception (King, 1981). If a nurse facilitates the ability of an individual or a group to be true to the self, both the nurse and the individual or group "grow in self-awareness and in understanding of human behavior" (King, 1981, p. 28).

Example: A client who was short and underweight acted as if he were tall and muscular. The nurse, recognizing the client's perception of self, responded to the perception, not the physical appearance.

Space

Space is a "function of area, volume, distance and . . . time" (King, 1981, p. 37). Space exists within all cultures but is perceived differently by each individual and depends upon the situation (King, 1981). "Space determines the transactions between human beings and the environment" (King, 1981, p. 37).

Space is an essential component in an open-system framework. Knowledge of space is important for nurses to understand both their own and a client's self in relation to personal space. Because personal space is associated with self identity, it is relevant when considering the distance involved in providing personal care to patients (King, 1981).

Example: When a nurse came too close to the newly admitted client, the client's muscles tensed. By increasing the personal space of the client, the nurse facilitated the client's relaxation.

Status

An individual's or group's status depends on the situation in which that individual or group exists. Status also depends on the position held within a situation. Because status is related to a position, the level of status can decrease when a position is changed.

Status can be considered as the "prestige attached to a role [and is] associated with individuals [or groups] who have the power and authority to make decisions" (King, 1981, pp. 129-130). Because these decisions often influence the attainment of client care goals, departments of nursing should have equal status with all other departments. Thus it is important for nurses to recognize the significance of status in the process of goal attainment (King, 1981).

Example: Within the health care setting, a nurse who has conducted research is perceived as more valuable to the Director of Nursing than are other nurses. This nurse has status.

Stress

All human beings experience stress, and the level of stress experienced by an individual or group constantly changes. Stress is experienced by human beings in a personal and subjective manner and "is not limited by time or place" (King, 1981, p. 97).

King (1981) views stress as an energy response of an individual to persons, objects, and events called "stressors" (p. 99). The level of stress experienced by an individual is influenced by a variety of factors. Individual or group factors include, but are not limited to:

- Age
- Cognition
- Environmental background
- Meaning of the event
- Motivation
- Personality
- Response
- Sex/predominant gender (group)
- Situation
- Stressors
- The time of the event (King, 1981)

An increase in stress lowers one's ability both to perceive events and to make rational decisions (King, 1981). This "may then lead to decreased interactions and goal setting between nurse and [client], and to ineffective nursing care. In addition, subsequent interference in each person's developmental tasks may occur" (King, 1981, p. 148). Nurses can decrease stress through various techniques, which may include:

1. Providing information
2. Assessing physiological change
3. Assisting clients (individuals or groups) to articulate concerns
4. Facilitating goal setting by clients (individuals or groups)
5. Suggesting alternative means to attain the goals (King, 1981)

Example: At the change of shift—a busy time for nurses—two clients were admitted. Arriving when they did, these admissions added stress to the nurses involved.

Time

Time is universal and exists in every culture. However, time is based on an individual's perceptions of the movement of life events (King, 1981).

"Time moves from the past to the future" (King, 1981, p. 43) and is measurable. However, time is to be viewed in relation to other concepts such as age, body temperature, order of events, sequence of events, and space.

There are several time perspectives: (a) biological, (b) psychological, which is perceived subjectively, (c) physical, as measured by clocks, and (d) relational, which connects the past with the present and the future. However, time is defined by each individual (King, 1981).

Example: Within 5 minutes, the nurse returned to the client with a pain medication. To the client, it seemed as though half an hour had passed. Each had a different perception of time.

Transaction

The concept of transaction was developed from a review of research literature that identified its characteristics. From these characteristics, a definition was formulated. A transaction involves the perceptions of individuals and is therefore unique. It concerns both verbal and nonverbal communication. Each transaction is a "series of events in time" used to achieve a goal (King, 1981, pp. 80-81).

Whereas communication is the informational component of interactions, transaction is the "valuational component" (King, 1981, p. 62). Transaction "involves bargaining, negotiating, and social exchange, and is influenced by role expectations and role performance" (King, 1981, p. 147).

A transaction "represents a life situation in which . . . each person enters the situation as an active participant, and each is changed in the process of these experiences"(King, 1981, p. 142). A transaction is affected by the actions, judgments, perceptions, and reactions of human beings (King, 1981). The "unit of analysis is the dyadic interactions of nurse and [client] who come together in a specific place called a nursing situation that is within a larger system called a health care system" (King, 1981, p. 83).

Goal attainment occurs as a result of a transaction between a nurse and a client (King, 1981). Transaction involves the process of mutual goal setting and the joint establishment of the means to achieve the goal.

Example: A nurse and a client discussed how they could work together to decrease the client's use of pain medications. They decide that the goal would be two pain pills per 24-hour period. They identified relaxation techniques that could be used to increase the length of time between pain pills and determined that they would increase the length of time between pain pills by half an hour each time. Together, they implemented this plan until, on the third day, the client was comfortable with only two pain pills in 24 hours.

Metaparadigm Concepts

Metaparadigm concepts identified in the nursing literature are (a) environment, (b) health, (c) nursing, and (d) person. Although there is controversy as to whether nursing should be included as a metaparadigm concept, the following section reviews King's writings about three of these four concepts. (Person was discussed in relation to personal systems.)

Health

Each culture defines health differently. King's definition of health is "a dynamic state of an individual in which change is [a] constant and an ongoing process" (1989a, p. 152); it is a "functional state in the life cycle" (King, 1981, p. 5).

According to King (1981, p. 4), health is a "process of human growth and development [and] relates to the way individuals deal with the stress of growth and development while functioning within the cultural pattern in which they were born and to which they attempt to conform." Health is needed in order to lead a "useful, satisfying, productive and happy life. The level of health depends on harmony and balance in each person's environment" (King, 1981, p. 4).

Health and illness are not part of a linear continuum. King has chosen not to address wellness because it is too abstract and would lend support to the continuum perspective (King, 1990). Whereas health is a "functional state in the life cycle, [illness is] some interference in the cycle" (King, 1981, p. 5). King (1981) defines illness as a "deviation from normal, that is, an imbalance in a person's biological structure or . . . psychological make-up, or a conflict in a person's social relationship" (p. 5).

Preventing illness is not the same as promoting health. Health of individuals and groups is "the goal for nursing" (King, 1975b, p. 37).

Environment

King does not discuss environment directly in her 1981 book. However, she does define the environment as the social system surrounding the concept in question (King, 1990). Hence the environment of a child could include family, school, peer, religious, and neighborhood social systems.

In addition, King determined that an environment can be both external and internal. In this holistic view of the environment, external and internal aspects are interrelated. For example, the "internal environment of human beings transforms energy to enable them to adjust to continuous external environmental changes" (King, 1981, p. 5).

Nursing

Nursing involves (a) "recognition of presenting conditions, (b) operations or activities related to the situation or conditions, and (c) motivation to exert some control over the events in the situation to achieve goals" (King, 1981, p. 144). Goal setting occurs in every nursing situation (King, 1981). Other important aspects of nursing are (a) listening, (b) communicating, (c) special knowledge, (d) professional skills and values, and (e) goal setting (King, 1981).

King (1989a, p. 150) wrote that the focus of nursing is the interaction of human beings with their environment "in ways that lead to self fulfillment and to maintenance of health" (King, 1981, p. 3)—the "care of human beings" (King, 1981, p. 10). What makes nursing unique, according to King (1981), is the way nurses use knowledge to perform their functions. Nursing goals are separate from the activities undertaken to attain them, and they are "distinct from the goals of other professions" (King, 1981, p. 97).

King (1981) defines the domain of nursing as promotion, maintenance, and restoration of health, and care of the sick, injured, and dying. The goal of nursing is to "help individuals maintain their health so they can function in their roles" (King, 1981, pp. 3-4).

The function of nursing is, in King's (1981) view, to "teach, guide and counsel individuals and groups to help them maintain health" (p. 8). This function includes the "interpretation of specific information to plan, implement and evaluate nursing care. Knowledge from natural and behavioral sciences and the humanities is integrated and applied in concrete situations" (p. 8). This knowledge is applied in relation to human behavior under normal and stressful conditions. Techniques used by nurses include (a) assessment, (b) communication, (c) systematic gathering of information, (d) interviews, (e) measurement, and (f) observation.

The basic unit of nursing behavior is a nursing act; an interaction between a nurse and client (King, 1989a). These interactions focus on the concerns of the client (King, 1981). It is "important to move toward reciprocally contingent interactions where the behavior of one person influences the behavior of the other, . . . which requires participation by both individuals" (King, 1981, p. 85). A nurse is responsible for initiating a relationship with a client. While attempting to understand a client's behavior, a nurse involves the client in decision making and provides information for determining means to achieve goals. Nurses must be aware of a client's right to make decisions, and must provide information in order for clients to make informed choices (King, 1981). While a nurse assists a client in better understanding the perception of self and "what is happening to interfere with life events, both [the nurse and the client] help each other increase their coping behavior, and they grow in the process" (King, 1981, p. 87).

There are essential variables in nursing situations. These include communication, expectations, interdependent roles of a nurse and client, location, mutual goals, and perceptions (King, 1981).

Propositions

A proposition is a statement that "identifies a relationship between concepts" (Catanzaro & Woods, 1988, p. 20). Although distinct relationships between concepts are not always distinguished within a conceptual framework, the following propositions were initially identified by King (1964). To assist the reader, concepts from the conceptual framework and metaparadigm are italicized.

- The *nursing* process is conducted within a *social system*. The dimensions include (a) *nursing* process, (b) the *individuals* involved in the *nursing* process, (c) the *individuals* involved in the *environment* within which the *nursing* process is activated, (d) the social organization within which the *nursing* process is activated, [and] (e) the community within which the social organization functions.
- The *nursing* process will differ, dependent upon the individual nurse and each recipient of *nursing* service.
- The *nursing* process will differ relative to all *individuals* in the *environment*.
- The *nursing* process will differ relative to the social organization in which the *nursing* process takes place.
- The relationships among the dimensions have an effect upon the *nursing* process.
- *Nursing* includes specific components: (a) *nursing* judgment, (b) nurse action, (c) *communication*, (d) evaluation, [and] (e) coordination.
- The *nursing* judgment will vary relative to each *nursing* action.
- The effectiveness of *nursing* action will vary with the extent to which it is *communicated* to those responsible for its implementation.

- *Nursing* action is more effectively assured if the goals are *communicated* and standards of *nursing* performance have been established.
- *Nursing* action is based on facts, which may change; thus *nursing* judgments and action are evaluated and revised as the situation changes.
- *Nursing* is a component of *health* care; thus *health* care is effected by the coordination of *nursing* with *health* services. (pp. 401-402)

9

Theory of Goal Attainment

King has derived one theory from her conceptual framework—the Theory of Goal Attainment. The focus of this theory is the interpersonal system because what nurses do with, and for, individuals is what "makes the difference between nursing and any other health profession. [The focus of the theory is on] holism—that is, the total human being interacting with another total human being in a specific situation" (King, 1989a, pp. 154-155).

The Theory of Goal Attainment is a "theory of nursing [that] deals with phenomena called process and outcome" (Smith, 1988, p. 82). The process that is the critical, independent variable is mutual goal setting. The theory "defines outcomes in the form of the goals to be attained" (King, 1989a, p. 156). If the goals are identified as client behaviors, then they become criteria by which the effectiveness of nursing care can be measured (King, 1989a).

Context

King characterized the context within which the Theory of Goal Attainment occurs as:

(a) Nurse and client do not know each other.
(b) Nurse is licensed to practice professional nursing.

(c) Client is in need of the services provided by the nurse.

(d) Nurse and client are in a reciprocal relationship in that the nurse has special knowledge and skills to communicate appropriate information to help client set goals. Client has information about self and perceptions of problems or concerns that, when communicated to nurse, will help in mutual goal setting.

(e) Nurse and client are in mutual presence, purposefully interacting to achieve goals.

(f) Interactions are in a two-person group.

(g) Interactions are limited to licensed professional nurse and to a client in need of nursing care.

(h) Interactions are taking place in natural environments. (King, 1981, p. 150)

Assumptions

The following are the assumptions on which the Theory of Goal Attainment is based:

(a) Individuals are social beings.

(b) Individuals are sentient beings.

(c) Individuals are rational beings.

(d) Individuals are reacting beings.

(e) Individuals are perceiving beings.

(f) Individuals are controlling beings.

(g) Individuals are purposeful beings.

(h) Individuals are action-oriented beings.

(i) Individuals are time-oriented beings.

(j) Perceptions of nurse and of client influence the interaction process.

(k) Goals, needs and values of nurse and client influence the interaction process.

(l) Individuals have a right to knowledge about themselves.

(m) Individuals have a right to participate in decisions that influence their life, their health, and community services.

(n) Health professionals have a responsibility to share information that helps individuals make informed decisions about their health care.

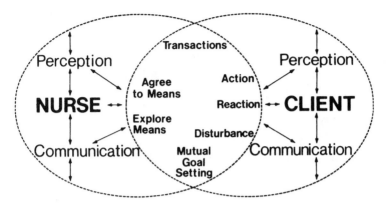

Figure 9.1. Schematic diagram of a theory of goal attainment.
SOURCE: King (1981, p. 157). Copyright 1981 by Delmar Publishers, Inc. Reprinted by permission.

    (o) Individuals have a right to accept or reject health care.

    (p) Goals of health professionals and goals of recipients of health care may be incongruent. (King, 1981, pp. 143-144)

Concepts

Major elements in the theory lie within the interpersonal system "in which two people . . . come together . . . to help and be helped to maintain a state of health that permits functioning in roles" (King, 1981, p. 142). The theory uses the concepts of communication, growth and development, interaction, perception, role, self, space, stress, time, and transaction.

The theory also identifies that "decision making is a shared collaborative process in which client and nurse give information to each other, identify goals, and explore means to attain goals; each moves forward to attain goals" (King, 1989a, p. 155). Figure 9.1 illustrates how goals are attained according to this theory.

The theory cannot be directly applied to practice because of its abstract nature. However, one can apply knowledge of the concepts in practice. If relationships among concepts within practice are identified and tested in research, the resulting knowledge can also then be applied (King, 1989a).

Propositions

The following are the propositions of the Theory of Goal Attainment. To assist the reader, the theory's concepts have been italicized.

(a) If *perceptual* accuracy is present in nurse-client *interactions, transactions* will occur.

(b) If nurse and client make *transactions,* goals will be attained.

(c) If goals are attained, satisfactions will occur.

(d) If goals are attained, effective nursing care will occur.

(e) If *transactions* are made in nurse-client *interactions, growth and development* will be enhanced.

(f) If *role* expectations and *role* performance as *perceived* by nurse and client are congruent, *transactions* will occur.

(g) If *role* conflict is experienced by nurse or client or both, *stress* in nurse-client *interactions* will occur.

(h) If nurses with special knowledge and skills *communicate* appropriate information to clients, mutual goal setting and goal attainment will occur. (King, 1981, p. 149)

Testing of the Theory of Goal Attainment

King (1981) states that "the first phase of testing the theory was to describe nurse-[client] interactions that lead to transactions in concrete nursing situations" (p. 151). A study was designed to answer three questions.

First, "What elements in nurse-[client] interactions lead to transactions?" (King, 1981, p. 151). King's research resulted in the following elements of interactions that may lead to transactions: (a) the client identifies a health concern; (b) the "nurse and [client] explore the situation, share information and mutually set goals" (King, 1981, p. 154); and (c) the nurse and client explore means by which the concern can be addressed, the goal attained, thus implementing the plan and achieving the goal.

Second, "What are the relationships between the elements in the interactions that lead to transactions?" (King, 1981, p. 151). King (1981) defined six relationships that were identified as predictors or independent variables:

1. One member of the nurse-client dyad initiates behavior.
2. Opposite member of the nurse-client dyad responds with behavior.
3. Disturbance (or problem) is noted in the dyadic situation if a state or condition is identified.
4. Some goal is mutually agreed upon by members of the dyad.
5. Exploration of means to achieve goals is initiated by one member of dyad, or behavior is exhibited by member of dyad that moves toward goals.
6. Other member agrees with means to achieve goal. (pp. 150-151)

The presence of these behaviors could predict the possibility of transactions. The seventh behavior was labeled as the dependent variable.

Third, "What are the essential variables in nurse-[client] interactions that result in transactions?" (King, 1981, p. 151). As a result of the research, the following variables are proposed as essential in nurse-[client] interactions. The first variable is that the perceptions regarding the situation of both a nurse and a client need to be congruent. The perceptions could relate to expectations, goals, health concerns, means to achieve goals, and roles. Relevant communication also must be present. Finally, if a transaction is to occur, mutual goal setting must be present. Together, a nurse and client collaborate in identifying goals to be achieved (for additional details about the method, procedure, sample, and outcome of the study, see King, 1981, pp. 153-156).

Hypotheses

The hypotheses of a theory are "tentative statements that can be tested empirically" (Woods & Catanzaro, 1988, p. 558). King (1981) derived the following hypotheses from the Theory of Goal Attainment:

(a) Perceptual accuracy in nurse-[client] interactions increases mutual goal setting.

(b) Communication increases mutual goal setting between nurses and [clients] and leads to satisfactions.

(c) Satisfactions in nurses and [clients] increase goal attainment.

(d) Goal attainment decreases stress and anxiety in nursing situations.

(e) Goal attainment increases [client] learning and coping ability in nursing situations.

(f) Role conflict experienced by [clients], nurses, or both decreases transactions in nurse-[client] interactions.

(g) Congruence in role expectations and role performance increases transactions in nurse-[client] interactions. (p. 156)

The following additional hypotheses have been developed and tested by other researchers:

1. Functional abilities will be greater in clients who participate in mutual goal setting than in clients who do not.

2. Goal attainment will be greater with clients who participate in mutual goal setting than with clients who do not.

3. There will be a positive relationship between a client's functional abilities and goal attainment.

4. Mutual goal setting will increase a client's functional abilities in activities of daily living.

5. Mutual goal setting will increase elderly clients' morale.

6. Mutual goal setting by client and nurse leads to goal attainment.

7. Mutual goal setting by client and nurse leads to increased satisfaction for both.

8. Mutual goal setting increases self esteem of the client. (King, 1990)

10

Utilization of the Conceptual Framework and the Theory of Goal Attainment

Whereas the conceptual framework provides nurses with a perspective from which to practice, the "Theory of Goal Attainment provides a theoretical base for nursing process as it demonstrates a way for nurses to interact purposefully with clients" (King, 1981, p. 176). Both the conceptual framework and the theory can be applied to various nursing contexts. These applications include the following:

- Assisting nurses to arrange facts into meaningful wholes
- Developing research hypotheses
- Providing a foundation for nursing care administration
- Developing curriculum
- Practice applications (King, 1989a)
- Delineating the Goal Oriented Nursing Record
- Measuring the effectiveness of nursing care through quality assurance activities (King, 1981)

The following uses of the conceptual framework and the Theory of Goal Attainment in nursing practice are discussed:

1. Use of the conceptual framework to guide the nursing process
2. Use of the theory related to the Goal Oriented Nursing Record (GONR)
3. Use of the theory related to the Criterion-Referenced Measure of Goal Attainment (CRMGA).

Nursing Process

The following discussion describes the nursing process as it could be conducted according to King's (1981) conceptual framework. In the assessment phase of the nursing process, nurses gather information about a nurse, a client, and a situation. To do this, nurses employ observation and measurement skills (King, 1989a). An assessment could include the following information that has been arranged based on King's (1981) framework:

1. Body image
2. Growth and development
   (a) Chronological age
   (b) Developmental age
   (c) Diet history
   (d) Education
   (e) Medication history
   (f) Initial assessment of a client's intact sensory system
   (g) Interference in any of the senses
   (h) Sex
   (i) Substance abuse history
3. Perceptions
   (a) Anxiety level
   (b) Current health status
   (c) Reason for seeking health care
   (d) Stress level
4. Self
   (a) Communication style between client and family, and client and health care providers
   (b) Culture
   (c) Learning needs

(d) Motivation for learning

(e) Space

(f) Personal space definition

5. Time

(a) Time orientation

(b) Time estimation

In the planning phase of nursing, a nurse determines client needs by communicating (verbally and nonverbally), observing, and interpreting information (King, 1981). A nurse and a client engage in mutual goal setting and identification of the means to achieve them.

Implementation occurs when a nurse and client work together in a unique relationship in a health care setting. In this relationship, a client has an active role in making decisions about the present and future and gains control and independence through this participation (King, 1981). Together, a nurse and client begin to implement mechanisms by which the mutually agreed upon goals can be attained, and the needs of a client can be met. For example, a client's need for personal space could be met by a nurse (a) controlling the client care environment, (b) explaining to a client why a nurse was in that client's room, (c) explaining procedures prior to their implementation, and (d) orienting a client to the health care setting (King, 1981).

Evaluation occurs when a nurse and client determine whether or not the mutually set goals were attained. Goals may then be revised, or new goals mutually established, to continue the process.

Goal Oriented Nursing Record (GONR)

The GONR records both the process (means used to achieve goals) and the outcomes (attainment of goals) (King, 1981). This documentation system demonstrates that quality assurance in nursing includes process and outcomes based on the Theory of Goal Attainment. The GONR has five major elements: database, nursing diagnoses, goal lists, nursing orders that accompany the goals, plans, and progress notes.

The database contains all assessment information regarding an individual client. Based on the information in the database, a nurse develops nursing diagnoses. These diagnoses are revised as they are resolved and as new information is obtained. The diagnoses serve as a guide for "continual assessment of subjective and objective signs and symptoms of a disturbance or interference in clients' ability to perform in usual roles, . . . [and] planning the immediate nursing care" (King, 1981, p. 170).

The goal list results from nurse-client interactions that focus on plans for the resolution of previously identified concerns. The goal list can serve several additional purposes:

1. Assist a nurse in monitoring the health concerns of a client
2. Serve as a mechanism for a nurse and client to transact
3. Foster the provision of continuity of care
4. Emphasize a client's involvement in health care decisions
5. "Provide a consistent and systematic approach to help individuals move toward a healthy state.
6. Facilitate nursing audits" (King, 1981, p. 171)

The plan is founded on the database. It includes the nursing diagnoses, goals, and actions used by the nurse and client to achieve those goals (King, 1981).

Progress notes provide the documentation of the nursing care and client involvement. Progress notes can be one of the following three types: (a) narrative, (b) flow sheet (could be designed like a table for the presentation of data) (King, 1990), and (c) final summary or discharge note that describes the status of the goals.

Criterion-Referenced Measure of Goal Attainment (CRMGA)

CRMGA is another application of the Theory of Goal Attainment to nursing practice. This measure estimates a client's "functional ability and goal attainment, [developed] to measure goal attainment . . . in nursing situations" (King, 1988, p. 198).

Nurses generally establish goals. However, they "have not always stated them in terms of expected client performance behavior that is observable and/or measureable" (King, 1988, p. 110). There are three objectives for the instrument related to a client's performance of daily living activities: (a) "assess physical ability of individuals . . . ,

(b) assess the behavioral response of individuals . . . , and (c) select a goal and measure goal attainment" (King, 1988, p. 111).

There are three scales in the instrument: Physical Abilities, Behavioral Responses, and Goals. Each scale has three subscales: Personal Hygiene, Movement, and Human Interactions.

Some initial reliability and validity estimates of the instrument have been obtained. Interrater reliability was established at 85% within a nursing home setting and 99% in a critical care setting (King, 1988) (for additional data regarding the reliability and validity estimates, refer to King, 1988).

11

Future Directions for Research

As evidenced by the hypotheses previously detailed, research about King's conceptual framework and Theory of Goal Attainment is ongoing. However, much work remains to be done. King (1990) has indicated that additional research should focus on the application of her theory to school, home health practice, occupational health, and transcultural settings. Additional research that uses the conceptual framework to develop theories within the three systems (personal, interpersonal, and social) would also aid in extending the application of King's work.

12

Summary

King's conceptual framework and theory focus on the mutual presence of a nurse and a client as they work together regarding the client's health concerns. By viewing both the nurse and client holistically, an emphasis is placed on verbal and nonverbal communication. As a nurse and client mutually set client goals and the means to achieve these goals, the focus remains on a client's active involvement in health care.

King's conceptual framework and theory can be used to develop (a) theory-based clinical nursing practice, (b) nursing administration within a social systems context, (c) nursing curriculums, (d) nursing knowledge, and (e) nursing theories. "The value of viewing nursing within this general system framework is a special way of looking at phenomena—holistically," wrote King (1989a), "yet within a specific focus based on the situation" (p. 154).

Glossary

Authority
Conceptual Framework: "transactional process characterized by active, reciprocal relations in which members' values, backgrounds, and perceptions play a role in defining, validating, and accepting the [directions] of individuals within an organization" (King, 1981, p. 124).

Body Image
Conceptual Framework: "an individual's perceptions of his/her own body, others' reactions to his/her appearance which results from others' reactions to self" (King, 1981, p. 33).

Communication
Conceptual Framework: "information processing, a change of information from one state to another" (King, 1981, p. 69).

Theoretical: "process whereby information is given from one person to another either directly in face-to-face meetings or indirectly through telephone, television, or the written word" (King, 1981, p. 146).

Decision Making
Conceptual Framework: "dynamic and systematic process by which a goal-directed choice of perceived alternatives is made, and acted upon, by individuals or groups to answer a question and attain a goal" (King, 1981, p. 132).

Growth and Development

Conceptual Framework: "the processes that take place in an individual's life that help the individual move from potential capacity for achievement to self actualization" (King, 1981, p. 31).

Theoretical: "continuous changes in individuals at the cellular, molecular, and behavioral levels of activities" (King, 1981, p. 148).

Health

Conceptual Framework: "dynamic life experiences of a human being which implies continued adjustment to stressors in the internal and external environment through optimum use of one's resources to achieve maximum potential for daily living" (King, 1981, p. 5).

Interaction

Conceptual Framework: "acts of two or more persons in mutual presence" (King, 1981, p. 85).

Theoretical: "process of perception and communication between person and environment and between person and person, represented by verbal and nonverbal behaviors that are goal-directed" (King, 1981, p. 145).

Nursing

Conceptual Framework: "process of action, reaction, and interaction whereby nurse and client share information about their perceptions in the nursing situation. A nursing situation is the immediate environment, spatial and temporal reality, in which nurse and client establish a relationship to cope with health states and adjust to changes in activities of daily living if the situation demands adjustment" (King, 1981, p. 2).

Theoretical: "process of human interactions between nurse and client whereby each perceives the other and the situation; and through communication, they set goals, explore means, and agree on means to achieve goals" (King, 1981, p. 144).

Organization

Conceptual Framework: "a system whose continuous activities are conducted to achieve goals" (King, 1981, p. 119).

Operational: "composed of human beings with prescribed roles and positions who use resources to accomplish personal and organizational goals" (King, 1981, p. 119).

Perception
Conceptual Framework: "process of organizing, interpreting, and transforming information from sense data and memory" (King, 1981, p. 24).

Theoretical: "each person's representation of reality; awareness of persons, objects, and events" (King, 1981, p. 146).

Power
Conceptual Framework: "capacity to use resources in organizations to achieve goals"; "process whereby one or more persons influence other persons in a situation"; "capacity or ability of a group to achieve goals" (King, 1981, p. 124).

Role
Conceptual Framework/Theoretical: "set of behaviors expected when occupying a position in a social system" (King, 1981, p. 93).

Self
Conceptual Framework: "the self is a composite of thoughts and feelings which constitute a person's awareness of his/her individual existence, his/her conception of who and what he/she is. A person's self is the sum total of all he/she can call his/hers. The self includes, among other things, a system of ideas, attitudes, values and commitments. The self is a person's total subjective environment. It is a distinctive center of experience and significance. The self constitutes a person's inner world as distinguished from the outer world consisting of all other people and things. The self is the individual as known to the individual. It is that to which we refer when we say 'I' " (Jersild, 1952, pp. 9-10).

Space
Conceptual Framework: "existing in all directions and is the same everywhere" (King, 1981, p. 37).

Theoretical: "the immediate environment in which nurse and client interact and move to goal attainment" (King, 1981, p. 149).

Status
Conceptual Framework: "the position of an individual in a group or a group in relation to other groups in an organization" (King, 1981, p. 129).

Stress

Conceptual Framework/Theoretical: "dynamic state whereby a human being interacts with the environment to maintain balance for growth, development, and performance which involves an exchange of energy and information between the person and the environment for regulation and control of stressors" (King, 1981, p. 98).

Time

Conceptual Framework: "duration between the occurrence of one event and the occurrence of another event" (King, 1981, p. 44).

Theoretical: "sequence of events moving onward to the future" (King, 1981, p. 148).

Transaction

Conceptual Framework: "process of interaction in which human beings communicate with the environment to achieve goals that are values" (King, 1981, p. 82).

Theoretical: "observable behaviors of human beings interacting with their environment" (King, 1981, p. 147).

Operational: "One member of the nurse-patient dyad initiates behavior. Opposite member of the nurse-patient dyad responds with behavior. Disturbance (or problem) is noted in the dyadic situation if a state or condition is identified. Some goal is mutually agreed upon by members of the dyad. Exploration of means to achieve goals is initiated by one member of dyad, or behavior is exhibited by member of dyad that moves toward goals. Other member agrees with means to achieve goal. Both move toward goal" (King, 1981, pp. 150-151).

References

Ackermann, M. L., Brink, S. A., Jones, C. G., Moody, S. L., Perlich, G. L., & Prusinski, B. B. (1986). Imogene King: Theory of goal attainment. In A. Marriner (Ed.), *Nursing theorists and their work* (pp. 231-245). St. Louis: C. V. Mosby.

Bertalanffy, L. von (1968). *General system theory: Foundations, development, applications.* New York: George Braziller.

Catanzaro, M., & Woods, N. F. (1988). Developing nursing theory. In N. F. Woods & M. Catanzaro (Eds.), *Nursing research: Theory and practice* (pp. 18-34). St. Louis: C. V. Mosby.

Daubenmire, M. J., & King, I. M. (1973). Nursing process models: A systems approach. *Nursing Outlook, 21*(8), 512-517.

Fawcett, J. (1984). *Analysis and evaluation of conceptual models of nursing.* Philadelphia: F. A. Davis.

Gulitz, E. A., & King, I. M. (1988). King's general systems model: Application to curriculum development. *Nursing Science Quarterly, 1*(3), 128-132.

Jersild, A. T. (1952). *In search of self.* New York: Teachers College Press.

King, I. M. (1964, October). Nursing theory: Problems and prospects. *Nursing Science*, pp. 394-403.

King, I. M. (1971). *Toward a theory for nursing: General concepts of human behavior.* New York: John Wiley.

King, I. M. (1975a). A process for developing concepts for nursing through research. In P. J. Verhovick (Ed.), *Nursing research I* (pp. 25-43). Boston: Little, Brown.

King, I. M. (1975b). Patient aspects. In L. J. Shuman, R. D. Speas, Jr., & J. P. Young (Eds.), *Operations research in health care: A critical analysis* (pp. 3-20). Baltimore: Johns Hopkins University Press.

King, I. M. (1981). *A theory for nursing: Systems, concepts, process.* New York: John Wiley.

King, I. M. (1988). Measuring health goal attainment in patients. In C. F. Waltz & O. L. Strickland (Eds.), *Measurement of nursing outcomes: Measuring client outcomes* (Vol. 1, pp. 108-127). New York: Springer.

King, I. M. (1989a). King's general systems framework and theory. In J. P. Riehl-Sisca (Ed.), *Conceptual models for nursing practice* (3rd ed., pp. 149-158). Norwalk, CT: Appleton & Lange.

King, I. M. (1989b). King's systems framework for nursing administration. In B. Henry, C. Arndt, M. Di Vincenti, & A. Marriner-Tomey (Eds.), *Dimensions of nursing administration: Theory, research, education, practice* (pp. 35-45). Cambridge: Blackwell Scientific.

King, I. M. (1990, July). Speech presented at the Wayne State University College of Nursing Summer Research Conference, Detroit, MI.

Meleis, A. I. (1985). *Theoretical nursing: Development and progress.* Philadelphia: J. B. Lippincott.

Smith, M. J. (1988). Perspectives on nursing science. *Nursing Science Quarterly, 1*(2), 80-85.

Woods, N. F., & Catanzaro, M. (1988). *Nursing research: Theory and practice.* St. Louis: C. V. Mosby.

Bibliography

Other Publications by Imogene King

1964, October. Nursing theory: Problems and prospects. *Nursing Science*, pp. 394-403.

1968. A conceptual frame of reference for nursing. *Nursing Research, 17*(1), 27-31.

1971. *Toward a theory for nursing: General concepts of human behavior.* New York: John Wiley.

1976. The health care systems: Nursing intervention subsystem. In H. H. Werley, A. Zuzich, M. Zajkowski, & A. D. Zagornik (Eds.), *Health research: The systems approach* (pp. 50-51). New York: Springer.

1978. The "why" of theory development. In *Theory development: What, why, how?* (pp. 11-16). New York: National League for Nursing.

1982. The effect of structured and unstructured pre-operative teaching: A replication. *Nursing Research, 31*(6), 324-329.

1984. Effectiveness of nursing care: Use of a goal oriented nursing record in end stage renal disease. *American Association of Nephrology Nurses and Technicians Journal, 11*(2), 11-17, 60.

1987. King's theory of goal attainment. In R. R. Parse (Ed.), *Nursing science: Major paradigms, theories, and critiques* (pp. 107-113). Philadelphia: W. B. Saunders.

1988. Concepts: Essential elements of theories. *Nursing Science Quarterly, 1*(1), 22-25.

1990. Health: The goal for nursing. *Nursing Science Quarterly, 3*(3), 123-128.

Publications About Imogene King

Austin, J. K., & Champion, V. L. (1983). King's theory for nursing: Explication and evaluation. In P. L. Chinn (Ed.), *Advances in nursing theory development* (pp. 49-61). Rockville, MD: Aspen Systems.

Brown, S. T., & Lee, B. T. (1980). Imogene King's conceptual framework: A proposed model for continuing nursing education. *Journal of Advanced Nursing, 5*(5), 467-473.

Elberson, K. (1989). Applying King's model to nursing administration. In B. Henry, C. Arndt, M. Di Vincenti, & A. Marriner-Tomey (Eds.), *Dimensions of nursing administration: Theory, research, education, practice* (pp. 47-53). Cambridge: Blackwell Scientific.

Fawcett, J. (1984). *Analysis and evaluation of conceptual models of nursing.* Philadelphia: F. A. Davis.

George, J. B. (1985). Imogene M. King. In J. B. George (Ed.), *Nursing theories: The base for professional nursing practice* (pp. 235-256). Englewood Cliffs, NJ: Prentice Hall.

Gonot, R. J. (1983). Imogene M. King: A theory for nursing. In J. Fitzpatrick & A. Whall (Eds.), *Conceptual models of nursing: Analysis and application.* Bowie, MD: Robert J. Brady.

Hanchett, E. S. (1988). *Nursing frameworks and community as client: Bridging the gap.* Norwalk, CT: Appleton & Lange.

Hanucharurnkul, S. (1989). Comparative analysis of Orem's and King's theories. *Journal of Advanced Nursing, 14*(5), 365-372.

Meleis, A. I. (1985). *Theoretical nursing: Development and progress.* Philadelphia: J. B. Lippincott.

Pearson, A., & Vaughan, B. (1986). *Nursing models for practice.* London: Heinemann Nursing.

Torres, G. (1986). *Theoretical foundations of nursing.* Norwalk, CT: Appleton-Century-Crofts.

PART III

Callista Roy

An Adaptation Model

LOUETTE R. JOHNSON LUTJENS

Biographical Sketch of the Nurse Theorist:
Sister Callista Roy, PhD, RN, FAAN

Born: October 14, 1939
BA: Nursing, Mount St. Mary's College, Los Angeles, 1963
MSN: University of California, Los Angeles, 1966
MA: Sociology, University of California, Los Angeles, 1975
PhD: Sociology, University of California, Los Angeles, 1977
Post Doctoral Fellow: Robert Wood Johnson Clinical Nurse
        Scholar Program (Neuroscience), University of
        California, San Francisco, 1983-1985
Fellow: American Academy of Nursing
Member: Sisters of St. Joseph of Carondolet
Position: Professor, School of Nursing, Boston College

Foreword

When you walk onto our unit at Montefiore Medical Center you often will not see a nurse. The nurses are with the patients and their families. Since the implementation of the Roy Adaptation Model for theory based practice, there is a new perspective of the nurse-patient relationship.

The evolution of nursing models has been rapid. Over the past five years, the development of nursing theory derived from these models has also grown dramatically, adding to the scientific base of nursing. Because nursing is a practice discipline, the ultimate goal of nursing theory is to guide and enhance that practice.

Each of the nursing models and related theories provides a particular lens for the nurse to use when viewing nursing situations. The Roy Adaptation Model provides one of these lenses. Roy's view of the person as an adaptive system is a particularly useful one given the complex nature of the problems nurses encounter in today's heath care arena.

The value of the Roy Model is in its ability to serve as a framework for practice, education, administration, and research. Dr. Louette Lutjens has masterfully presented the model in a way that emphasizes its value for contributing to each of these areas. She also demonstrates how the Roy Adaptation Model provides a viable framework for organizing and providing nursing care as well as for building nursing knowledge through theory development.

91

As nursing educators increasingly include nursing models in the beginning education levels of the profession, as well as in graduate studies, nurses will increasingly depend on nursing conceptual models in their practice. The use of works such as this will serve nursing well by providing a guide for nurses to make informed and assertive demands for theory-based practice.

Through this section, Dr. Lutjens offers the next generation of nurses an enhanced pride of membership in a truly scientific profession.

KEVILLE FREDERICKSON, RN, EDD
Professor of Nursing
Lehman College of the City University of New York
and Clinical Nurse Scientist
Montefiore Medical Center
Bronx, NY

Preface

The nursing profession is fortunate to have many nurse theorists who have provided the discipline with conceptual models with which to view the world of nursing. The various models capture the diversity inherent in nursing while at the same time shaping its unique body of knowledge.

Sister Dr. Callista Roy is a well-known nurse theorist whose conceptual model is based on the concept of adaptation. This volume presents a current, succinct description of the Roy Adaptation Model, as well as the theory of Person as an Adaptive System and the Theory of Adaptive Modes. Serving as a summary of the basic concepts of the model and derived theories, this section supplements the original primary sources primarily Roy and Roberts (1981), Roy (1984), Andrews and Roy (1986), and Roy and Andrews (1991).

This section is intended primarily for undergraduate students who are studying several nursing models with their differing terms, language, and theory-specific definitions of common concepts. It could also be used as a brief review by nursing faculty and graduate students.

A bibliography is provided to direct readers to appropriate sources for in-depth information on the Roy model, including use of the nursing process, applications to practice and education, and analysis and critique of the conceptual model. It is hoped that this description of the Roy Adaptation Model will entice readers to make use of the references provided.

I would like to acknowledge the careful and thoughtful critique of this text by Dr. Patricia Underwood, Associate Professor and Coordinator of the Graduate Program at Kirkhof School of Nursing, Grand Valley State University, Allendale, MI. Dr. Underwood is also the current president of the Michigan Nurses' Association. Also, I would like to thank Sister Callista Roy for her review of an earlier draft of this text and her encouragement and support over the past several years.

—Louette R. Johnson Lutjens

13

Origin of the Model

While a graduate student at the University of California, Los Angeles (1964-1966), Sister Dr. Callista Roy was challenged in a seminar by another nurse theorist, Dorothy E. Johnson, to develop a theory of nursing. Subsequently, in 1964, the Roy Adaptation Model (RAM) was born as a derivation of Bertalanffy's General Systems Theory and Harry Helson's Adaptation-Level Theory. Other experts in the field of adaptation who influenced Roy in the development of her model included Dohrenwend, Lazarus, Mechanic, and Selye. Rapoport's ideas in the area of systems and Maslow's thoughts on human needs also contributed to the model.

The adaptation concept was introduced to Roy in a psychology class. In her clinical work in pediatric nursing, she had been impressed with the ability of children to bounce back when faced with illness. The adaptation concept seemed to be a suitable concept upon which to base a conceptual model of nursing. Roy's ultimate goal was "to demonstrate that the practice of nursing, based on the science of nursing, makes a difference in the health status of the population" (Roy & Roberts, 1981, xv). Roy estimates that more than 1,500 faculty and students have contributed to the theoretical development of the Roy Model (Andrews & Roy, 1991a).

The Roy Adaptation Model was first formally used in 1968 as the conceptual framework for the baccalaureate nursing curriculum at Mount St. Mary's College in Los Angeles, where Roy was chair of the

Department of Nursing. Roy is a prolific writer who has spent much time and effort over the years developing and refining the model. The seminal and classic theory text on the Roy Adaptation Model is *Theory Construction in Nursing: An Adaptation Model* written by Roy and Sharon Roberts and published in 1981. Roy works extremely well with other nurse scholars on a national and international basis, mentoring them in the use of her model in education, service, practice, and research. Roy's contributions to nursing science are commendable and significant.

14

Assumptions of the Model

Assumptions are "givens"—that is, statements assumed to be true without proof. With any conceptual model or theory, students must be able to accept the assumptions before adopting the specific model or theory.

Scientific Assumptions

Roy's scientific assumptions have received much attention in the literature. These eight assumptions, which are based on systems and adaptation-level theories, are as follows:

1. The person is a bio-psycho-social being.
2. The person is in constant interaction with a changing environment.
3. To cope with a changing world, the person uses both innate and acquired mechanisms, which are biologic, psychologic, and social in origin.
4. Health and illness are one inevitable dimension of life.
5. To respond positively to environmental changes, the person must adapt.
6. The person's adaptation is a function of the stimulus exposed to and one's adaptation level.

7. The person's adaptation level is such that it comprises a zone that indicates the range of stimulation that will lead to a positive response.

8. The person is conceptualized as having four modes of adaptation: physiologic, self-concept, role function, and interdependence. (Roy, 1980, pp. 180-182)[1]

Philosophical Assumptions

Until recently, the philosophical assumptions of the RAM had not been as explicit, specific, and organized as the scientific assumptions. Roy (1988) addressed this limitation by a thoughtful explication of eight philosophical assumptions, four based on the philosophical principle of humanism and four based on the philosophical principle of "veritivity" (a word coined by Roy).

Humanism. Humanism "recognizes the person and subjective dimensions of human experience as central to knowing and to valuing" (Roy, 1988, p. 29). Roy credits Maslow with influencing her thoughts on humanism. The four philosophical assumptions based on the humanist principle are as follows. The individual

1. Shares in creative power
2. Behaves purposefully, not in a sequence of cause and effect
3. Possesses intrinsic holism
4. Strives to maintain integrity and to realize the need for relationships

Veritivity. The term veritivity, derived from the Latin *veritas,* meaning truth, was coined by Roy. The premise underlying Roy's term is that there is an absolute truth. Roy (1988) defines veritivity "as a principle of human nature that affirms a common purposefulness of human existence" (p. 30). The four philosophical assumptions based on the veritivity principle are as follows. The individual is viewed in the context of

1. Purposefulness of human existence
2. Unity of purpose of humankind

3. Activity and creativity for the common good
4. Value and meaning of life (p. 32)

The eight scientific and eight philosophical assumptions provide a basis for theorizing and research within the RAM.

Note

1. Slight revisions have been made in the scientific assumptions to reflect changes made by Roy over the years.

15

Concepts of the Model

Roy's model is a systems model that focuses on outcomes. The major features of systems models are the system and its environment. According to Andrews and Roy (1991a), "a system is a set of parts connected to function as a whole for some purpose and does so by virtue of the interdependence of its parts" (p. 7). A system is open, nonmechanistic; behavior is determined by the free interplay of changing forces (Roy & Anway, 1989).

Roy views adaptation as both a process and a product or end-state. The process of adaptation is described as one in which stressors produce, at least in part, an interaction called stress. Stress triggers the use of coping behaviors to assist persons to reduce or alleviate the stress. The ways or methods of coping produce adaptive or ineffective responses. Adaptation is a process that "involves a systematic series of actions directed toward some end" (Roy, 1990). The result of the process of adaptation is the end-state or outcome of adaptation. Adaptation as a state is "the condition of the person with respect to the environment" (Roy, 1990).

In the Roy Adaptation Model, the person is conceptualized as an open adaptive system engaging in interchange with the environment. Roy and McLeod (1981) described adaptation for the open system of an individual as "the person's response to the environment which promotes the general goals of the person including survival, growth, reproduction, and mastery" (p. 53). Major factors influencing the adaptation of the person throughout life are culture, family, and growth and development (Sato, 1984).

Person

Key concepts in the Roy Adaptation Model are person, goal, health, environment, and nursing activities. Roy uses person in her model as a concept to identify the recipient of nursing care. Critical to the model is the description of recipients of nursing care as holistic adaptive systems. The term *adaptive* "means that the human system has the capacity to adjust effectively to changes in the environment and, in turn, affect the environment" (Andrews & Roy, 1991a, p. 7). Persons employ coping mechanisms to assist them in adapting to their environment. Roy has identified four major areas in which the activities of the coping mechanisms can be seen. She refers to these areas as adaptive modes. Together the coping mechanisms and the modes reflect the integration of the individual.

Goal

The goal of nursing within this model is to promote adaptation in four adaptive modes (physiologic, self-concept, role function, and interdependence) and thereby contribute to health. When people are in an adaptive state, they are free to respond to other stimuli. "This freeing of energy links the concept of adaptation to the concept of health" (Roy, 1984, p. 38).

Health

Health has been defined as "a state and a process of being and becoming an integrated and whole person" (Andrews & Roy, 1991a, p. 19). Holism and integrated functioning are not only basic premises

of systems theory (Roy & Anway, 1989) but are also congruent with
the philosophical assumptions of Roy's model (Roy, 1988).

Health as a state reflects the adaptation process and is demonstrated by adaptation in each of four integrated adaptive modes:
physiologic, self-concept, role function, and interdependence. The
integration of these four adaptive modes reflects wholeness.

Health is a process whereby individuals are striving to achieve their
maximum potential. This process can be readily seen in healthy
people who exercise regularly, do not smoke, and pay attention to
their dietary habits. The process of health can also be seen in persons
in the terminal stages of cancer as they seek control over symptoms,
such as pain, and strive for integration within themselves and in
relation to significant others.

Environment

Roy has broadly defined environment as "all conditions, circumstances, and influences that surround and affect the development and
behavior of the person" (Andrews & Roy, 1991a, p. 18) or group (Roy,
1984, p. 39). Thus all stimuli, whether internal or external, are part of
the person's environment. Within her model, Roy specifically catego-
rizes stimuli as focal, contextual, and residual. (The categories of
stimuli are discussed later.) Changes in the environment act as cata-
lysts, stimulating persons to make adaptive responses.

Nursing Activities

The last key concept in the Roy Adaptation Model is nursing
activities, which have been described as the nursing process. The
nursing process, according to the Roy model, consists of six steps:
assessment of behavior, assessment of stimuli, nursing diagnosis,
goal setting, intervention, and evaluation. Roy describes two levels
of assessment. The first level consists of an assessment of behavior in
each of the adaptive modes. Behavior is an indicator of how well
persons are adapting to or managing to cope with changes in their
health status. Areas of concern or adaptive problems evolve through

a mutual (nurse and patient) process in the form of ineffective behaviors needing modification or adaptive behaviors needing reinforcing. An initial tentative nursing judgment is made at this level as to whether the patient behaviors are adaptive or ineffective. Andrews and Roy (1991b) have developed typologies of commonly recurring adaptation problems (pp. 41-42) and indicators of positive adaptation (pp. 38-39) associated with each of the four modes. (Examples of adaptation problems and indicators of positive adaptation are given in the sections on adaptive modes.)

The second level of assessment involves the identification of focal, contextual, and residual stimuli that have influenced those behaviors that are of concern to the nurse and the patient. Common contextual stimuli that have an effect on behavior in all adaptive modes are culture, family, developmental stage, integrity of adaptive modes, effectiveness of the cognator processes, and other environmental factors, such as the use of drugs, alcohol, and tobacco (Andrews & Roy, 1991b). Nursing diagnoses are made based on the nurse's interpretation of assessment data. The diagnoses are clinical judgments conveying the person's adaptation status that may be stated in one of three ways: as a summary label (e.g., anxiety) for behaviors in one mode (self-concept), as a statement of the behaviors within one mode with the most relevant influencing stimuli (e.g., symptoms of anxiety from medical treatment of cancer), or as a label that summarizes a behavioral pattern when more than one mode is being affected by the same stimuli (e.g., depression related to loss of a breast) (Andrews & Roy, 1991b).

Goals are stated in terms of patient outcomes after they have been mutually agreed upon by patient and nurse. Nursing interventions are selected and directed toward the management of stimuli to produce adaptive responses that promote health and well-being. Nursing management is directed toward altering the focal stimulus or broadening the adaptation level by changing the other stimuli present. "When energy is freed from ineffective coping attempts, this energy can promote healing and enhance health" (Roy, 1984, p. 38). The relationships among the major concepts in the Roy Adaptation Model (RAM) are presented in Figure 15.1.

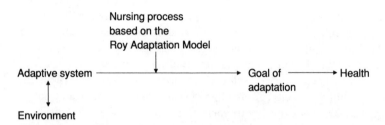

Figure 15.1. Relationships between the key concepts of the Roy model.
SOURCE: Roy (1984, p. 40). Reprinted by permission.

16

Theory of Person
as an Adaptive System

In 1981, Roy and McLeod developed a Theory of Person as an Adaptive System from the Roy Adaptation Model. In addition to the concepts of person, goal of nursing, health, environment, and nursing activities in the model, the Theory of Person as an Adaptive System employs additional concepts.

Focal, Contextual,
and Residual Stimuli

The Roy Adaptation Model describes the environment as comprising external and internal stimuli that act as stressors. These stimuli serve as input to the person, provoking a response (behavior). The stimuli have been categorized as focal, contextual, and residual. Each of the three categories can include stimuli from external and internal sources. The focal stimulus is the provoking situation or event immediately confronting persons that demands attention and prompts persons to seek relief. Contextual stimuli are all other stimuli present in the situation, or surrounding the event, that contribute to the effect of the focal stimulus. Residual stimuli are those general, vague, ambiguous factors that may be affecting a person, but their influence cannot be immediately ascertained or validated. After residual stimuli are validated, they become either focal or contextual stimuli.

More important than making fine-line distinctions about what to label a stimulus (focal, contextual, residual) is to understand which stimuli are influencing a situation and what individual factors determine how a person perceives and responds to the influencing stimuli. A given factor is not automatically a focal or contextual stimulus. It may be a focal stimulus in one situation and a contextual stimulus in another.

Adaptation Level

Helson first used the term adaptation level to label the combined effect of the three classes of stimuli (focal, contextual, and residual). In addition to the influence of the particular stimuli, the adaptation level, or combination of stimuli, influences the person. Adaptation level is a constantly changing point that represents the person's ability to cope with the changing environment in a positive manner. Adaptation level sets up a zone or range within which stimulation will lead to adaptive responses. Stimuli falling outside this adaptive zone lead to ineffective responses. Suicide due to inability to cope with the death of a child is an extreme example of an ineffective response.

If one accepts that people can be taught coping skills and can learn coping skills from life experiences, then it follows that people can change their own adaptation level to more positively deal with the challenges of everyday life. Thus the person is not passive in relation to the environment. People are active participants interacting with the environment and formulating adaptive responses—those responses contributing to general goals of survival, growth, reproduction, and mastery. Roy views these goals in a broad sense. Growth as a goal is more than an increase in physical size; individuals grow cognitively, psychologically, emotionally, and spiritually. Reproduction as a general goal is viewed as generating or "bringing forth" through a variety of human accomplishments, such as producing a pictorial or literary work of art, in addition to producing children (Roy, 1990).

Coping Mechanisms

Within the process of adaptation, coping refers to the use of behavior in response to stimuli. Defined broadly, coping refers to the use of both routine and nonroutine behaviors (Roy & McLeod, 1981). In a routine sense, coping refers to the use of accustomed patterns of behavior employed by individuals in dealing with daily situations. Roy also uses coping to refer to the use of new behaviors in response to unusual or drastic situations wherein accustomed responses are ineffective. Meeting the challenges of the unexpected allows for creative, novel responses. Inherited (genetically determined) or acquired ways of responding to the changing environment, are referred to as coping mechanisms.

According to Roy, coping mechanisms are of two types: regulator and cognator. The regulator is used primarily as a mechanism to cope with physiological stimuli, while the cognator is used mainly as a mechanism to cope with psychosocial stimuli, dealing primarily in areas of cognition, judgment, and emotion. Regulator and cognator mechanisms are linked through the process of perception. Frequently, the regulator mechanism operates at a level below cognitive awareness. At times, however, outputs from the regulator subsystem are translated into perceptions in the cognator subsystem. While the initial processing of stimuli within the regulator and cognator mechanisms cannot be observed, cognitive perceptions and the behavioral outcomes of these coping mechanisms are amenable to assessment. The behaviors will generally fall into one of four adaptive modes, each contributing to the "promotion of the adaptive goals of the total person system—survival, growth, reproduction, and mastery" (Roy & McLeod, 1981, p. 67).

Adaptive Modes

The concept of adaptive modes did not appear in the literature until 1971. Adaptive modes evolved at the request of students who felt a need for a way to organize assessment data. In 1970, approximately 500 samples of patient behaviors from all clinical areas were collected

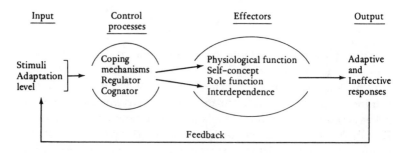

Figure 16.1. The person as an adaptive system.
SOURCE: Roy (1984, p. 30). Reprinted by permission.

by baccalaureate nursing students (Roy, 1971). These behaviors were then categorized into what came to be known as adaptive modes. An example of a pediatric history and assessment based on adaptive modes can be found in Andrews and Roy (1986, pp. 173-177).

Roy has identified four adaptive modes: physiological, self-concept, role function, and interdependence. Although these modes are discussed further under the section on Theory of Adaptive Modes, it is important to recognize that it is the *manifestation* of the coping mechanisms that can be observed and measured within the adaptive modes. Thus the adaptive modes are often referred to as effectors.

Adaptive Responses

Behaviors that contribute to the general goals of persons (i.e., survival, growth, reproduction, and mastery) are considered adaptive responses. Behaviors not contributing to general goals are considered ineffective responses. Adaptive responses bring about a state of adaptation. A diagram depicting the relationships among the concepts of the Theory of Person as an Adaptive System is presented in Figure 16.1.

Propositions

A proposition is a statement about a particular concept or the relationship between concepts. Roy and Roberts (1981) use the term "to describe the initial relationship between variables asserted by the theory" (p. 12). Propositions are important because we can use them to develop hypotheses that can be tested in the clinical area. Roy has developed many propositions from her theories.

Regulator Subsystem Propositions. The first set of propositions is related to the role of the regulator subsystem in the adaptation of persons. The regulator subsystem comprises inputs, major parts, processes, effectors, and feedback loops. Figure 16.2 depicts the regulator subsystem.

Roy's background as a neuroscience postdoctoral fellow is clearly evident in her conceptualization of the regulator subsystem. Inputs consist of external stimuli and internal stimuli from changes in the person's dynamic equilibrium, commonly known as homeostasis. "The inputs are chemical in nature or have been transduced into neural information" (Roy & McLeod, 1981, p. 60). As readers can see from the middle of Figure 16.2, the major parts of the regulator are neural, endocrine, and perception/psychomotor. The propositions that have been developed for the regulator subsystem are related to Figure 16.2 by numbers and are as follows:

1.1. Internal and external stimuli are basically chemical or neural; chemical stimuli may be transduced into neural inputs to the central nervous system.

1.2. Neural pathways to and from the central nervous system must be intact and functional if neural stimuli are to influence body responses.

2.1. Spinal cord, brainstem, and autonomic reflexes act through effectors to produce automatic, unconscious effects on the body responses.

3.1. The circulation must be intact for chemical stimuli to influence endocrine glands to produce the appropriate hormone.

3.2. Target organs or tissues must be able to respond to hormone levels to effect body responses.

4.1. Neural inputs are transformed into conscious perceptions in the brain (process unknown).

4.2. Increase in short-term or long-term memory will positively influence the effective choice of psychomotor response to neural input.

4.3. Effective choice of response, retained in long-term memory, will facilitate future effective choice of response.

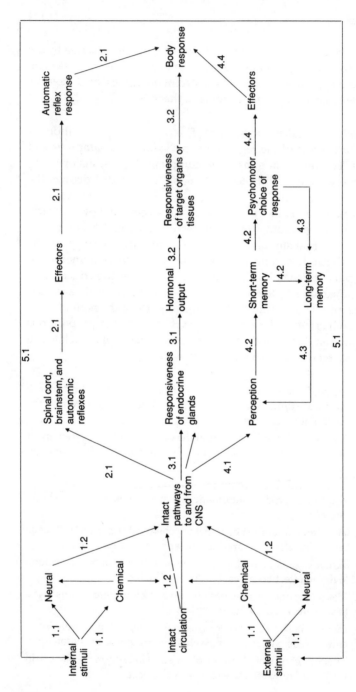

Figure 16.2. The regulator subsystem.
SOURCE: Roy & Roberts (1981, p. 61). Reprinted by permission.

4.4. The psychomotor response chosen will determine the effectors activated and the ultimate body response.

1.1 through 2.1, 3.2, 4.4. The magnitude of the internal and external stimuli will positively influence the magnitude of the physiological response of an intact system.

3.1 through 2.1, 4.4. Intact neural pathways will positively influence neural output to effectors.

1.1 through 3.2. Chemical and neural inputs will influence normally responsive endocrine glands to hormonally influence target organs in a positive manner to maintain a state of dynamic equilibrium.

1.1 through 5.1. The body's response to external and internal stimuli will alter those external and internal stimuli.

1.1 through 5.1. The magnitude of the external and internal stimuli may be so great that the adaptive systems cannot return the body to a state of dynamic equilibrium. (Roy & McLeod, 1981, p. 62)

Cognator Subsystem Propositions. Figure 16.3 depicts the cognator subsystem. A little less complex than the regulator subsystem, the cognator comprises input, parts, processes, and effectors. Inputs are positive and negative internal and external stimuli that include physiological, psychological, social, and spiritual factors. Internal stimuli include the output of the regulator subsystem. Parts consist of apparatus and pathways that enable processes, thereby bringing about a psychomotor choice of response. Effectors are internal and external verbalizations. As with the regulator mechanism, the numbers in the figure correspond to the propositions, which are as follows:

1.1. The optimum amount and clarity of input of internal and external stimuli positively influence the adequacy of selective attention, coding, and memory.

1.2. The optimum amount and clarity of input of internal and external stimuli positively influence the adequacy of imitation, reinforcement, and insight.

1.3. The optimum amount and clarity of input of internal and external stimuli positively influence the adequacy of problem solving and decision making.

1.4. The optimum amount and clarity of input of internal and external stimuli positively influence the adequacy of defenses to seek relief, and affective appraisal and attachment.

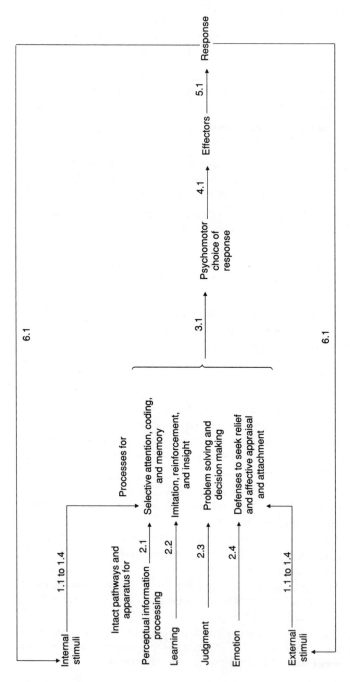

Figure 16.3. The cognator subsystem.

SOURCE: Roy & Roberts (1981, p. 64). Reprinted by permission.

112

2.1. Intact pathways and perceptual/information-processing apparatus positively influence the adequacy of selective attention, coding, and memory.

2.2. Intact pathways and learning apparatus positively influence imitation, reinforcement, and insight.

2.3. Intact pathways and judgment apparatus positively influence problem solving and decision making.

2.4. Intact pathways and emotional apparatus positively influence defenses to seek relief, and affective appraisal and attachment.

3.1. The higher the level of adequacy of all the cognator processes, the more effective the psychomotor choice of response.

4.1. The psychomotor response chosen will be activated through intact effectors.

5.1. Effector activity produces the response that is at an adaptive level, determined by the total functioning of the cognator subsystem.

6.1. The level of adaptive responses to internal and external stimuli will alter those internal and external stimuli. (Roy & McLeod, 1981, p. 65)

17

Theory of Adaptive Modes

The Theory of Adaptive Modes was developed in 1981 and has undergone substantial revision. The theory consists of four parts, each focusing on one of four adaptive modes: physiological, self-concept, role function, and interdependence. It is important to remember that each adaptive mode represents a grouping of behaviors that promote the individual's movement toward the general goals (survival, growth, reproduction, and mastery). A basic need has been identified in relation to each adaptive mode.

Physiological Mode

The basic human need within the physiological mode is for physiological integrity. Physiological wholeness (integrity) is "achieved by adapting to changes in physiological needs" (Andrews & Roy, 1991c, p. 58). The regulator coping mechanism is primarily responsible for attaining and maintaining this integrity. Five primary needs have been identified as necessary for physiological integrity: oxygen, nutrition, elimination, activity and rest, and protection. Other complex processes that influence regulator activities are the senses, fluids and electrolytes, neurological function, and endocrine function.

An adaptation problem in relation to the physiological need for protection would be pressure sores. The focal stimulus might be prolonged pressure over a bony area. Poor nutrition, incontinence, and edema would be examples of possible contextual stimuli. Residual stimuli might include the nurse's hunch that the way in which bed sheets are washed may contribute to the problem.

In Roy's Theory of Adaptive Modes, physiological propositions developed for the regulator mechanism were used to develop additional relational statements within the physiological adaptive mode (Roy & Roberts, 1981). An example of a hypothesis in the activity/rest need category initially generated from a regulator proposition is: "If the nurse helps the patient maintain muscle tone through proper exercising, the patient will experience fewer problems associated with immobility" (Roy & Roberts, 1981, p. 90).

Self-Concept Mode

Self-concept is one of three psychosocial modes. The basic human need within this mode is psychic integrity, which means "people need to know who they are so that they can exist with a sense of unity" (Roy & Andrews, 1991, p. 267). A person's level of self-esteem reflects the self-concept. Thus nursing diagnoses indicating adaptation problems and indicators of positive adaptation with regard to self-esteem are commonly found in the self-concept mode. Self-concept is "the composite of beliefs and feelings that one holds about oneself at a given time, formed from perceptions particularly of others' reactions, and directing one's behavior" (Driever, cited in Andrews, 1991a, p. 270). Self-concept has been categorized into physical self and personal self.

Physical self. Physical self is an "appraisal of one's physical attributes, appearance, functioning, sensation, sexuality, and wellness-illness status" (Buck, 1991a, p. 282). Physical self has been further divided into body sensation (how one feels about one's self) and body image (how one thinks one's body looks and how one feels about how one's body looks). An example of a disturbance in the body image component of the physical self might be verbalizations by an anorexic patient that she is fat and wants to lose 10 pounds within the next month. Other nursing diagnoses, identified by Buck (1991a), that indicate adaptation problems in the physical self are sexual dysfunction and rape trauma syndrome.

Personal self. Personal self is an "appraisal of one's own characteristics, expectations, values, and worth" (Andrews, 1991a, p. 270). Personal self has been subdivided into the moral-ethical-spiritual self, self-consistency, and self-ideal/self-expectancy. The moral-ethical-spiritual self is the individual's morals and belief system. "I believe God will help me through this surgery" is an example of a verbalization behavior in a belief system. Spiritual distress is an example of a nursing diagnosis resulting from a disruption of the moral-ethical-spiritual self.

Self-consistency is the individual's actual performance and/or personality traits. "I'm usually a pretty even-tempered person" is a statement about an individual's self-consistency. Anxiety is a nursing diagnosis arising from an adaptation problem in this area of the self.

Self-ideal/self-expectancy is what one would like to do or become relative to one's capabilities. "I would like to finish high school by taking the GED" is a verbalization about self-ideal/self-expectancy. Powerlessness is a nursing diagnosis indicating a disruption in this part of the self-concept mode. Other adaptation problems in the self-concept mode have been identified by Buck (1991a, 1991b).

Self-Concept Mode Propositions

For the self-concept adaptive mode, separate propositions were developed using the same format as for the coping mechanisms. Figure 17.1 depicts the parts of the self-concept subsystem.

The propositions corresponding to Figure 17.1 are as follows:

1.1. The positive quality of social experience in the form of others' appraisals positively influences the level of feelings of adequacy.

1.2. Adequacy of role taking positively influences the quality of input in the form of social experience.

1.3. The number of social rewards positively influences the quality of social experience.

1.4. Negative feedback in the form of performance compared with ideals leads to corrections in levels of feelings of adequacy.

1.5. Conflicts in input in the form of varying appraisals positively influences the amount of self-concept confusion experienced.

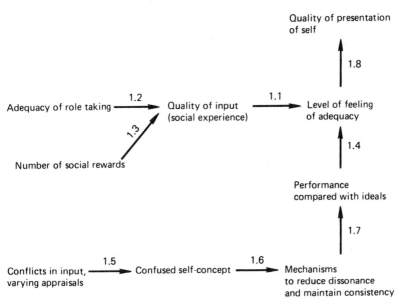

Figure 17.1. Linking of parts of the self-concept mode.
SOURCE: Roy & Roberts (1981, p. 255). Reprinted by permission.

1.6. Confused self-concept leads to activation of mechanisms to reduce dissonance and maintain consistency.

1.7. Activity of mechanisms for reducing dissonance and maintaining consistency (e.g., choice) tends to lead to feelings of adequacy.

1.8. The level of feelings of adequacy positively influences the quality of presentation of self. (Roy & Roberts, 1981, p. 255)

Roy and Roberts (1981) give an example of a hypothesis generated from these propositions: "If the nurse helps the new mother to practice role taking, the mother will develop a higher level of feelings of adequacy" (p. 258).

Role Function Mode

The basic need in the role function adaptive mode is for social integrity. This means that people need to know who they are in relation to others so that they can act. All people have roles in society. With each role, there are expected behaviors (i.e., societal norms). A common nursing diagnosis of an adaptation problem in this mode would be altered role performance. Roles have been divided into primary, secondary, and tertiary.

Roles. The primary role is determined by the majority of behaviors that are engaged in by persons during specific periods in life; it is determined by age, gender, and developmental stage (e.g., 24-year-old female young adult). Secondary roles are those that persons assume to complete tasks associated with the primary role and developmental stage. Secondary roles are normally achieved and stable (e.g., wife, mother, and nurse). Tertiary roles are related primarily to the secondary roles, usually temporary, and are freely chosen. These roles represent ways in which people meet the obligations associated with their other roles. Hobbies also are included in tertiary roles. Examples of tertiary roles might be Scout leader, part-time graduate nursing student, and reader of mysteries. Some roles may change from tertiary to secondary: During an acute illness, for example, the person assumes a tertiary sick role; if the illness becomes chronic, the sick role becomes secondary.

Behaviors associated with roles. Instrumental and expressive behaviors are associated with each role. Instrumental behaviors are usually of a physical and long-term nature. The goal is role mastery for these action-oriented behaviors. An example of instrumental behavior in the secondary role is acquisition of psychomotor skills by nursing students. Expressive behaviors are usually of an emotional nature. They are expressions of feelings or attitudes for which the goal is direct or immediate feedback. The novice nurse discussing a patient care situation with an expert nurse is an example of expressive behavior.

Role performance requirements associated with roles. Four requirements for role performance are necessary before a person can engage in instrumental or expressive behaviors. To perform the role, there needs to be a consumer, a reward to the performer, facilities within which to perform the role, and cooperation. Questions that clarify the role requirements for instrumental behavior are as follows:

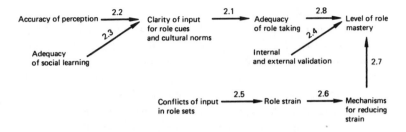

Figure 17.2. Linking of parts of the role function mode.
SOURCE: Roy & Roberts (1981, p. 267). Reprinted by permission.

1. Consumer: Who or what benefits from the performance of the behavior?
2. Reward: What is the reward for the behavior?
3. Access to facilities/set of circumstances: What equipment, supplies, or tools are needed to perform the role?
4. Cooperation/collaboration: Is time allowed to perform the role behaviors?

Questions related to the role performance requirements for expressive behaviors are similar to those for instrumental behavior:

1. Consumer: Is there an appropriate and receptive person who will provide feedback?
2. Reward: Is there a network to provide feedback on role performance?
3. Access to facilities/set of circumstances: Do I have what I need to accomplish my task?
4. Collaboration/cooperation: Will the setting provide the circumstances and climate needed to fulfill the role? (Andrews, 1991b; Roy, 1984)

Role Function Mode Propositions

The relationships among concepts in the second psychosocial adaptive mode of role function are depicted in Figure 17.2, and the numbered propositions correspond to the numbers in that figure.

2.1. The amount of clarity of input in the form of role cues and cultural norms positively influences the adequacy of role taking.

2.2. Accuracy of perception positively influences the clarity of input in the form of role cues and cultural norms.

2.3. Adequacy of social learning positively influences the clarity of input in the form of role cues and cultural norms.

2.4. Negative feedback in the form of internal and external validations leads to corrections in adequacy of role taking.

2.5. Conflicts in input in the form of conflicting role sets positively influence the amount of role strain experienced.

2.6. Role strain leads to activation of mechanisms for reducing role strain and for articulating role sets.

2.7. Activity of mechanisms for reducing role strain and for articulating role sets (e.g., choice) leads to adequacy of role taking.

2.8. The level of adequacy of role taking positively influences the level of role mastery. (Roy & Roberts, 1981, p. 267)

Again, Roy and Roberts (1981) offer an example of a hypothesis derived from the propositions: "If the nurse orients the patient to the sick role, the patient will perform at a higher level of role mastery in the sick role" (p. 270).

Interdependence Mode

Interdependence is a social adaptive mode. The basic need is affectional adequacy or the "feeling of security in nurturing relationships" (Tedrow, 1991, p. 386). Interdependence means "the close relationships of people that involve the willingness and ability to love, respect, and value others, and to accept and respond to love, respect, and value given by others" (p. 386). Servonsky and Tedrow (1991) identified loneliness as a common adaptation problem resulting from a disruption in this mode.

Behaviors. There are two types of behaviors within the interdependence adaptive mode: receptive and contributive. Receiving, taking in, and/or assimilating nurturing behaviors offered by significant others or support systems are receptive behaviors. Contributive behaviors are those that give or supply nurturing to significant

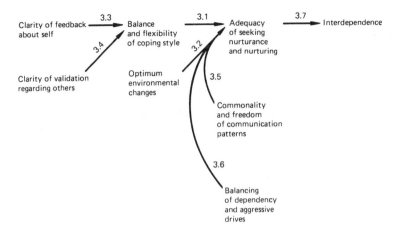

Figure 17.3. Linking of parts of the interdependence mode.
SOURCE: Roy & Roberts (1981, p. 278). Reprinted by permission.

others or support systems. Significance may be assigned to another person or inherent in an interaction. Significant others have the most meaning or importance in a person's life. Support systems are continuing social collectives such as groups, organizations, and networks.

Interdependence Mode Propositions

Figure 17.3 depicts the schematic model that illustrates the propositions for this social mode, which are:

3.1. The balance and flexibility of coping style positively influence the adequacy of seeking nurturance and nurturing.

3.2. The optimum amount of environmental changes positively influences the adequacy of seeking nurturance and nurturing.

3.3. Clarity of feedback about self positively influences the balance and flexibility of coping style.

3.4. Clarity of validation regarding others positively influences the balance and flexibility of coping style.

3.5. Commonality and freedom of communication patterns positively influence the adequacy of seeking nurturance and nurturing.

3.6. The balancing of dependency and aggressive drives positively influences the adequacy of seeking nurturance and nurturing.

3.7. Adequacy of seeking nurturance and nurturing positively influences interdependence. (Roy & Roberts, 1981, p. 277)

An example of a hypothesis relevant for practice might be, "If the nurse provides the time and space for private family visits, the patient will demonstrate more appropriate attention-seeking behavior" (Roy & Roberts, 1981, p. 280).

More recently, Roy and Anway (1989) developed propositions for the Roy Adaptation Model to be applied to nursing administrative practice. Those propositions will not be listed here because it would be important to first understand the theory upon which the propositions are based.

18

Clinical Example

Many examples illustrating the use of the Roy Adaptation Model in various clinical settings have been published, some of which are described in the publications listed in the bibliography. Another example of how the RAM could be used in the clinical setting follows.

A woman in her mid-40s recently has been diagnosed with breast cancer. Having undergone a unilateral modified radical mastectomy, she is now faced with the prospect of chemotherapy. The nurse encounters the patient on her first postoperative day. The patient is alert and oriented and denies pain or acute discomfort. The nurse observes facial tension, however, and a slight trembling of the patient's hands. The nurse asks the patient if she has had an opportunity to talk with the surgeon since her operation. The patient replies that the surgeon had visited her earlier that day and informed her that the medical oncologist would be in later to introduce herself and give an overview of the chemotherapy treatment. The patient states that, although she had been told she would also have "chemo" in addition to surgery, the news today was "final." She admits she had secretly hoped that the surgery "would be it." The tone of her voice is apprehensive. She expresses feelings of "being scared, jittery inside, and nervous." Having heard about the side effect of hair loss, she finds that upsetting. She has nice hair and has always been complimented on its color and body. She considers it one of her best features and so does her husband.

We can tentatively determine from a first-level assessment of the subjective and objective behaviors in the scenario that one nursing diagnosis is anxiety. The patient is experiencing a subjective awareness of information. In assessing the stimuli (second-level assessment), the nurse identifies the focal stimulus as concern over the chemotherapy side effect of hair loss. Contextual stimuli influencing how the patient deals with the focal stimulus are identified as the unknown experience of chemotherapy, the diagnosis of cancer, and concern over the husband's response to her hair loss. Residual stimuli would be the cultural norm of hair on the head of females and the general societal feeling about female appearance relative to hair. This patient's behaviors can be categorized in the physical self component of the self-concept adaptive mode. Her basic need is for psychic integrity, specifically with regard to body image.

Within the context of the discussion, both nurse and patient agree that a goal is to decrease patient anxiety. The nurse then selects interventions to manage the stimuli confronting the patient, thereby promoting adaptation of the patient to the environmental situation at hand (i.e., chemotherapy). The interventions include allowing the patient's verbalization; educating with regard to the chemotherapy, principally in terms of the power of drugs that destroy hair follicles in addition to cancer cells and the temporary nature of the hair loss; and reassuring with regard to the availability of attractive, well-fitting wigs that can be matched to her natural hair color and the fact that turbans are an "in" fashion item. The nurse and patient could also discuss how the husband could be involved in components of her care in a way that would be comfortable for both of them. The coping mechanism of cognator will assist the patient in processing information, learning about chemotherapy and wigs, selecting wigs and turbans, and talking with her husband about the imminent, yet temporary, hair loss. The effect from the activity of the patient's cognator coping mechanism will be observed principally in the body-image physical self component of the self-concept adaptive mode. Successful nursing interventions will result in a decrease or elimination of signs and symptoms of the patient's anxiety and an increase in necessary coping skills. Adaptive responses would include a more confident person with a positive body image regardless of the presence of a wig.

Research could be conducted on interventions used to promote adaptation of patients. The Tulman, Fawcett, Groblewski, and Silverman (1990) article is one example of recent research using Roy's model.

19

Conclusion

The Roy Adaptation Model and its derived theories of Person as an Adaptive System and Adaptive Modes have been discussed in this section in relation to origin, assumptions, key concepts, and propositions. Several schematic diagrams have been included to visually present major concepts and linkages within the theories. Finally, an example was presented of the use of Theory of Person as an Adaptive System in an application of the Roy model to medical-surgical patients in the hospital.

The Roy Adaptation Model has demonstrated utility in nursing practice, education, and, in a more limited fashion, research. A distinct advantage of the theories generated from Roy's model is their broad scope. They are applicable to all clinical settings. A limitation is the complexity of the regulator and cognator subsystems. The Theory of Adaptive Modes also has become increasingly complex since its initial development in 1981. The quantity and quality of the literature illustrating the Roy model are noteworthy and helpful to those desiring to learn more about the model and its relationship to the practice of nursing.

Glossary

Adaptation
"A process of responding positively to environmental changes in such a way as to decrease responses necessary to cope with the stimuli and increase sensitivity to respond to other stimuli" (Roy, 1984, p. 37); "the person's response to the environment which promotes the general goals of the person including survival, growth, reproduction, and mastery" (Roy & McLeod, 1981, p. 53); "a process of coping with stressors as well as the end state produced by this process" (Roy & McLeod, 1981, p. 57).

Adaptation level
"A changing point, influenced by the demands of the situation and the person's internal resources including capabilities, hopes, dreams, aspirations, motivations, and all that makes the person constantly move toward mastery" (Andrews & Roy, 1991a, p. 6); "focal, contextual, and residual stimuli pool to make up the person's adaptation level" (Andrews & Roy, 1991a, p. 10).

Adaptive
"The capacity to adjust effectively to changes in the environment and, in turn, affect the environment" (Andrews & Roy, 1991a, p. 6).

Adaptive behavior
See Adaptive responses.

126

Adaptive modes
"Ways of coping that show the activity of the regulator and cognator mechanisms" (Andrews & Roy, 1986, p. 7); "ways of categorizing the effects of cognator and regulator activity" (Roy, 1984, p. 22); "classification of ways of coping that manifest regulator and cognator activity, that is, physiologic, self-concept, role function, and interdependence" (Roy, 1984, p. 28); "provide the particular form or manifestation of cognator and regulator activity" (Roy & Roberts, 1981, p. 43, 67); "effectors of adaptation" (Roy & Roberts, 1981, pp. 43, 67).

Adaptive responses
"Promote the integrity of the person in terms of the goals of adaptation: survival, growth, reproduction, and mastery" (Andrews & Roy, 1991a, p. 12).

Adaptive zone
"Range of coping" (Andrews & Roy, 1986, p. 31); "stimulation [within the zone] will lead to a positive or adaptive response; stimuli that fall outside the zone lead to negative or ineffective responses" (Roy, 1984, p. 37).

Behavior
"Responses of the adaptive system" (Andrews & Roy, 1991a, p. 12); "actions and reactions under specified circumstances" (Andrews & Roy, 1986, p. 32).

Client of nursing
"A person, a family, a group, a community, or society" (Roy & Roberts, 1981, p. 42).

Cognator
Mechanism that "responds through four cognitive-emotive channels: perception and information processing, learning, judgment, and emotion" (Andrews & Roy, 1991a, p. 14); "involves the psychological processes for dealing cognitively and emotionally with the changing environment" (Roy, 1984, p. 22); one of two "ways or methods of adapting or coping" (Roy & McLeod, 1981, p. 66).

Contextual stimuli
"All the environmental factors that present to the person from within or without, but which are not the center of the person's attention and/or energy" (Andrews & Roy, 1991a, p. 9); "all other stimuli present, either within persons as their internal condition or coming

as input from the environment" (Roy, 1984, p. 37); "all other stimuli present that contribute to the behavior caused or precipitated by the focal stimulus" (Roy & Roberts, 1984, p. 43); "all other stimuli present in the situation of the stressor" (Roy & McLeod, 1981, p. 55); a mediating factor that contributes to the effect of the stressor (focal stimulus) (Roy & McLeod, 1981, p. 55).

Coping
"Routine, accustomed patterns of behavior to deal with daily situations as well as the production of new ways of behaving when drastic changes defy the familiar responses" (Roy & McLeod, 1981, p. 56); "operating to produce adaptive responses" (Roy & McLeod, 1981, p. 56).

Coping mechanism
"Innate or acquired ways of responding to the changing environment" (Andrews & Roy, 1991a, p. 13).

  Innate: "genetically determined or common to a species"; "automatic process"

  Acquired: "developed through processes such as learning" (Andrews & Roy, 1991a, p. 13).

Environment
"All conditions, circumstances, and influences that surround and affect the development and behavior of the person" (Andrews & Roy, 1991a, p. 18).

First-level assessment
"Gathering data about behavior in each adaptive mode by skillful observation, accurate measurement of responses, and communicative interviewing" (Roy, 1984, p. 43).

Focal stimulus
"The internal or external stimulus most immediately confronting the person; the object or event that attracts one's attention" (Andrews & Roy, 1991a, p. 8); "degree of change that precipitates adaptive behavior; stimulus most immediately confronting the person, the one to which he must make an adaptive response; stressor" (Roy & McLeod, 1981, p. 55).

Goal of nursing
"Promotion of adaptation in each of the four modes, thereby contributing to the person's health, quality of life, and dying with dignity" (Andrews & Roy, 1991a, p. 20); "to promote patient adaptation in regard to the four [adaptive] modes" (Roy & Roberts, 1981, p. 44).

Health
"A state and a process of being and becoming an integrated and whole person . . . a reflection of adaptation" (Andrews & Roy, 1991a, p. 19).

Holistic
"Pertains to the idea that the human system functions as a whole and is more than the mere sum of its parts" (Andrews & Roy, 1991a, p. 6).

Humanism
"Recognizes the person and subjective dimensions of human experience as central to knowing and to valuing" (Roy, 1988, p. 29).

Ineffective response
Behavior that "does not promote integrity nor contribute to the goals of adaptation" (Andrews & Roy, 1991a, p. 12); "behavior that does not lead to [goal attainment] or that disrupts the integrity of the individual" (Roy & McLeod, 1981, p. 57).

Integrity
"Degree of wholeness achieved by adapting to changes in needs" (Andrews & Roy, 1991c, p. 59).

Interdependence
"The close relationships of people that involve the willingness and ability to love, respect, and value others, and to accept and respond to love, respect, and value given by others" (Tedrow, 1991, p. 386).

Living system
"A whole made up of parts or subsystems that function as a unity for some purpose" (Roy & McLeod, 1981, p. 53).

Nursing activities
"Assess behavior and factors that influence adaptation level and intervene by managing the focal, contextual, and residual stimuli" (Roy, 1984, p. 13); nursing process.

Nursing diagnosis
"Judgment process resulting in a statement conveying the person's adaptation status" (Andrews & Roy, 1991b, p. 37); "interpretation of assessment data stated as a summary label for one mode, as a statement of the behaviors within one mode, with the most relevant influencing factors, or as a label that summarizes a behavioral pattern with more than one mode being affected by the same stimuli" (Roy, 1984, p. 43).

Nursing intervention
Management of stimuli that "involves altering, increasing, decreasing, removing, or maintaining" focal, contextual, and residual stimuli (Andrews & Roy, 1991b, p. 44); "selection and carrying out of an approach to change or stabilize adaptation by managing stimuli" (Roy, 1984, p. 43); "carried out in the context of the nursing process" (Roy & Roberts, 1981, p. 46).

Person
"Holistic adaptive system" (Andrews & Roy, 1991a, p. 6); "an adaptive system with cognator and regulator acting to maintain adaptation in regard to the four adaptive modes" (Roy & Roberts, 1981, pp. 44, 48); biopsychosocial being in constant interaction with a changing environment (Roy, 1980).

Regulator
"Responds automatically through neural, chemical, and endocrine coping processes" (Andrews & Roy, 1991a, p. 14).

Residual stimuli
Factors "having an indeterminate effect on the person's behavior; their effect has not or cannot be validated" (Andrews & Roy, 1991b, p. 35); "environmental factors within or [outside] the person whose effects in the current situation are unclear, possible, yet uncertain, influencing stimuli" (Andrews & Roy, 1986, p. 29); includes beliefs, attitudes, experience, or traits (Roy, 1984); mediating factors that contribute to the effect of the stressor (focal stimulus); "presumed to effect the current situation, although this effect cannot be validated or measured" (Roy & McLeod, 1981, p. 56).

Second-level assessment
"Identification of the focal, contextual, and residual factors that influence the person" (Roy, 1984, p. 43).

Self-concept
"Composite of beliefs and feelings that one holds about oneself at a given time, formed from perceptions particularly of others' reactions, and directing one's behavior" (Driever cited in Andrews, 1991a, p. 270).

Significant other
"The individual to whom the most meaning or importance is given. It is a person who is loved, respected, and valued; and who, in turn, loves, respects, and values the other to a degree greater than in all other relationships" (Tedrow, 1991, p. 386).

Stimuli
"That which provokes a response" (Andrews & Roy, 1991b, p. 33); "inputs for the person . . . [that] come from the [outside] environment (external stimuli) and internally from the self (internal stimuli)" (Andrews & Roy, 1986, p. 21).

Stressor
"Demand for an adaptive response" (Roy & McLeod, 1981, p. 55); focal stimuli mediated by contextual and residual factors (Roy & McLeod, 1981).

Veritivity
"A principle of human nature that affirms a common purposefulness of human existence" (Roy, 1988, p. 30).

References

Andrews, H. A. (1991a). Overview of the self-concept mode. In C. Roy & H. A. Andrews, *The Roy adaptation model: The definitive statement* (pp. 269-279). Norwalk, CT: Appleton & Lange.

Andrews, H. A. (1991b). Overview of the role function mode. In C. Roy & H. A. Andrews, *The Roy adaptation model: The definitive statement* (pp. 347-361). Norwalk, CT: Appleton & Lange.

Andrews, H. A., & Roy, C. (1986). *Essentials of the Roy adaptation model.* Norwalk, CT: Appleton-Century-Crofts.

Andrews, H. A., & Roy, C. (1991a). Essentials of the Roy adaptation model. In C. Roy & H. A. Andrews, *The Roy adaptation model: The definitive statement* (pp. 3-25). Norwalk, CT: Appleton & Lange.

Andrews, H. A., & Roy, C. (1991b). The nursing process according to the Roy adaptation model. In C. Roy & H. A. Andrews, *The Roy adaptation model: The definitive statement* (pp. 27-54). Norwalk, CT: Appleton & Lange.

Andrews, H. A., & Roy, C. (1991c). Overview of the physiological mode. In C. Roy & H. A. Andrews, *The Roy adaptation model: The definitive statement* (pp. 57-66). Norwalk, CT: Appleton & Lange.

Buck, M. (1991a). The physical self. In C. Roy & H. A. Andrews, *The Roy adaptation model: The definitive statement* (pp. 281-310). Norwalk, CT: Appleton & Lange.

Buck, M. (1991b). The personal self. In C. Roy & H. A. Andrews, *The Roy adaptation model: The definitive statement* (pp. 311-355). Norwalk, CT: Appleton & Lange.

Roy, C. (1971). Adaptation: A basis for nursing practice. *Nursing Outlook, 19,* 254-257.

Roy, C. (1980). The Roy adaptation model. In J. P. Riehl & C. Roy (Eds.), *Conceptual models for nursing practice* (2nd ed., pp. 179-192). New York: Appleton-Century-Crofts.

Roy, C. (1984). *Introduction to nursing: An adaptation model* (2nd ed.). Englewood Cliffs, NJ: Prentice Hall.

Roy, C. (1988). An explication of the philosophical assumptions of the Roy adaptation mode. *Nursing Science Quarterly, 1*(1), 26-34.

Roy, C. (1990). Strengthening the Roy adaptation model through conceptual clarification: Response. *Nursing Science Quarterly, 3*(2), 64-66.

Roy, C., & Andrews, H. A. (1991). *The Roy adaptation model: The definitive statement.* Norwalk, CT: Appleton & Lange.

Roy, C., & Anway, J. (1989). Roy's adaptation model: Theories for nursing administration. In B. Henry, C. Arndt, M. Di Vincenti, & A. Marriner-Tomey (Eds.), *Dimensions of nursing administration: Theory, research, education, practice* (pp. 75-88). Boston: Blackwell Scientific.

Roy, C., & McLeod, D. (1981). Theory of person as an adaptive system. In C. Roy & S. L. Roberts, *Theory construction in nursing: An adaptation model* (pp. 49-69). Englewood Cliffs, NJ: Prentice Hall.

Roy, C., & Roberts, S. L. (1981). *Theory construction in nursing: An adaptation model.* Englewood Cliffs, NJ: Prentice Hall.

Sato, M. K. (1984). Major factors influencing adaptation. In C. Roy, *Introduction to nursing: An adaptation model* (2nd ed., pp. 64-87). Englewood Cliffs, NJ: Prentice Hall.

Servonsky, J., & Tedrow, M. P. (1991). Separation anxiety and loneliness. In C. Roy & H. A. Andrews, *The Roy adaptation model: The definitive statement* (pp. 405-422). Norwalk, CT: Appleton & Lange.

Tedrow, M. P. (1991). Overview of the interdependence mode. In C. Roy & H. A. Andrews, *The Roy adaptation model: The definitive statement* (pp. 385-403). Norwalk, CT: Appleton & Lange.

Tulman, L., Fawcett, J., Groblewski, L., & Silverman, L. (1990). Changes in functional status after childbirth. *Nursing Research, 39,* 70-75.

Bibliography

Theory

Andrews, H. A., & Roy, C. (1986). *Essentials of the Roy adaptation model*. Norwalk, CT: Appleton-Century-Crofts.

Blue, C. L., Brubaker, K. M., Fine, J. M., Kirsch, M. J., Papazian, K. R., & Riester, C. M. (1989). Sister Callista Roy: Adaptation model. In A. Marriner-Tomey (Ed.), *Nursing theorists and their work* (2nd ed., pp. 325-411). St. Louis: C. V. Mosby.

Buck, M. H. (1984). Self-concept: Theory and development. In C. Roy, *Introduction to nursing: An adaptation model* (2nd ed., pp. 255-283). Englewood Cliffs, NJ: Prentice Hall.

Chinn, P. L., & Kramer, M. K. (1991). *Theory and nursing: A systematic approach* (3rd ed., p. 187). St. Louis: C. V. Mosby.

DeFeo, D. J. (1990). Change: A central concern of nursing. *Nursing Science Quarterly, 3*, 88-94.

Galbreath, J. G. (1990). Sister Callista Roy. In J. B. George, *Nursing theories: The base for professional nursing practice* (3rd ed.). Norwalk, CT: Appleton & Lange.

Nuwayhid, K. A. (1984). Role function: Theory and development. In C. Roy, *Introduction to nursing: An adaptation model* (2nd ed., pp. 284-305). Englewood Cliffs, NJ: Prentice Hall.

Roy, C. (1970). Adaptation: A conceptual framework for nursing. *Nursing Outlook, 18*(3), 42-45.

Roy, C. (1971). Adaptation: A basis for nursing practice. *Nursing Outlook, 19*, 254-257.

Roy, C. (1983). Roy adaptation model. In I. W. Clements & F. B. Roberts (Eds.), *Family health: A theoretical approach to nursing care* (pp. 255-277). New York: John Wiley.

Roy, C. (1984). *Introduction to nursing: An adaptation model* (2nd ed.). Englewood Cliffs, NJ: Prentice Hall.

Roy, C. (1987). Roy's adaptation model. In R. R. Parse (Ed.), *Nursing science: Major paradigms, theories, and critiques* (pp. 35-45). Philadelphia: W. B. Saunders.

Roy, C. (1988). An explication of the philosophical assumptions of the Roy adaptation model. *Nursing Science Quarterly, 1,* 26-34.

Roy, C. (1989). The Roy adaptation model. In J. P. Riehl-Sisca (Ed.), *Conceptual models for nursing practice* (3rd ed., pp. 105-114). Norwalk, CT: Appleton & Lange.

Roy, C., & Andrews, H. A. (1991). *The Roy adaptation model: The definitive statement.* Norwalk, CT: Appleton & Lange.

Roy, C., & McLeod, D. (1981). Theory of person as an adaptive system. In C. Roy & S. L. Roberts, *Theory construction in nursing: An adaptation model* (pp. 49-69). Englewood Cliffs, NJ: Prentice Hall.

Roy, C., & Roberts, S. L. (1981). *Theory construction in nursing: An adaptation model.* Englewood Cliffs, NJ: Prentice Hall.

Sato, M. K. (1984). Major factors influencing adaptation. In C. Roy, *Introduction to nursing: An adaptation model* (2nd ed., pp. 64-87). Englewood Cliffs, NJ: Prentice Hall.

Tedrow, M. P. (1984). Interdependence: Theory and development. In C. Roy, *Introduction to nursing: An adaptation model* (2nd ed., pp. 306-322). Englewood Cliffs, NJ: Prentice Hall.

Tiedeman, M. E. (1989). The Roy adaptation model. In J. Fitzpatrick & A. Whall, *Conceptual models of nursing: Analysis and application* (2nd ed., pp. 185-204). Bowie, MD: Brady.

Analysis and Evaluation of the Roy Adaptation Model

Artinian, N. T. (1990). Strengthening the Roy adaptation model through conceptual clarification: Commentary. *Nursing Science Quarterly, 3,* 60-64.

Fawcett, J. (1989). Roy's adaptation model. In J. Fawcett, *Analysis and evaluation of conceptual models of nursing* (2nd ed., pp. 307-353). Philadelphia: F. A. Davis.

Giger, J. N. (1990). Nightingale and Roy: A comparison of nursing models. *Today's OR Nurse, 12*(4), 25-28, 30-33.

Huch, M. H. (1987). A critique of the Roy adaptation model. In R. R. Parse (Ed.), *Nursing science: Major paradigms, theories, and critiques* (pp. 47-66). Philadelphia: W. B. Saunders.

Mastal, M. F., & Hammond, H. (1980). Analysis and expansion of the Roy adaptation model: A contribution to holistic nursing. *Advances in Nursing Science, 2*(4), 71-81.

Meleis, A. I. (1985). Sister Callista Roy. In A. I. Meleis, *Theoretical nursing: Development and progress* (pp. 206- 218). Philadelphia: J. B. Lippincott.

Roy, C. (1990). Strengthening the Roy adaptation model through conceptual clarification: Response. *Nursing Science Quarterly, 3,* 64-66.

Extensions of the Roy Adaptation Model to Groups

DiIorio, C. K. (1989). Application of the Roy model to nursing administration. In B. Henry, C. Arndt, M. Di Vincenti, & A. Marriner-Tomey (Eds.), *Dimensions of nursing administration: Theory, research, education, practice* (pp. 89-104). Boston: Blackwell Scientific.

Hanchett, E. S. (1988). Callista Roy—Focus: Adaptive systems. In E. S. Hanchett, *Nursing frameworks and community as client: Bridging the gap* (pp. 49-78). Norwalk, CT: Appleton & Lange.

Hanchett, E. S. (1990). Nursing models and community as client. *Nursing Science Quarterly, 3,* 67-72.

Roy, C. (1983a). Analysis and application of the Roy adaptation model. In I. W. Clements & F. B. Roberts (Eds.), *Family health: A theoretical approach to nursing care* (pp. 298-303). New York: John Wiley.

Roy, C. (1983b). Analysis and application of the Roy adaptation model. In I. W. Clements & F. B. Roberts (Eds.), *Family health: A theoretical approach to nursing care* (pp. 375-378). New York: John Wiley.

Roy, C., & Anway, J. (1989). Roy's adaptation model: Theories for nursing administration. In B. Henry, C. Arndt, M. Di Vincenti, & A. Marriner-Tomey (Eds.), *Dimensions of nursing administration: Theory, research, education, practice* (pp. 75-88). Boston: Blackwell Scientific.

Applications to Practice and Research

Barnfather, J. S., Swain, M. A. P., & Erickson, H. C. (1989). Evaluation of two assessment techniques for adaptation to stress. *Nursing Science Quarterly, 2,* 172-182.

Calvert, M. M. (1989). Human-pet interaction and loneliness: A test of concepts from Roy's adaptation model. *Nursing Science Quarterly, 2,* 194-202.

DiMaria, R. A. (1989). Posttrauma responses: Potential for nursing. *Journal of Advanced Medical Surgical Nursing, 2*(1), 41-48.

Downey, C. (1974). Adaptation nursing applied to an obstetric patient. In J. P. Riehl & C. Roy (Eds.), *Conceptual models for nursing practice* (pp. 151-159). New York: Appleton-Century-Crofts.

Farkas, L. (1981). Adaptation problems with nursing home application for elderly persons: An application of the Roy adaptation nursing model. *Journal of Advanced Nursing, 6,* 363-368.

Fawcett, J. (1981a). Assessing and understanding the cesarean father. In C. F. Kehoe (Ed.), *The cesarean experience: Theoretical and clinical perspectives for nurses.* New York: Appleton-Century-Crofts.

Fawcett, J. (1981b). Needs of cesarean birth parents. *Journal of Obstetric, Gynecologic, and Neonatal Nursing, 10,* 371-376.

Fawcett, J., & Tulman, L. (1990). Building a programme of research from the Roy adaptation model of nursing. *Journal of Advanced Nursing, 15,* 720-725.

Galligan, A. C. (1979). Using Roy's concept of adaptation to care for young children. *The American Journal of Maternal Child Nursing, 4*(1), 24-28.

Giger, J. A., Bower, C. A., & Miller, S. W. (1987). Roy adaptation model: ICU adaptation model. ICU application. *Dimensions of Critical Care Nursing, 6,* 215-224.

Gordon, J. (1974). Nursing assessment and care plan for a cardiac patient. In J. P. Riehl & C. Roy (Eds.), *Conceptual models for nursing practice* (pp. 144-150). New York: Appleton-Century-Crofts.

Hoch, C. C. (1987). Assessing delivery of nursing care. *Journal of Gerontological Nursing, 13*, 10-17.

Janelli, L. M. (1980). Utilizing Roy's adaptation model from a gerontological perspective. *Journal of Gerontological Nursing, 6*, 140-150.

Kehoe, C. F. (1981). Identifying the nursing needs of the postpartum cesarean mother. In C. F. Kehoe (Ed.), *The cesarean experience: Theoretical and clinical perspectives for nurses*. New York: Appleton-Century-Crofts.

Leuze, M., & McKenzie, J. (1987). Preoperative assessment: Using the Roy adaptation model. *AORN Journal, 46*, 1122-1134.

Limandri, B. J. (1986). Research and practice with abused women: Use of the Roy adaptation model as an explanatory framework. *Advances in Nursing Science, 8*(4), 52-61.

Logan, M. (1990). The Roy adaptation model: Are nursing diagnoses amenable to independent nurse functions? *Journal of Advanced Nursing, 15*, 468-470.

Mastal, M., Hammond, H., & Roberts. M. (1982). Theory into hospital practice: A pilot implementation. *The Journal of Nursing Administration, 12*(6), 9-15.

Mitchell, G. J., & Pilkington, B. (1990). Theoretical approaches in nursing practice: A comparison of Roy and Parse. *Nursing Science Quarterly, 3*, 88-94.

Norris, S., Campbell, L., & Brenkert, S. (1982). Nursing procedures and alternations in transcutaneous oxygen tension in premature infants. *Nursing Research, 31*, 330-336.

Pollock, S. E., Christian, B. J., & Sands, D. (1990). Responses to chronic illness: Analysis of psychological and physiological adaptation. *Nursing Research, 39*, 300-304.

Randell, B., Tedrow, M. P., & Van Landingham, J. (1982). *Adaptation nursing: The Roy conceptual model applied*. St. Louis: C. V. Mosby.

Roy, C. (1967). Role cues and mothers of hospitalized children. *Nursing Research, 16*, 178-182.

Roy, C. (1971). Adaptation: A basis for nursing practice. *Nursing Outlook, 19*, 254-257.

Roy, C. (1975). A diagnostic classification system for nursing. *Nursing Outlook, 23*, 90-94.

Silva, M. C. (1987). Needs of spouses of surgical patients: A conceptualization within the Roy adaptation model. *Scholarly Inquiry for Nursing Practice: An International Journal, 1*(1), 29-44.

Schmitz, M. (1980). The Roy adaptation model: Application in a community setting. In J. P. Riehl & C. Roy (Eds.), *Conceptual models for nursing practice* (2nd ed., pp. 193-206). New York: Appleton-Century-Crofts.

Smith, M. C. (1988). Roy's adaptation model in practice. *Nursing Science Quarterly, 1*, 97-98.

Starn, J., & Niederhauser, V. (1990). An MCN model for nursing diagnosis to focus intervention. *MCN, 15*, 180-183.

Starr, S. L. (1980). Adaptation applied to the dying patient. In J. P. Riehl & C. Roy (Eds.), *Conceptual models for nursing practice* (2nd ed., pp. 189-192). New York: Appleton-Century-Crofts.

Tulman, L., & Fawcett, J. (1990a). A framework for studying functional status after diagnosis of breast cancer. *Cancer Nursing, 13*, 95-99.

Tulman, L., & Fawcett, J. (1990b). Functional status during pregnancy and the postpartum: A framework for research. *Image, 22,* 191-194.

Tulman, L., Fawcett, J., Groblewski, L., & Silverman, L. (1990). Changes in functional status after childbirth. *Nursing Research, 39,* 70-75.

Wagner, P. (1976). Testing the adaptation model in practice. *Nursing Outlook, 24,* 682-685.

Applications to Education

Brower, H. T. F., & Baker, B. J. (1976). The Roy adaptation model: Using the adaptation model in a practitioner curriculum. *Nursing Outlook, 24,* 686-689.

Camooso, C., Green, M., & Reilly, P. (1981). Students' adaptation according to Roy. *Nursing Outlook, 29,* 57-65.

Morales-Mann, E. T., & Logan, M. (1990). Implementing the Roy model: Challenges for nurse educators. *Journal of Advanced Nursing, 15,* 720-725.

Roy, C. (1973). Adaptation: Implications for curriculum change. *Nursing Outlook, 21,* 163-165.

Roy, C. (1975). Adaptation: Implications for curriculum change. *Nursing Outlook, 23,* 90-94.

Roy, C. (1979). Relating nursing theory to education: A new era. *Nurse Educator, 4*(2), 16-20.

PART IV

Dorothea Orem
Self-Care Deficit Theory

DONNA L. HARTWEG

Biographical Sketch of the Nurse Theorist: Dorothea Elizabeth Orem

Born: 1914, Baltimore, Maryland

Education: Diploma (early 1930s), Providence Hospital School of Nursing, Washington, DC; BSN Ed. (1939) and MSN Ed. (1945) from the Catholic University of America, Washington, DC.

Honorary Doctorates: Doctor of Science from Georgetown University (1976) and Incarnate Word College in San Antonio, Texas (1980); Doctor of Humane Letters from Illinois Wesleyan University, Bloomington, Illinois (1988).

Special Award: Catholic University of America Alumni Achievement Award for Nursing Theory (1980)

Current Position: Consultant in Nursing, Savannah, Georgia

Foreword

Thinking about nursing is as important as doing nursing. The conceptual structure of the discipline of nursing must be known by those nurses who practice nursing and those who teach nursing. Nurses in practice must be able to identify the phenomena that are of concern to them and must have a framework for reflecting on their practice. The meaning given to data is a direct result of the conceptual frame the nurse brings to the practice situation. Dorothea Orem's general theory of nursing, referred to as the Self-Care Deficit Nursing Theory, provides such a framework for nurses. The elements of the theory and their elaboration in the form of propositions and descriptions provide the starting point for the development of the nurse's understanding of the conceptual framework practice.

The theory is both simple and complex. Its simplicity is found in the basic structure of the theory; its complexity in the development and implementation of those conceptual elements in practice. To make full use of the theory, it is necessary to comprehend the theory. This can only be done through extensive study and reflection on the original work.

This section complements that work, providing the reader with information about the basic structure of the theory from the viewpoint of the user. The author is well qualified to do this. She has studied the theory and has used it in teaching baccalaureate students for nearly a decade. The author draws upon this background to provide examples and interpretations, and our understanding of the theory is enhanced. As theory-based nursing becomes the norm, the expectation will be that nurses be conversant with one or more theories of nursing.

SUSAN G. TAYLOR, RN, PHD
Associate Professor
School of Nursing
University of Missouri—Columbia

Preface

The purpose of this section is to present a descriptive overview of Dorothea Orem's Self-Care Deficit Theory of Nursing. It is not intended to replace the primary works of Orem but to provide direction for their use. It is hoped that the reader will be enticed to search the writings of Orem and others for further understanding. A detailed reference list and bibliography of classic works and critiques are included to facilitate the reader's further exploration. Orem (1991), the most recent primary work at the time of this writing, is cited unless other editions or works have greater historical or substantive significance.

This section is primarily intended for use by beginning students of Orem's theory, including undergraduate students, graduate students encountering their first nursing theory course, and educators, researchers, and practitioners who are unfamiliar with Orem's work. Those familiar with the theory will find that selected sections present a view of the Orem literature not found in other sources. For example, the first section, which deals with the origins of the theory, incorporates not only the writings of Orem but also selected remarks by Orem at conferences and on videocassettes. The second presents the assumptions, three theories, concepts, and propositions, with use of examples for clarification. The third presents a summary of application to practice, research, and education. No attempt was made to be comprehensive but to provide diverse examples of theory application. As this work is descriptive, no critique of Orem's work was included, although the reader should note critiques listed in the bibliography.

Teaching Orem's Self-Care Deficit Theory to undergraduate students at Illinois Wesleyan University, and subsequent doctoral study at Wayne State University, served as the impetus for an in-depth study of Orem's work. I am grateful to undergraduate students who challenged me to explain the theory in practical terms and to doctoral faculty who stimulated me to analyze, critique, and propose ideas and methods for theory development. My dissertation chair, Mary J. Denyes, served as a role model, supporting and challenging me throughout the process. The Orem Research Study group at Wayne State University provided a rich forum for further collective exploration. Self-care conferences, particularly those sponsored by the University of Missouri, have been invaluable to my own understanding and clarification. I am hopeful that this description of Orem's work will entice others to study and apply this emerging practical nursing science. I feel the product of Orem's genius is yet to be fully realized but is indeed a means for nursing to truly make a difference in the health care of people.

— DONNA L. HARTWEG

Acknowledgment

The author wishes to acknowledge the contribution of Susan G. Taylor, Associate Professor of Nursing at the University of Missouri, Columbia, who reviewed the manuscript and made valuable suggestions for revision.

20

Origin and Development

Dorothea Orem's general theory of nursing evolved over a period of four decades from individual work and through collaboration with students, practitioners, researchers, educators, administrators, and scholars. She began her work by looking for the uniqueness of nursing. How was it different from other disciplines? How was it similar? This search for distinctive nursing knowledge was directed toward answering one question, "What is the domain and what are the boundaries of nursing as a field of practice and a field of knowledge?" (Orem & Taylor, 1986, p. 39). Orem searched for the meaning of nursing, using reflection and questioning as the primary method. Today, as a consultant, Orem continues to clarify and refine her work through interaction with nurses committed to theory development. She regularly publishes new insights and gives presentations at regional, national, and international conferences.

Orem describes the model development in all primary sources. However, writings by Orem and Taylor (1986) and a video presentation, "The Nurse Theorists. Portraits of Excellence: Dorothea Orem" (Helene Fuld Health Trust, 1988), provide interesting reflections and descriptions. Eben, Gashti, Nation, Marriner-Tomey, and Nordmeyer (1989) summarize personal and professional background information based on communication and interviews with Orem.

Origins of the Model (1949-1959)

The original ideas for the model developed while Orem served as a nurse consultant with the Indiana State Board of Health between 1949 and 1957. As she traveled around the state, she became aware of the ability of nurses to do nursing, but their inability to talk about nursing. After much observation and questioning, she summarized her initial ideas about nursing in an Indiana State Board of Health report (Orem, 1956). These ideas were further developed while Orem was serving as a consultant in the Office of Education, U.S. Department of Health, Education, and Welfare. Her task was to improve the nursing component of a vocational nursing curriculum. She realized that the curriculum could not be determined until there was an understanding of the subject matter of nursing in general. Vocational nursing was a "piece of a pie" called nursing.

As a result of reflecting on her own experiences, Orem completed her search for the answer to the question "What is nursing?" through a statement about the proper object or the focus of nursing—that is, "What condition exists when judgments are made that people need nursing?" (Helene Fuld Health Trust, 1988). The answer she found was stated as follows: "The inabilities of people to care for themselves at times when they need assistance because of their state of personal health" (Orem, 1959, p. 5). This definition of nursing's focus was similar to one posed by Henderson (1966); however, Orem clearly stated that her own notions evolved from her unique experiences and observations, and were not derived from Henderson's work (Orem & Taylor, 1986).

Early nursing experiences that impacted Orem's ideas about nursing included practice roles of staff nurse in medical-surgical and pediatric nursing and assistant director of nursing in a general hospital. Additional positions in nursing education were those of teacher of biological sciences in a nursing program and assistant director of a school of nursing. Orem credits her ability to reflect and search for meaning in nursing both to these experiences in nursing and the study of formal logic and metaphysics and to the use of resources from many fields, including human organization and action theory. Specific literature related to action theory included the "works of Aristotle and Thomas Aquinas, as well as modern works by logicians, philosophers, psychologists, physiologists, sociologists, and industrialists" (Orem, 1987, p. 73). Important to her thinking were the works of Barnard (1962), Kotarbinski (1965), Macmurray (1957), and Parsons, Bales, and Shils (1953) (Helene Fuld Health Trust, 1988). Orem cited B. J. F. Lonergan's *Insight* (1958) as critical to her reflective thinking, and essays by Wallace (1979, 1983) as impacting more recent clarifications (Orem & Taylor, 1986). Her ideas evolved from observations in practice, with formalization coming from her extensive reading and self-reflection. Orem credits her ability to see the "whole in nursing situations" as important to her conceptualization of the theory (Helene Fuld Health Trust, 1988).

Formalization of the Model (1960-1980)

For 20 years, Orem continued to formalize her general theory of nursing with increased input from students, scholars, and colleagues. Two groups contributed significantly to the development and refinement of ideas. The Nursing Model Committee of the Nurse Faculty of the Catholic University of America, chaired by Orem, initiated its work in 1965. The impetus for the work of the committee was the inability of graduate students and faculty to identify unanswerable nursing research questions. Because the faculty identified that nursing seemed different from other disciplines, they decided to come together as a committee and develop ideas about nursing as a "mode of thought as well as a mode of doing" (Helene Fuld Health Trust, 1988).

The work of the Nursing Model Committee was continued in 1968 by the Nursing Development Conference Group (NDCG). This group comprised Orem and 10 other nurses with specialties in practice, education, and administration. Five of the members were from the Nursing Model Committee. The NDCG members "came together one by one because of dissatisfaction and concern due to the absence of an organizing framework for nursing knowledge and with the belief that a concept of nursing would aid in formalizing such a framework" (NDCG, 1973, p. ix). The NDCG was committed to the development of structured nursing knowledge and to nursing as a practice discipline. Group ideas refined those of Orem and formalized earlier work. This group process and the resulting product were published in two volumes, *Concept Formalization in Nursing: Process and Product* (1973, 1979). These books, now out of print, provided rich descriptions of the work of the NDCG. Other publications appeared during the decade from group members, such as Allison (1973), Backscheider (1974), and Kinlein (1977a, 1977b). Other publications during the 1970s reflected the initial impact of Orem's work on education and practice. Piemme and Trainor (1977) described the effect of the curriculum on first-year nursing students at Georgetown University. Nowakowski (1980) described its practical application to a community-based program at Georgetown University.

Nursing: Concepts of Practice (Orem, 1971) was the original publication of the conceptual framework. A revision in 1980 presented more formalized concepts and propositions, reflecting input of the NDCG. The three theories within the general theory of nursing were an addition to the second edition. The title of the book clearly reflected Orem's practice philosophy. Concepts were developed for nursing practice to clarify the legitimate role of the nurse in practice situations. The NDCG continued the emphasis on practice by using case studies to refine ideas.

Dissemination, Verification, and Current Development (1980-1991)

During the 1980s, Orem revised *Nursing: Concepts of Practice* (Orem, 1985b). Changes were limited to the addition of assumptions and definitions of selected concepts, such as health. The fourth edition, published in 1991, included several substantive changes, such as new propositions in the Theory of Self-Care. Also, selected components of *Concept Formalization in Nursing: Process and Product* (1979) not previously included in *Nursing: Concepts of Practice* (Orem, 1971, 1980, 1985b) were integrated throughout the book.

Clarification of components in the model continued throughout the decade, partially in response to analysis and critiques of the theory. For example, Meleis (1985) questioned the model's utility in promoting health and well-being. Hartweg (1990) subsequently described a conceptualization of health promotion self-care within the model. Health promotion self-care was defined as self-care to promote well-being rather than health as a physical and functional state. Orem (1985b) defined health as the integrity of human structure and functioning. In contrast, well-being was described as happiness, contentment, and fulfillment of one's self-ideal. Hartweg viewed this clarification of health promotion self-care as a necessary step for specific health promotion self-care practice and research.

The decade was also one of increased application, testing, and refinement through nursing practice and research. As numerous scholars, educators, researchers, practitioners, and administrators encountered the model, communication became essential. Susan Taylor of the University of Missouri, Columbia, facilitated dissemination through initiation of a *Self-Care Deficit Theory Curriculum Network Directory* (1980) and later as newsletter coordinator of the *Self-Care Deficit Nursing Theory Newsletter* (available through the School of Nursing, University of Missouri, Columbia). With Taylor's leadership, the University of Missouri, Columbia, began sponsoring biannual conferences in 1982 that facilitated communication and promoted development of selected concepts. For example, the Sixth Annual Self-Care Deficit Theory Conference, held in 1987, examined two concepts within the model, nursing agency and nursing systems. Work sessions were held with scholars, practitioners, and researchers who shared ideas regarding concept development. Proceedings of the conferences were published. Other conferences were held regularly in Toronto, Ontario, and Vancouver, British Columbia. The First International Self-Care Deficit Nursing Theory (S-CDNT) Conference was held in Kansas City in 1989, with participants from Sweden, Netherlands, Canada, Thailand, Australia, Japan, and the United States. This participation reflected the global impact of the theory. Examples of the international application and development of the model are included throughout Chapter 22.

In addition to conferences, scholarly groups developed in institutions. An Orem Research Study Group was organized in 1984 at Wayne State University in Detroit, Michigan. Doctoral students and faculty regularly meet to facilitate model development and testing. Publications have resulted from the group's work (Denyes, O'Connor, Oakley, & Ferguson, 1989; Gast et al., 1989).

During this period, journals increasingly focused on articles about the theory. Fawcett (1989) provided a detailed summary of articles and personal communications on its application and use in practice, education, research, and administration. Examples of application included all clinical areas and nursing settings. Numerous articles appeared in international journals (e.g., Rosenbaum, 1989). Orem was named to an advisory panel for *Nursing Science Quarterly: Theory,*

Research, and Practice. Theory-based computer software for bedside care was developed within Orem's general theory of nursing by Nursing Systems International. The Self-Care model linked the patient assessments with nursing diagnosis, expected patient outcomes, discharge planning, quality assurance variables, clinical research, and external agency reports.

Future Directions for Theory Development

Continued development will distinguish among variations in the concepts, develop rules for nursing practice, and finally establish rules for nursing specific populations. Orem dreams of a time when a general theory of nursing is no longer needed but is replaced by practice models and rules specific to populations and subgroups in need of nursing (Orem, 1988b). Orem (1987, 1988a) proposed future directions by identifying five stages for model development. Stage 1 includes the development of the theory, with identification of the concepts and their relationships. This stage has been completed. Stage 2 is an investigation of variations in nursing situations. The development and testing of the concept of self-care agency in various populations and settings is an example of this stage, which is in progress. Stage 3 is the development of models and rules for nursing practice. Examples of such models are those by Horn and Swain (1977), who created standards for determining nursing's effectiveness, and the preliminary work by Orem (1984, 1985b) on application to families and communities. Stage 4 includes the development of nursing cases by practitioners within the nursing model. Some case studies are now recorded (Orem & Taylor, 1986), but many others need to be observed and recorded. Stage 5 is the development of models and rules for providing nursing to populations. Orem suggests this includes nursing provided to entire populations, such as those in a hospital. She views this as important to nursing administration and nursing economics. Stages 3 through 5 need much development.

The stages suggested by Orem for model development clearly reflect her beliefs about the importance of nursing practice. She believes that this development will facilitate the understanding of nursing as a "practical science" (Orem, 1988a).

21

Assumptions, Theories, Concepts, and Propositions

Orem's theory has been called a general theory of nursing, Self-Care Deficit Theory of Nursing, Self-Care Deficit Nursing Theory, and Self-Care Theory of Nursing. Orem (1980) described her work as a general theory of nursing comprising three "articulating" or interrelated theories: theory of self-care, theory of self-care deficit, and theory of nursing systems. The specific name for Orem's general theory of nursing, however, is Self-Care Deficit Theory of Nursing, or S-CDTN (Orem, 1991). She chose the name "deficit" as it describes and explains a relationship between abilities of individuals to care for themselves and the self-care needs or demands of the individual, their children, or the adults for whom they care. The notion of "deficit" does not refer to a specific type of limitation, but to the relationship between the capabilities of the individual and the needs for action. Although Orem focuses on the individual throughout the major works, the model can be used with families (Orem, 1983b, 1983c; Tadych, 1985; Taylor, 1989), and communities (Orem, 1984; Hanchett, 1988, 1990).

Assumptions in
Self-Care Deficit Theory of Nursing

Orem (1991) described several sets of assumptions. The first and most basic are general assumptions that relate to the entire general theory of nursing. There are also assumptions that Orem called presuppositions, which relate to each of the three interrelated theories. Assumptions are also identified that relate to specific concepts, such as the concept of self-care requisites. These assumptions throughout S-CDTN serve to guide thinking about the many component parts of the theory.

Five general assumptions or generalizations about human beings relate to all three theories and have been implicit in Orem's thinking from the beginning. These "principles of nursing," as she called them in the early years, were initially presented in 1973 in a paper given by Orem at the Fifth Annual Post-Masters Conference of Marquette University's School of Nursing (Orem, 1987). They were not published until 1985 in *Nursing: Concepts of Practice*. More recently, she referred to the five assumptions as the underlying premises of the general theory (Orem, 1991, pp. 66-67).

These premises or general assumptions about individual human beings, their capabilities and their relationships, provided an important foundation for the future development of specific concepts of the general theory. For example, two assumptions that describe human agency were important to the later development of the concepts of self-care agency and nursing agency. These assumptions describe the relationship of requirements for human action (demand) and human agency, as well as the sociocultural basis for nursing.

Three Interrelated Theories

Each of the interrelated theories of self-care, self-care deficit, and nursing systems has a central idea, propositions, and presuppositions (Orem, 1991, pp. 67-73). The central idea describes the focus of the theory. The set of propositions are statements that describe concepts or relationships among concepts in the theory; refer to Table 21.2 for a list of propositions. Presuppositions are assumptions, or "givens," that are more specific to each of the three theories than the general assumptions. Orem explained that these sets of presuppositions help link the three theories to one another. For example, Set 1 of the presuppositions under the theory of self-care deficit (or dependent-care deficit) provides the link to the theory of self-care. Set 2 links the theory of self-care deficit to the theory of nursing system. Orem (1987) also identified specific questions to be addressed by each theory.

Theory of Self-Care Deficit (or Dependent-Care Deficit)

The central idea, six propositions, and two sets of presuppositions in the theory of self-care deficit (Orem, 1991, pp. 70-71) propose an answer to the question "When and why do people require the health service nursing?" (Orem, 1987, p. 72). The central idea is that individuals are affected from time to time by limitations that do not allow them to meet their self-care needs. These limitations may occur because of a health condition, such as an accident or diabetes, or because of factors that are internal or external to the individual. For example, an internal factor is age. Certain self-care limitations may occur with age, such as those of a geriatric client, that place the person in need of nursing. An example of an external factor is a specific life experience, such as an unexpected death in the family. This event may incapacitate a person and limit the ability to meet general or specific human needs. Orem is clear that nursing must be "legitimate"—that is, the relationship between the person-nurse and the person-patient is based on the condition that establishes a need for nursing and not some other condition such as a medical condition.

Theory of Self-Care (Dependent-Care)

The central idea, six propositions, and four presuppositions in the theory of self-care (Orem, 1991, pp. 69-70) propose to answer the question "What is self-care and what is dependent care?" (Orem, 1987, p. 72). Orem (1991) made substantive changes in the propositions of this theory, replacing 10 principles with 6 new propositions.

Two ideas about self-care are emphasized in the theory: self-care as learned behavior and self-care as deliberate action. Self-care is described as behavior that is learned from interaction and communication in larger social groups. A presupposition is that self-care actions vary by the cultural and social experiences of the individual. In other words, the self-care actions performed in response to needs created by respiratory illness will vary among individuals who have been raised in different social or cultural environments. *Cao gio*, or coin rubbing, is a self-care action learning within the Vietnamese culture and initiated in response to respiratory illness (Hautman, 1987).

Self-care and dependent care are performed "purposively," or with purpose. A related phrase throughout the theory is "deliberate action." Self-care is not instinctive or reflexive but is performed rationally in response to a known need. One such need for women, which is known through our knowledge of medical science, is to perform breast self-examination. Some women will take deliberate action to gain the knowledge and subsequently perform the action every month. Other women will not seek the knowledge or take action. Orem explains this through two presuppositions. All individuals have the potential ability and motivation necessary to provide care for themselves and dependents. However, having the ability or potential does not mean that all will seek knowledge or take action.

Dependent care is explained indirectly though the theory of self-care. Orem (1991) states that self-care is performed by mature and maturing individuals. If self-care is learned and performed deliberately in response to a need, it assumes that the individual has had time for interaction and communication to learn about the necessary action. It also assumes that the physical and intellectual development are present to perform the action. But self-care cannot be performed if the abilities have not had time to develop and mature or if developed abilities have become inoperable. Infants and children cannot meet the requirements necessary for life, health, and well-being because they are not developed. Adults who have matured and developed are at times unable to meet their needs. The abilities of a 20-year-old comatose, motorcycle accident victim have developed over time. But because of a comatose state, the abilities are not "operable"—that is, the patient cannot use that which has been learned. In these situations where all or some abilities are underdeveloped and inoperable, someone must perform the self-care. When a family member or responsible adult performs such care, it is termed "dependent care."

Theory of Nursing System

Understanding Orem's theory of nursing system is the key to understanding her general theory of nursing. The major components of the theory of self-care and the theory of self-care deficit are incorporated within the theory of nursing system (Orem & Taylor, 1986). Orem (1987) therefore called this the "unifying theory." The "theory of nursing system subsumes the theory of self-care deficit, which subsumes the theory of self-care" (Orem, 1991, p. 66). It is through this theory that the relationship between nursing actions and role and patient actions and role are explained. The central idea, eight propositions, and two presuppositions propose an answer to three questions: "What do nurses do when they nurse?", "What is the product made by nurses?", and "What results are sought by nurses?" (Orem, 1987, p. 72). These questions are similar to those that guided Orem's initial development of the general theory and provide understanding of why she views it as the unifying theory.

The central idea is that nurses have abilities that they use to determine if nursing help is necessary or "legitimate." The process involves the nurse determining an existing or potential deficit relationship between the abilities and demands for action in situations involving the health of an individual. If the deficit relationship exists, then the nurse should design a plan of care that clearly identifies what is to be done and by whom: the nurse, the patient, or the family member. These actions of the nurse and of the patient and/or dependent-care giver are collectively called the nursing system. The goal of the nursing system is to increase the patient's capabilities to meet a need, or requisite, or to decrease the demand. The two presuppositions assume that nursing is a practical service that has its own domain and boundaries. It is composed of deliberate actions over a period of time. If a nurse is performing an injection in a doctor's office as a one-time function, a nursing system for that patient may not be developed unless the nurse and patient together determine that follow-up on the injection or further nursing intervention is necessary.

Summary

The three theories of self-care, self-care deficit, and nursing system are interrelated through the presuppositions. Researchers and practitioners select one or all of the theories to guide their work. However, sometimes nurses focus their care primarily within one theory. For example, a nurse in an acute care setting may use the theory of self-care deficit, whereas the nurse in an ambulatory care setting may function primarily within the theory of self-care (Taylor, 1990). However, the key to understanding is through the theory of nursing system, which describes and explains the nursing role.

Concepts

S-CDTN is composed of six basic concepts and one related, or peripheral, concept. The basic, or core, concepts are self-care, self-care agency, therapeutic self-care demand, self-care deficit, nursing agency, and nursing system. The first four—self-care, self-care agency, therapeutic self-care demand, and self-care deficit—are related to the patient, or the person in need of nursing, whereas the latter two—nursing agency and nursing system—are related to the nurses and their actions. The concept of basic conditioning factors is related to selected patient and nurse concepts. Within the set of patient concepts, basic conditioning factors relate to self-care agency and to therapeutic self-care demand. Within the set of nurse concepts, they relate to nursing agency. Basic conditioning factors influence selected concepts. These include "age, gender, developmental state, health state, sociocultural orientation, health care system factors . . . family system factors, pattern of living, . . . environmental factors, resource availability and adequacy" (Orem, 1991, p. 136). Additional conditioning factors, such as nursing educational preparation and nursing experience, influence nursing agency (see Figure 21.1).

The assumptions, definitions, and relationships of each of the concepts are presented below. Historical context is presented where relevant.

Self-Care (Dependent Care)

Orem defines self-care as "the practice of activities that individuals initiate and perform on their own behalf in maintaining life, health, and well-being" (Orem, 1991, p. 117). This definition has been used consistently since the earliest descriptions of self-care by Orem (1956; 1959).

The general assumptions about self-care evolved from Orem's original papers and through the work of the Nursing Model Committee and the Nursing Development Conference Group (NDCG). Members of the groups spent 2 years clarifying the concept through analysis of specific practice situations and through subsequent validation of self-

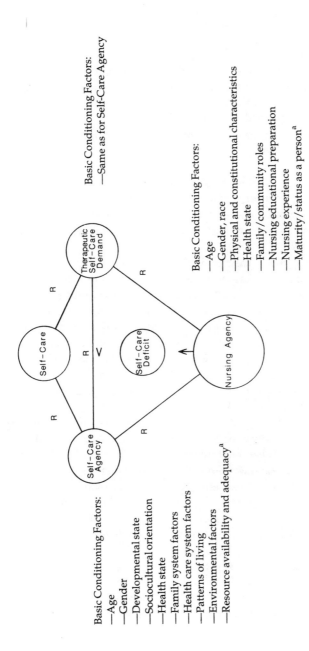

Figure 21.1. Conceptual Structure of the Self-Care Deficit Theory of Nursing.

SOURCE: Adapted from Orem (1987, p. 70) by permission of W. B. Saunders.
NOTE: R = relationship; < means that a self-care deficit exists when self-care agency is less than the therapeutic self-care demand.
a. From Orem (1991).

Basic Conditioning Factors:
—Age
—Gender
—Developmental state
—Sociocultural orientation
—Health state
—Family system factors
—Health care system factors
—Patterns of living
—Environmental factors
—Resource availability and adequacy[a]

Basic Conditioning Factors:
—Same as for Self-Care Agency

Basic Conditioning Factors:
—Age
—Gender, race
—Physical and constitutional characteristics
—Health state
—Family / community roles
—Nursing educational preparation
—Nursing experience
—Maturity / status as a person[a]

care conduct through group analysis of case study films (NDCG, 1973). Basic assumptions of the concept that have been consistent throughout development of the model include the following:

1. Self-care is ego-processed activity, which is learned through the individual's interpersonal relations and communications.
2. Each adult person has both the right and responsibility to care for self; this may include responsibilities for others, such as infants, children, the aged, or an adolescent.
3. An adult may need assistance from time to time to accomplish self-care. (NDCG, 1973, p. 99)

Self-care is not assumed to contribute to the positive nature of the health state. However, it is assumed that at the time when the individual first selected and performed the self-care action, it was done with the understanding that it was related in some way to health or well-being (NDCG, 1973).

Orem refers to self-care as "deliberate action." As learned behavior, it is a goal directed with a purpose in mind. A person consumes water, knowing that life and health cannot continue without it. A person with hypertension takes prescribed medication, knowing its importance in maintaining blood pressure within a healthy range. A 50-year-old woman increases the intake of calcium in her diet, knowing its importance in the prevention of osteoporosis in later life. Each of these instances is an example of a learned, goal-directed self-care action in which the prerequisite of "knowing" and "deciding" is presented. This emphasizes that self-care has phases. To perform a self-care action for a specific purpose one must first have knowledge of the action and how it relates to continued life, health, or well-being. The woman must seek and find information about the special calcium needs of middle-aged women and then reflect on the information. She then must make a decision either to change her food habits to obtain additional calcium or not to change food habits to meet the increased calcium needs for middle-aged women. These phases of seeking knowledge and decision making must precede the obvious self-care action of consuming or not consuming selected foods with increased calcium. Therefore one self-care action is composed of a series of operations, or phases. The early development of two series was developed by Backscheider (1974) and Pridham (1971). The phases of self-care are described by Orem (1991) as estimative, transitional, and productive operations. The phases of deliberate action are detailed by Orem (p. 85), with subsequent elaboration of phases of the three types of operations (pp. 85, 163-167).

The related concept of dependent care is within definitions of self-care. Dependent care is "actions performed by responsible adults to meet the components of their dependents' therapeutic self-care demands" (Orem & Taylor, 1986, p. 49). Orem is clear that the focus in dependent care given by families, friends, or other adults to other persons is related to the dependent's inability to provide the care needed because of a health state and not because of needs related to age or development (Orem, 1985b). That is to say, the term dependent care is not used for the normal care provided by a mother to her infant. But when the needs of the child change due to health state, such as an episode of pneumonia, then dependent care becomes relevant.

Self-Care Agency (Dependent-Care Agency)

Orem describes self-care agency as the power of individuals to engage in self-care and the capability for self-care (NDCG, 1979, p. 181). The person who uses this power or self-care ability is the self-care agent. Assumptions about self-care agency (p. 183) are inherent in these definitions. Self-care agency is an acquired ability that is affected by conditions and factors in the environment. For example, an individual who is educationally deprived may have less ability to seek information about health care than will one who has had many educational opportunities. Self-care agency is an ability to engage in self-care that develops from childhood, reaches maturity in adulthood, and declines with old age. Dependent-care agency is the ability of responsible adults to meet the continuing demands for self-care of their dependents.

Self-care agency, as a theoretical concept, has evolved from the early work of the NDCG as power and ability. It is described as a complex, hierarchical three-part structure (Orem & Taylor, 1986); see Figure 21.2. As one progresses from the base upward, the components relate more specifically to abilities needed for specific self-care action.

Part 1: Foundational Capabilities and Dispositions. The base of the structure includes the foundational capabilities and dispositions necessary for persons to engage in all types of deliberate action, not only self-care. For example, an individual may "deliberately

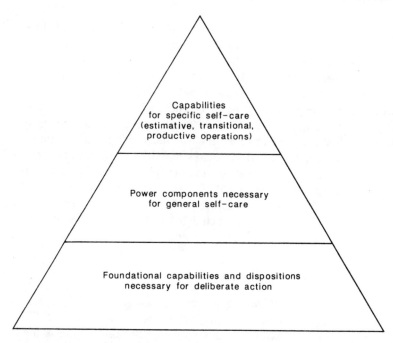

Figure 21.2. The three-part hierarchical structure of self-care agency.
SOURCE: Reprinted from *Advances in Nursing Science*, Vol. 12, No. 1, pp. 26-38, with permission of Aspen Publishers, Inc., © 1989.

act" to fix the car. Foundational capabilities are necessary, such as ability to work, to regulate position and movement of the body, and to remember directions for the repair. Dispositions affecting the goal of the action are also required, such as awareness of one's ability to make the repairs. Other capabilities and dispositions are components of this foundation, such as interests and values of the individual (NDCG, 1979, p. 212).

Part 2: Power Components. Ten power components comprise the middle portion of the hierarchy and relate specifically to self-care (see Table 21.1). Capabilities, such as motivation to engage in self-care, are clearly necessary for the individual to take action. To perform self-care, these "empowering capabilities" for self-care must be developed and operating. If a patient is comatose, the ability to maintain attention is not present. The ability may have been developed over time, but is clearly not operating at the

TABLE 21.1 Power Components of Self-Care Agency

---

1. Ability to maintain attention and exercise requisite vigilance with respect to (a) self as self-care agent and (b) internal and external conditions and factors significant to self-care

2. Controlled use of available physical energy that is sufficient for the initiation and continuation of self-care operations

3. Ability to control the position of the body and its part in the execution of the movements required for the initiation and completion of self-care operations

4. Ability to reason within a self-care frame of reference

5. Motivation (i.e., goal orientations for self-care that are in accord with its characteristics and its meaning for life, health, and well-being)

6. Ability to make decisions about care of self and to operationalize these decisions

7. Ability to acquire technical knowledge about self-care from authoritative sources, to retain it, and to operationalize it

8. A repertoire of cognitive, perceptual, manipulative, communication, and interpersonal skills adapted to the performance of self-care operations

9. Ability to order discrete self-care actions or action systems into relationships with prior and subsequent actions toward the final achievement of regulatory goals of self-care

10. Ability to consistently perform self-care operations, integrating them with relevant aspects of personal, family, and community living

---

SOURCE: Reprinted from Nursing Development Conference Group (1979, pp. 195-196) by permission of Little, Brown, and Company.

present. In the absence of the operability of self-care agency, nursing or dependent-care agents will need to provide compensatory care. Orem states that the 10 power components can be summarized as knowledge, attitudes, and skills that enable the individual to engage in self-care (Orem, 1990).

Part 3: Capabilities for Estimative, Transitional, and Productive Operations. The level in the hierarchy closest to the concrete self-care action is composed of three specific types of power and abilities: ability to determine what needs to be done to regulate one's health and well-being; ability to judge and decide what to do from the information that has been obtained; and ability to actually perform the self-care actions once the knowledge is obtained and the decision to act has been made. These three capabilities are related to three types of action necessary to meet specific self-care demands:

estimative, transitional, and productive operations or actions, respectively (NDCG, 1979; Orem, 1991). Estimative actions are those the individual performs when determining what self-care is to be performed; that is, the 50-year-old woman reads books and asks her nurse practitioner or physician about the special calcium needs of middle-aged women. Transitional operations or actions include reflecting on the course of action to be taken and then making a decision. The middle-aged woman must reflect on a variety of options related to the need for calcium. Should she change her daily food habits to obtain additional calcium or maintain the same food habits and consume calcium tablets daily? Productive operations relate to preparing the self to add this new self-care action to the daily routine, monitoring the effects of the new self-care action, and deciding the effectiveness of the action. If the middle-aged woman decides to take calcium tablets, productive operations would include purchasing the tablets, integrating the action into the daily routine, and determining their effect on her health and well-being. Specific abilities are necessary for each of these three types of actions.

Although the complexity of the concept was apparent in the early work, efforts to develop instruments to measure self-care agency have revealed its many dimensions or elements (Gast et al., 1989). Orem (1987) refers to self-care agency as the "summation of all the human capabilities needed for performing self-care" (p. 76) in actual situations. It combines those necessary for deliberate action, those required for general self-care, and those relevant to specific self-care.

Therapeutic Self-Care Demand

Therapeutic self-care demand (TSCD) is a concept that developed from the work of the NDCG over a 3-year period. It can be thought of as a collection of actions to be performed, or a "program of action" (NDCG, 1979, p. 184). It addresses this question: What are *all* the self-care actions that *should be performed* by the individual over time to maintain life, health, and well-being? Orem (1991) more recently described these as the "summation of measures of self-care required at moments in time and for some duration" (p. 65). This summation or totality of care actions is performed to meet what Orem calls self-care requisites, or generalized purposes for which the individual performs self-care. The self-care requisite is the general purpose. For example, a person deliberately drinks a quantity of water each day to maintain a sufficient intake of water, a basic self-care requisite. When a person deliberately selects and eats food, the self-care action is meeting the requisite for "maintenance of sufficient intake of food."

Each individual has only one therapeutic self-care demand that must be calculated from extensive knowledge and skill to meet the many known requirements or requisites that promote life, health, and well-being. Through experience, the individual learns about the specific requirements that must be met. As new events occur, such as illness or pregnancy, health care workers inform the individual of new requirements for action. Therefore, there is an interlinking of scientific knowledge and knowledge inherent within the person and the environment (NDCG, 1979).

Orem identified three types of self-care requisites, or requirements, for action: universal, developmental, and health deviation. Universal self-care requisites are those of all human beings throughout all stages of the life cycle and can be adjusted for age, environment, and other factors. There are eight universal self-care requisites:

1. The maintenance of sufficient intake of air
2. The maintenance of a sufficient intake of water
3. The maintenance of a sufficient intake of food
4. The provision of care associated with elimination processes and excrements
5. The maintenance of a balance between activity and rest
6. The maintenance of a balance between solitude and social interaction
7. The prevention of hazards to human life, human functioning, and human well-being
8. The promotion of human functioning and development within social groups in accord with human potential, known human limitations, and the human desire to be normal. *Normalcy* is used in the sense of that which is essentially human and that which is in accord with the genetic and constitutional characteristics and the talents of individuals.[1]

Normalcy relates to the development of a realistic self-concept. Developmental self-care requisites are of two types, the first being maturational and related to the universals but adjusted for age or developmental stage. For example, needs for food and interaction in adulthood are different from needs for food and interaction as a neonate. The second type of developmental requisite is situational and related to self-care that prevents or overcomes effects of life events or experiences that can impact human development. Examples are the tragedy of death, a change of residence, or those experiences related to social conditions, such as educational deprivation or oppressive living conditions. Each of these creates new requirements that must be met by the individual for life, health, and well-being.

Six health deviation self-care requisites exist for individuals who are "ill, are injured, have specific forms of pathology including defects and disabilities, and who are under medical diagnosis and treatment" (Orem, 1991, p. 132). Both genetic and acquired defects from health and well-being bring about needs for actions to prevent further problems or to control and overcome the effects of the existing deviations from normal. Because knowledge of these conditions emanates from medical science and technology, many of these needs are not known by individuals and must be learned through interaction with health care professionals. For example, the first health deviation self-care requisite cited by Orem suggests a need for women at risk for breast cancer, an example of "evidence of genetic conditions known to produce pathology" (p. 134), to seek assistance to learn self-breast examination and to seek resources and monitoring through mammography. The frequency of such self-care actions may be different from those who are not at risk.

Ideal sets of actions to be taken by patients with specific health conditions are being identified and are forming the basis for assessment in health care institutions where Orem's model is being used as the framework for practice. For example, ideal sets of actions have been identified for patients with laryngectomies and angina (Harry S. Truman Veteran's Administration, 1986, p. 131).

The ability to "calculate" all the self-care actions to be performed to meet all the universal, developmental, and health deviation self-care requisites requires much knowledge about health, illness, and human development. It also requires much information about individuals and groups, including specific cultures. Orem is clear that the therapeutic self-care demand or component of self-care demand must be known before the individual can engage in self-care. Once the requirements are known, then the adequacy of self-care agency can be assessed in relationship to the known self-care demand. It is, therefore, the TSCD that is much like a standard and "sets the specifications for self-care agency as well as for self-care" (NDCG, 1979, p. 181).

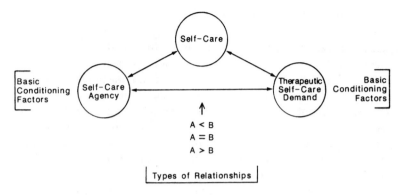

Figure 21.3. The three types of relationships between self-care agency and therapeutic self-care demand.
SOURCE: Adapted from Orem (1991, p. 146) by permission of Mosby-Year Book, Inc.

Self-Care Deficit (Dependent-Care Deficit)

Self-care deficit is a patient-focused concept that expresses a qualitative and quantitative relationship between two concepts, self-care agency and therapeutic self-care demand. There are three possible relationships: greater than, equal to, or less than/not adequate (see Figure 21.3).

A self-care deficit is the "relationship between self-care agency and therapeutic self-care demands of individuals in which capabilities for self-care, because of existent limitations, are not equal to meeting some or all of the components of their therapeutic self-care demands" (Orem, 1991, p. 173). A dependent care deficit is an unequal relationship between capabilities (agency) of responsible adults and the dependent person's required therapeutic self-care demand. A self-care deficit or dependent-care deficit may exist with a current inadequacy or may be predicted for the future as changes in either self-care agency (dependent-care agency) or therapeutic self-care demand are anticipated (Orem, 1987). Orem is clear that the deficit itself is not a disorder or problem but an expression of this relationship between the two concepts. This self-care deficit, or potential for a self-care deficit, must exist for nursing to be legitimate. If the nurse and the patient determine that no current or potential self-care deficit exists, then there is no role for the nurse in this situation.

Self-care deficit is a conceptual element and is described as complete or partial—that is, after determining the sum of all self-care actions necessary to meet the requisites (the therapeutic self-care demand), and an assessment of the adequacy of self-care agency in relationship to the therapeutic self-care demand, the nurse can determine whether a self-care deficit exists and whether it is partial or complete. A complete self-care deficit means "no capability to meet a therapeutic self-care demand" (Orem, 1991, p. 173). A partial deficit exists when the individual has some capabilities to meet part of the therapeutic self-care demand but not all. A mother with an infant has the capability to carry out most of the self-care actions to meet universal self-care requisites but may need assistance with new developmental demands, such as care of breasts if she is breast-feeding.

Nursing Agency

Nursing agency, or collective nursing capabilities, is defined as the "complex property or attribute of persons educated and trained as nurses that is enabling when exercised for knowing and helping others know their therapeutic self-care demands, for helping others meet or in meeting their therapeutic self-care demands, and in helping others regulate the exercise or development of their self-care agency or their dependent-care agency" (Orem, 1991, p. 64). This theoretical concept has a three-part structure similar to self-care agency (refer to Figure 21.2). There are also necessary foundational capabilities and dispositions, such as positive attitudes and willingness to act. The power components of nursing agency are similar to self-care agency but are specific to providing nursing, such as motivation to provide nursing care and the ability to control body parts as developed nursing skills. The third and most specific capabilities include those necessary for steps of the nursing process, such as diagnosis, prescription, and regulation or development of the person's self-care agency, or meeting of the therapeutic self-care demand (Orem & Taylor, 1986). Within these specialized abilities, Orem (1991) identified three types of desired nursing characteristics: social, interpersonal, and technological (pp. 261-263). These characteristics suggest the need for knowledge and skill that includes not only specific nursing knowledge but also a strong foundation in the humanities, sciences, and arts.

Like self-care agency, nursing agency is a complex, acquired ability of adults to engage in deliberate action; that is, it is learned and performed with a goal in mind. It is specialized ability that varies in nurses through their educational experiences, their practice situations, their mastery of skills, and their ability to work with and care for others (Orem, 1985b). Capabilities of a new graduate nurse will differ from those of an experienced clinician. Orem (1991) elaborated on other factors important to the ultimate delivery of nursing care. Factors such as age, gender, race, culture, status, and maturity as a person may affect the relations with patients. The focus of nursing agency differs from self-care agency as follows: Nursing agency is "developed and exercised for the benefit and well-being of others and self-care agency is developed and exercised for the benefit and well-being of oneself" (Orem, 1991, p. 255).

Orem (1985b) described nursing agency as "activated or unactivated." Activated agency produces diagnosis, prescription, and regulation of self-care for persons with self-care deficits associated with their health state. When nursing agency is activated as such, a nursing system is produced.

Nursing System

Orem (1985b) defined nursing system generally as "all the actions and interactions of nurses and patients in nursing practice situations" (p. 148). This concept emerged from the early work of the Nursing Model Committee of Catholic University in 1970 as the "creative end product of nursing" (NDCG, 1973, p. 69). More recently, Orem (1991) described the concept as "something constructed through actions of nurses and nurses' patients . . . a product that should be beneficial to persons with patient status in nursing practice situations when the time frame for production fits the time of occurrence of requirements for nursing" (p. 63).

Nursing system is viewed as tridimensional, including a hierarchy of interlocking systems: social, interpersonal, and technological (see Figure 21.4). The social and interpersonal dimensions are common to all helping services. The technological dimension is specific to nursing and gives direction to the form and substance of nursing. It is within this component that the elements of therapeutic self-care demand, self-care agency, and nursing agency are interrelated. The

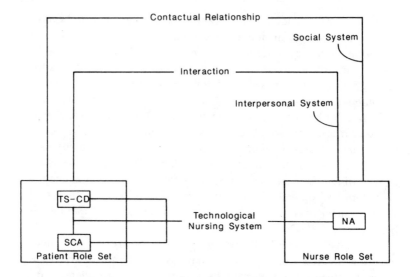

Figure 21.4. A hierarchy of interlocking systems.
SOURCE: Reprinted from Nursing Development Conference Group (1979, p. 112) by permission of Little, Brown, and Company.
NOTE: TS-CD = therapeutic self-care demand; SCA = self-care agency; NA = nursing agency.

efforts of the nurse are directed toward the "ability of others to engage in self-care effectively and continuously and . . . the continuous and effective meeting of the existing self-care requisites of others in the event of health-derived or health-related self-care deficits" (Orem, 1985b, pp. 147-148). However, Figure 21.4 clarifies assumptions of Orem and the NDCG that social and interpersonal aspects of nursing are also essential to the nursing system.

The social system is considered enabling of the interpersonal and technological systems (NDCG, 1973). The social system must exist or there is no basis for establishing the interpersonal relationship. The social system clarifies the role of the person as patient and the role of the nurse as the provider of care. If a self-care deficit exists, the person may become a patient of the nurse. If a person has nursing agency and the willingness to provide helping methods, a person may become the nurse of the patient. However, a critical element is also necessary: the establishment of a contractual relationship within the social system. This includes a contract or a formal agreement that clarifies the boundaries of the nursing care, the length of time for the care, and remuneration for the care. In such institutions as hospitals, this agreement may be implied when the patient signs an admission contract for care by nurses who are employed by the institution. Orem (1985b) emphasized the importance of the contractual nature of nurse-patient relationships in the following statement: "If nurses would accept the purpose of nursing and the contractual nature of nursing relationships, the deleterious practices of viewing patients as objects to be acted on and of processing patients through a system of routinized measures regardless of their conditions and needs might be eliminated" (p. 226).

Two factors produce the necessary interaction that occurs between the nurse and the patient in the interpersonal system: contact and association. The notion of association suggests that time is necessary for the relationship within the nursing system. Deliberate communication is mandated, making communication skills an important characteristic of nursing agency.

Types of Nursing Systems

There are three types of nursing systems: wholly compensatory, partly compensatory, and supportive–educative. These types can be clarified by answering one question in each nursing situation: "Who can or should perform those self-care actions . . . that require movement in space and controlled manipulation?" (Orem, 1991, p. 287; see Figure 21.5).

If the patient is unable to perform actions or control actions, the system is wholly compensatory; that is, the nurse performs all necessary actions. Examples are nursing systems for persons in a coma, in complete traction, or with a disease, such as severe Alzheimer's, where ambulation is possible but continuous supervision is necessary. If the nurse and patient share the responsibility for manipulative tasks and ambulation, the system is partly compensatory. Nursing systems may include those in which the patient performs most of the self-care actions related to universal requirements but needs assistance with those related to health-deviation requirements, such as techniques required in preparation for diagnostic tests. When a patient provides all self-care requiring movement in space and controlled manipulation and the nurse performs supportive and educative action, the system is supportive-educative or supportive-developmental. In this type of nursing system, the patient performs all

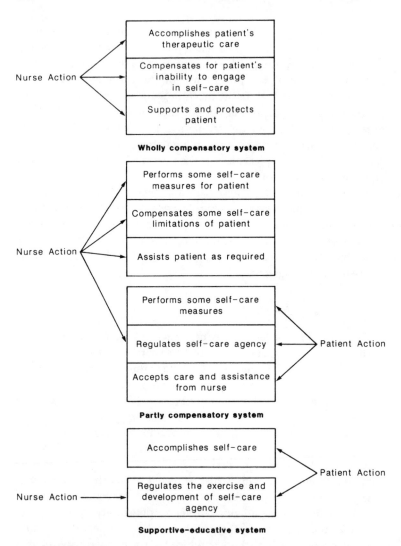

Figure 21.5. Basic nursing systems.
SOURCE: Reprinted from Orem (1991, p. 288) by permission of Mosby-Year Book, Inc.

self-care actions requiring ambulation and movement. For example, the nurse may provide information about breast-feeding to a new mother and support the mother psychologically during early feeding experiences. A patient may need all three types of nursing systems but at different times throughout one health condition. A patient suffering a stroke may initially need a wholly compensatory nursing system and progress to a supportive-educative nursing system. Combinations of types of systems occur at one point in time when nursing is provided to multiperson groups, such as families. The nurse may design a partly compensatory system for a home-care hospice patient and a supportive educative system for the grieving family member.

Methods of Assisting

Orem (1991) identified five general methods that persons use to assist or help others: acting for or doing for another; guiding another; supporting another, physically or psychologically; providing for a developmental environment; and teaching another (p. 286). Although these methods are not unique to nursing, they clarify the type of nursing system needed and the related roles for the nurse and patient. A grieving patient may need a supportive-educative system in which providing psychological support is the primary general method. The nurse's role is to listen in an understanding manner, whereas the patient's role is to actively confront and resolve a difficult situation (p. 286). Nurses tend to use the five different methods in combination within one type of nursing system. For example, a nurse may use acting and doing for to provide physical care to a postsurgical patient. Supporting another may be used to encourage the same patient to perform postoperative deep breathing and coughing exercises. Guiding another may be the general method in assisting the patient to make decisions about further medical interventions, such as chemotherapy. Teaching and providing a developmental environment may also be used within this one situation. In general, it is not appropriate to use "acting for" in the supportive-educative system. The determination of the supportive-educative system is based on the judgment that the nurse's patient is able to perform these self-care actions.

Basic Conditioning Factors

Orem (1987) describes the concept of basic conditioning factors (BCFs) as one that is peripheral to the six core, or major, concepts. It is related to two patient concepts (self-care agency and therapeutic self-care demand) and to one nurse concept (nursing agency). The BCFs, recently expanded by Orem (1991) from 8 to 10, are age, gender, developmental state, health state, sociocultural orientation, health care system elements (e.g., medical diagnosis and treatment modalities), family system elements, patterns of living, environmental factors, and resource availability and adequacy.

These factors, which are interrelated, actively influence both the quality and the quantity of self-care agency, therapeutic self-care demand, and nursing agency at instances in time. For example, age and patterns of living are BCFs that impact the universal self-care requisites of maintenance of a sufficient intake of food and water. An 18-year-old male athlete's requirements for quantity and types of nutrients and water is different from those of a 40-year-old sedentary woman. In addition, the BCFs affect self-care agency. For example, sociocultural orientation impacts a person's capability to engage in self-care. Values, folk beliefs, and practices affect the individual's self-care agency (Anna, Christensen, Hohon, Ord, & Wells, 1978; Brauch, 1985; Chamorro, 1985; Hammonds, 1985). Careful assessment of each of the BCFs is therefore necessary and serves as a critical component of the database for determining the presence or absence of the self-care deficit. There are other factors that impact nursing agency, such as nursing education and experience (see Figure 21.1).

Propositions

A theoretical proposition is a statement that describes a concept or explains and predicts the relationship between concepts. These statements are foundational to theory and serve as the basis for theory testing and theoretical application to practice. The three types of statements are existence, definition, and relational (Walker & Avant, 1988). These serve to purport the existence of a concept, define concepts generally or theoretically, and describe the relationships among concepts, respectively. Each statement can be developed into a hypothesis for a research study. As propositions or statements are supported by research findings, the theory becomes credible and is validated. Those not supported lead to refinement or disconfirmation of the theory.

Orem's theoretical propositions are presented within the theories of self-care deficit, self-care, and nursing system. The majority of the statements further define and describe concepts in the theory. Although limited testing of propositions in the theory has been conducted (Silva, 1986), selected statements have served as the basis for research studies and will be used as examples.

Theory of Self-Care Deficit (Dependent-Care Deficit)

The first set of propositions is related to the Theory of Self-Care Deficit (or Dependent-Care Deficit) (see Table 21.2). Concepts of self-care agency (capabilities), basic conditioning factors (age, developmental state, etc.), the relationship between self-care agency and demand, a definition of the type of relationship, and nursing as a legitimate service are further described and explained through these statements. Relationships are clarified by the use of figures. For example, Proposition 2 can be expressed through Figure 21.3 by examining the relationship between self-care agency and the basic conditioning factors of age, developmental state, sociocultural orientation, and health state. Because each of these factors can be considered a variable, this one proposition can become many research hypotheses. For example, Denyes (1988) studied the impact of health state on self-care ability. Health state was defined as health problems to examine the relationship between health state and self-care agency of adolescents. The significant relationship found between these two concepts provided support for Proposition 2 within the theory of self-care deficit (see Table 21.2). A subsequent study by Frey and Denyes (1989) provided further support for the relationship.

Theory of Self-Care (Dependent Care)

Six propositions within the theory of self-care provide further descriptions about the concepts of self-care and self-care system (see Table 21.2). These six propositions are a major change in the most recent edition of Orem (1991). Previously, 10 propositions provided descriptions of several concepts, including self-care requisites and dependent care (Orem, 1980, 1985b). The relationships of concepts to the BCFs were described. The revised propositions are limited to descriptions of the self-care concept, with further explanation of self-care systems and external and internal self-care actions.

Selected studies have provided initial support for Orem's earlier propositions (1980, 1985b). For example, studies by Dodd (1983, 1984a, 1984b) and Harper (1984) supported the original Proposition 1, that self-care is learned behavior within the context of social groups.

TABLE 21.2 Propositions in the Three Theories

Theory of Self-Care Deficit (Dependent-Care Deficit)

1. Persons who take action to provide their own self-care or care for dependents have specialized capabilities for action.
2. The individual's abilities to engage in self-care or dependent care are conditioned by age, developmental state, life experience, sociocultural orientation, health, and available resources.
3. The relationship of individuals' abilities for self-care or dependent care to the qualitative and quantitative self-care or dependent-care demand can be determined when the value of each is known.
4. The relationship between care abilities and care demand can be defined in terms of *equal to, less than, more than.*
5. Nursing is a legitimate service when
   (a) Care abilities are less than those required for meeting a known self-care demand (a deficit relationship).
   (b) Self-care or dependent-care abilities exceed or are equal to those required for meeting the current self-care demand, but a future deficit relationship can be foreseen because of predictable decreases in care abilities, qualitative or quantitative increases in the care demand, or both.
6. Persons with existing or projected care deficits are in, or can expect to be in, states of social dependency that legitimate a nursing relationship. (p. 71)

Theory of Self-Care (Dependent-Care)

1. Self-care is intellectualized as a human regulatory function deliberately executed with some degree of completeness and effectiveness.
2. Self-care in its concreteness is directed and deliberate action that is responsive to persons' knowing how human functioning and human development can and should be maintained within a range that is compatible with human life and personal health and well-being under existent conditions and circumstances.
3. Self-care in its concreteness involves the use of material resources and energy expenditures directed to supply materials and conditions needed for internal functioning and development and to establish and maintain essential and safe relationships with environmental factors and forces.
4. Self-care in its concreteness when externally oriented emerges as observable events resulting from performed sequences of practical actions directed by persons to themselves or their environments. Self-care that has the form of internally oriented self-controlling actions is not observable and can be known by others only by seeking subjective information. Reasons for the actions and the results being sought from them may or may not be known to the subject who performs the actions.

TABLE 21.2 (Continued)

5. Self-care that is performed over time can be understood (intellectualized) as an action system—a self-care system—whenever there is knowledge of the complement of different types of actions sequences or care measures performed and the connecting linkages among them.

6. Constituent components of a self-care system are sets of care measures or tasks necessary to use valid and selected means (i.e., technologies to meet existent and changing values of known self-care requisites). (pp. 69-70)

Theory of Nursing System(s)

1. Nurses relate to and interact with persons who occupy the status of nurse's patient.

2. Legitimate patients have existent and projected continuous self-care requisites.

3. Legitimate patients have existent or projected deficits for meeting their own self-care requisites.

4. Nurses determine the current and changing values of patients' continuous self-care requisites, select valid and reliable processes or technologies for meeting these requisites, and formulate the courses of action necessary for using selected processes or technologies that will meet identified self-care requisites.

5. Nurses determine the current and changing values of patients' abilities to meet their self-care requisites using specific processes or technologies.

6. Nurses estimate the potential of patients to (a) refrain from engaging in self-care for therapeutic purposes or (b) develop or refine abilities to engage in care now or in the future.

7. Nurses and patients act together to allocate the roles of each in the production of patients' self-care and in the regulation of patients' self-care capabilities.

8. The actions of nurses and the actions of patients (or nurses' actions that *compensate for the patients' action limitations*) that regulate patients' self-care capabilities and meet patients' therapeutic self-care needs constitute nursing systems. (pp. 72-73)

SOURCE: Reproduced by permission from Orem, Dorothea E.: *Nursing: Concepts of practice*, ed. 4, St. Louis, 1991, Mosby-Year Book, Inc.

However, each used different populations to explore the same statement. Dodd used cancer patients receiving chemotherapy, and Harper studied Black, elderly, hypertensive women attending an inner-city clinic. New studies will be needed to test propositions in revised works (Orem, 1991).

Theory of Nursing System(s)

Eight propositions within the theory of nursing systems provide description of legitimate patients and nursing systems and clarify the concept of roles for patient and nurse (see Table 21.2). Propositions 1, 4, 5, and 6 clarify the expectations for the individual in the role of nurse. Proposition 1 establishes the importance of interpersonal operations, and Propositions 4 and 5 describe the methods for determining the therapeutic self-care demand and self-care agency, respectively. Propositions 2 and 3 define and describe legitimate patients; Propositions 7 and 8 explain how the nurse and patient work together to determine roles and actions that become nursing systems. These propositions have served more to guide practice than as the basis for specific research studies. Taylor (1988) used the S-CDTN to organize and structure nursing practice, with the theory of nursing system providing structure for the nursing process. Propositions were presented and applied to the specific case study of Mr. Kay, a patient with amyotrophic lateral sclerosis, and Ms. Lee, the nurse. Proposition 7 provided clear direction to determining the roles of Mr. Kay, Ms. Lee, and others in the system before the self-care actions were assigned to any individual. Further examples of applications of research and practice are presented in the next section.

Note

1. Reproduced by permission from D. E. Orem, *Nursing: Concepts of Practice,* 4th ed., 1991. St. Louis: Mosby-Year Book, Inc.

22

Application to
Practice, Education, and Research

The varying applications of Orem's model to practice and nursing education as well as the use of the model in nursing research are described in the following pages.

Application to Nursing Practice

The application of Orem's model to practice takes many forms in the nursing literature. For example, it has been applied to patients with specific diseases, to specific age groups, and used in a variety of settings (see Table 22.1). Each article varies in its level of application. Some authors use the model as a philosophical guide to nursing practice, often citing self-care beliefs or building on Orem's definition of self-care (e.g., Fitzgerald, 1980). Others use Orem's concepts with precision and develop guides to nursing practice (e.g. Backscheider, 1974). Many provide examples of the nursing process using a case study to develop a plan of care for an individual client (e.g. Orem & Taylor, 1986; Smith, 1989; Taylor, 1988). Applications to families have also been made (Orem, 1983a, 1983b, 1983c; Tadych, 1985; Taylor, 1989), as well as to communities (Hanchett, 1988, 1990; Orem, 1984). These applications of case examples often vary depending on the primary work used by the author. For example, Joseph (1980) pre-

TABLE 22.1 Examples of Applications to Nursing Practice

Use as framework in a variety of settings
Acute care units (Mullin, 1980; Weis, 1988)
Ambulatory clinics (Alford, 1985; Allison, 1973; Backscheider, 1974)
College student health program (Hedahl, 1983)
Community health promotion program (Nowakowski, 1980)
Critical care units (Fawcett et al., 1987)
High-rise senior center (Neufeld & Hobbs, 1985)
Hospices (Murphy, 1981; Walborn, 1980)
Nursing homes (Anna, Christensen, Hohon, Ord, & Wells, 1978)
Obstetrical units (Woolery, 1983)
Pediatric units (Titus & Porter, 1989)
Psychiatric units (Davidhizar & Cosgray, 1990; Moscovitz, 1984)
Rehabilitation settings (Orem, 1985a)

Application to patients with specific diseases or conditions
Adolescent alcohol abusers (Michael & Sewall, 1980)
Adolescents with chronic disease (McCracken, 1985)
Alcoholics (Williams, 1979)
The chronically ill (Gulick, 1986)
Coronary bypass surgery (Campuzano, 1982)
Diabetes (Allison, 1973; Backscheider, 1974; Fitzgerald, 1980)
End stage renal disease (Michos, 1985)
Enterostomies (Bromley, 1980)
Head and neck surgery (Dropkin, 1981)
Hypertension (Galli, 1984)
Myocardial infarction (Garrett, 1985)
Neurological dysfunction (Perry & Sutcliffe, 1982)
Treatment with peritoneal dialysis (Perras & Zappacosta, 1982)
Rheumatoid arthritis (Smith, 1989)

Application to selected age groups
The aged (Bower & Patterson, 1986; Eliopoulos, 1984; Hankes, 1984; Hewes
& Hannigan, 1985; Sullivan & Munroe, 1986)
Children (Eichelberger, Kaufman, Rundahl, & Schwartz, 1980; Facteau, 1980;
Koster, 1983)
Mothers with newborns (Dunphy & Jackson, 1985)

sented an overview of Orem's nursing process using Orem (1971). This edition did not include the concept of developmental self-care requisites. Nurses using this primary source will find variation from the current model of nursing process described in Orem (1980, 1985b, 1991). Taylor's (1988) work exemplifies a current application of nursing process.

The practice literature also includes works that are modifications of Orem, such as Kinlein (1977a, 1977b) and Sullivan (1980). Chang (1980) presented a conceptual model that modified the theory for use with health care professionals promoting self-care. There are also self-care references in the nursing literature that are cited in Orem bibliographies that are not applications of Orem (e.g., Harris, 1980). The reader must distinguish between application of Orem's self-care model to practice and general application of other self-care models. Some authors combine theories or propose a blending of theoretical ideas, such as those of Orem, Leininger, and Rogers (Steiger & Lipson, 1985) and Orem and King (Swindale, 1989).

Orem's self-care model is increasingly used as a framework for practice in specific institutions. This has significant implications for nursing service administration. Newark Beth Israel Medical Center became the first acute-care hospital in the northeastern United States to base the nursing practice for the institution on Orem's model. Their library and media center are a resource for Orem's works (NLN News, 1987). Mississippi Methodist Hospital and Rehabilitation Center in Jackson, Mississippi (Allison, 1985), and Harry S Truman Hospital in Columbia, Missouri (Kunz, personal communication, 1987), have developed practical structures for implementation in their respective settings. Many Canadian health care institutions, such as those in Toronto, Scarborough, and Vancouver, use Orem's self-care theory as a model for nursing care delivery. Practical guides have been developed to facilitate implementation in their respective settings (e.g., Scarborough General Hospital, 1987). Other institutions, such as the Veterans Administration Center in Palo Alto, California, use the model on selected units. The literature is just emerging that demonstrates the effects of such application. Faucett, Ellis, Underwood, Naqvi, and Wilson (1990) found that nurses using Orem's model differ from control nurses in their assessments and goals of care for patients in a nursing home setting.

The application to nursing service administration has been described by several authors (Miller, 1980; Nickle-Gallagher, 1985). Allison (1985) described an administrator's perspective on structuring of nursing practice based on Orem's theory of nursing. Elements of the nursing system for a patient with a spinal cord injury were developed. Self-care capabilities and limitations, self-care requisites, and related nursing actions were identified for this one-patient population. Using Orem's concept of nursing agency, Allison further identified how the role and function of the professional, technical, and vocational nurse were defined in relationship to each of these components. Others (Clinton, Denyes, Goodwin, & Koto, 1977; Horn & Swain, 1977) have used Orem's concepts to develop instruments that measure patient outcomes, a method to determine the quality of nursing care.

Application to Nursing Education

Orem's framework has been used as a conceptual guide to nursing curricula in associate degree, diploma, and baccalaureate nursing programs. The number of schools currently using the model is unknown. Fawcett (1989) presented a partial listing of schools identified by Orem in personal communication. Examples are the following: Georgetown University, Washington, D.C.; Incarnate Word College in San Antonio, Texas; Medical College of Ohio in Toledo; Wichita State University in Wichita, Kansas; Catholic Education College in Melbourne, Australia; and Centennial College in Scarborough, Ontario. The University of Missouri-Columbia has been a leader in promoting theory development through educational and research programs. They have expanded conferences from regional to international ones in less than a decade (Eben, Gashti, Nation, Marriner-Tomey, & Nordmeyer, 1989).

The application of Orem's theory to nursing education also takes many forms. Fenner (1979) described how faculty used the model to identify curricular content that differentiated the role and function of the technical nurse from that of the professional nurse at Thornton Community College in South Holland, Illinois. Piemme and Trainor (1977) presented a rationale for exposing baccalaureate nursing students at Georgetown University to the theory early in the program. They proposed that an early understanding of Orem's theory broadened their perspective of nursing. Biehler (1987) described the development of the curricular structure at Illinois Wesleyan University in Bloomington, Illinois. The revised curriculum used seven nursing situations (Orem, 1980) to structure the clinical portion of the program. The seven disciplines of nursing knowledge identified by Orem provided an additional framework for the curricular content.

Many schools use Orem's nursing process in clinical practice, developing extensive assessment tools, teaching packets, and evaluation models. Herrington and Houston (1984) described the assessment tool and care plan forms used by students at the University of Southern Mississippi. The authors suggested the model and related application of Orem's process contributed to a stronger nursing focus.

The impact of a curricular structure using Orem's model is in early testing. Hartweg and Metcalfe (1986) studied the changes in self-care attitudes experienced by baccalaureate nursing students exposed to Orem's model. Using a longitudinal design, they compared attitude changes of nursing students to those of students in the general university. Self-care attitudes of nursing students increased significantly over those of general university students during the 3-year period. What is not known is the impact of general nursing knowledge, not self-care knowledge, on that change. Wagnild, Rodriguez, and Pritchett (1987) surveyed nurses who had graduated from a curriculum based on the Self-Care Deficit Theory of Nursing to determine if graduates used the model subsequently in their individual practice settings. Although limited by the response rate, the research suggested possible outcomes of such curricular structures and the variables that impact the ability of graduates to apply the self-care framework in their respective clinical settings following graduation.

Utilization in Nursing Research

Orem's conceptual framework has been used increasingly as a guide for nursing research. As with practice and education, there has been much variation in the application by researchers. Some researchers use the beliefs or definitions in the model as a basis for research (e.g. Brock & O'Sullivan, 1985). Others cite Orem's concepts but build on the ideas of others. For example, Stollenwerk (1985) referred to supportive-educative roles of Orem but used Gordon (1982) as a framework. Many researchers use several theories within one study (e.g., Allan, 1990). Other investigators select theoretical concepts, such as self-care or therapeutic self-care demand, to guide the research. These studies are descriptive, with a goal of describing or exploring concepts. Woods (1985) described the self-care practices of young adult married women. Kubricht (1984) used a descriptive survey to identify the therapeutic self-care demands of cancer patients having external radiation. Patterson and Hale (1985) used

grounded theory to determine types of self-care practices of menstru-
ating women.

The methods used in these studies are consistent with the recom-
mendation of a consultant hired in the early years of the Nursing
Model Committee of Catholic University (Nursing Development
Conference Group, 1973). The suggestion was to refrain from using
the research methods of the experimental sciences. Studies in these
disciplines use precise experiments that vary one factor in a situation
while holding others constant. This approach was viewed as inconsistent with Orem's model, which is based on the complexity of
human systems, the patient and the nurse. The approaches recommended by the consultant were the natural history method and the
hypothetical-deductive approach. The natural history approach gath-
ers data from individuals in their natural settings, often from interviews, diaries, or through observation. Woods (1985) and Patterson
and Hale (1985) are examples of this method. The hypothetical-
deductive method derives hypotheses from the propositions in the
theories. Recently, research using Orem's framework is appearing
that uses this method for theory-testing. Harper (1984) tested four
hypotheses deduced from propositions in Self-Care Deficit Theory of
Nursing using a population of elderly, Black, hypertensive patients.
Three of these hypotheses were derived specifically from the Theory
of Self-Care. The findings supported several of Orem's (1980) propositions, including the following: Self-care systems result from use of
knowledge and skills to meet known requisites; and self-care is
learned within the context of social groups through human interaction and communication.

Other theory-testing research continues to clarify and support the
theories within the model. Hartley (1988) tested the relationship
between the nursing system and self-care behavior in women learning breast self-examination. The proposition tested the relationship
between a supportive-educative nursing system and self-care behavior. Frey and Denyes (1989) studied insulin-dependent adolescents
and found support for the relationships between universal self-care
and global health state, and health deviation self-care and control of
pathology. Using aggregate data on adolescents, Denyes (1988) had
previously found support for distinctions between the two types of
self-care. Both studies were testing the relationship between basic
conditioning factors, particularly health state, and abilities to engage

in self-care. Although Orem (1991) recently made changes in propositions in the Theory of Self-Care, such testing by researchers contributes to knowledge development and further refinement of the theory. Other investigators have not explicitly identified propositions but have contributed to theory development by building on previous knowledge. Dodd's sequence of studies on self-care behavior of patients experiencing chemotherapy (1982, 1983, 1984a, 1984c, 1988b) and radiation therapy (1984b) included efforts to build on previous knowledge from prior studies through addressing limitations in other studies or through replication. Dodd used both descriptive (1982) and experimental (1983, 1984a) approaches. These studies supported Orem's proposition that self-care is learned within the context of social groups through human interaction and communication. Examples of other experimental studies are Ewing (1989) with stoma patients and Williams et al. (1988) with preparation of mastectomy/hysterectomy patients. Dodd (1987, 1988a) investigated the efficacy of proactive information on self-care of radiation therapy and chemotherapy patients. However, other theories were cited besides Orem's.

When research is conducted on theoretical concepts within a model, such as self-care agency, it is critical that a measuring instrument be valid and reliable. Much of the research within Orem's Self-Care Deficit Theory of Nursing has been directed to developing instruments to measure concepts in the model. Self-care agency is the concept most frequently operationalized by instruments. Gast et al. (1989) summarized the elements of self-care agency and described the instruments available for measurement. Other tools are in the process of development (Taylor & Geden, 1991). Jirovec and Kasno (1990) described the use of an instrument in development in both the Netherlands and the United States. The following authors have developed instruments frequently used to measure self-care agency: Denyes (1982), Hanson and Bickel (1985), and Kearney and Fleischer (1979). Kearney and Fleischer's instrument has been used to measure self-care agency of persons in East Germany (Whetstone, 1987) and Sweden (Whetstone & Hansson, 1989). Critiques and further development of the instruments have been conducted by Cleveland (1989), MacBride (1987), Riesch and Hauck (1988), and Weaver (1987). These studies are important as they raise important questions about the validity and reliability of the measurement tools. A further example of a modification of self-care agency was developed by Campbell (1986). Using Orem's framework, she developed the Danger Assessment as a measure of self-care agency of women at risk for battering.

Other investigators have developed instruments to measure self-care behaviors related to specific illnesses: side effects from cancer chemotherapy (Dodd, 1982); multiple sclerosis (Gulick, 1987); self-care medication behaviors (Harper, 1984); self-care responses to respiratory illnesses of Vietnamese (Hautman, 1987); mothers' performance of self-care for children (Moore & Gaffney, 1989); and self-care management in school-aged children with diabetes (Saucier, 1984).

Although this partial review reveals much research using Orem's model, its popularity for guiding research can be further demonstrated through a search of *Dissertation Abstracts*. Fawcett (1989) cited numerous examples of master's theses and dissertations that abound in the unpublished literature.

Glossary

Agency
ability, capability, or power to engage in action

Agent
the person who has the ability (agency) to perform the action or who actually performs the action

Basic conditioning factors (BCFs)
For the patient: factors that influence, at points in time, the individual's health-related needs/demands (therapeutic self-care demand) and the individual's ability (self-care agency) to engage in self-care. Examples are age, gender, health state, and family patterns.
For the nurse: factors that influence, at points, in time, the nurse's ability (nurse agency) to form interpersonal relationships and to assist with or perform self-care. Special note: In addition to the general BCFs, such nurse-specific factors as nursing experience and education influence nursing agency.

Deliberate action
"purposeful goal- or result-seeking activity" (Orem, 1991, p. 162)

Dependent care
activities performed by responsible adults for socially dependent individuals, children, or adults to meet portions of their therapeutic self-care demands

Dependent-care agency
ability, capability, or power of a responsible adult to meet the demands of the dependent individual

Dependent-care agent
the provider of dependent care, such as a parent, family member, or friend. These providers can be mature adults or maturing adults, such as adolescents.

Developmental self-care requisite
needs or goals for self-care that arise from either maturational changes in the life cycle, such as pregnancy, or from situational events that occur throughout human development, such as death of a significant other

Estimative self-care operations
process of seeking knowledge about the self-care that needs to be done (NDCG, 1979, p. 189)

Foundational capabilities and dispositions
general capabilities of self-care agency to engage in deliberate action (NDCG, 1979)

Health
structural and functional soundness and wholeness of the individual (Orem, 1991)

Health deviation self-care requisites
needs or goals for self-care that arise when persons are ill, injured, have defects or disabilities, or are undergoing diagnosis or treatment

Methods of assisting
general ways of helping that can be used by one person to give assistance to others, such as teaching, acting or doing for, guiding, supporting, or providing for a developmental environment

Nursing agency
specialized abilities of nurses for diagnosing, prescribing, and producing nursing care that result in meeting the individual's therapeutic self-care demand or in increasing self-care agency

Nursing system
the totality of the actions and interactions of nurses and patients and/or family in a nursing situation at a point in time

Partly compensatory nursing system
"when both nurse and patient perform care measures or other actions involving manipulative tasks or ambulation" (Orem, 1985b, p. 156)

Power components
enabling capabilities of self-care agency that must be developed and operational for individuals to perform self-care (Orem, 1987)

Productive self-care operations
process of making and doing, including the performance of the actions, monitoring the effects, and deciding to continue the actions (NDCG, 1979, p. 194)

Self-care
"practice of activities that individuals initiate and perform on their own behalf in maintaining life, health, and well-being" (Orem, 1991, p. 117)

Self-care agency
the complex, learned ability or power to perform self-care that is described as knowledge, skill, and motivation for self-care actions that promote life, health, and well-being

Self-care deficit
self-care ability of the person is not adequate to meet the therapeutic self-care demand

Self-care requisite
purposes or goals to be achieved through self-care

Supportive-educative nursing system
a nursing system in which the patient performs the actions, and the nurse guides and assists using methods of helping, such as supporting, guiding, providing for a developmental environment, and teaching. The patient is able to perform all self-care actions requiring controlled ambulation and manipulative movement.

Therapeutic self-care demand
all the self-care actions that should be performed by the individual at a point in time to maintain health and promote well-being

Transitional self-care operations
process of making judgments or decisions about what self-care should be performed; includes use of knowledge, experience, and values of the individual (NDCG, 1979, p. 194)

Universal self-care requisites
common human needs or goals of self-care that promote structural and functional integrity of the person and well-being. These include maintenance of air, food, water, and elimination; balance between activity and rest; solitude and social interaction; the prevention of hazards; and the promotion of normalcy.

Well-being
an "individual's perceived condition of existence . . . a state characterized by experiences of contentment, pleasure, and kinds of happiness; by spiritual experiences; by movement toward fulfillment of one's self-ideal; and by continuing personalization" (Orem, 1991, p. 184)

Wholly compensatory nursing system
a nursing system in which the nurse performs all the self-care actions that require controlled ambulation and manipulative movement

References

Alford, D. M. (1985). Self-care practices in ambulatory nursing clinics. In J. Riehl-Sisca (Ed.), *The science and art of self-care* (pp. 253-261). Norwalk, CT: Appleton-Century-Crofts.

Allan, J. D. (1990). Focusing on living, not dying: A naturalistic study of self-care among seropositive gay men. *Holistic Nursing Practice, 4*(2), 56-63.

Allison, S. E. (1973). A framework for nursing action in a nurse-conducted diabetic management clinic. *Journal of Nursing Administration, 3*(4), 53-73.

Allison, S. E. (1985). Structuring nursing practice based on Orem's theory of nursing: A nurse administrator's perspective. In J. Riehl-Sisca (Ed.), *The science and art of self-care* (pp. 225-235). Norwalk, CT: Appleton-Century-Crofts.

Anna, D. J., Christensen, D. G., Hohon, S. A., Ord, L., & Wells, S. R. (1978). Implementing Orem's conceptual framework. *Journal of Nursing Administration, 8*(11), 8-11.

Backscheider, J. E. (1974). Self-care requirements, self-care capabilities and nursing systems in the diabetic nurse management clinic. *American Journal of Public Health, 64*(12), 1138-1146.

Barnard, C. (1962). *The functions of the executive*. Cambridge, MA: Harvard University Press.

Biehler, B. (1987). Nursing situations as focus for curriculum design. In S. G. Taylor & E. A. Geden (Eds.), *Proceedings of the Fifth Annual Self-Care Deficit Theory Conference: Theory-based nursing process and product usin Orem's self-care theory of nursing in practice, education, research* (pp. 41-47). St. Louis: Curators of the University of Missouri.

Bower, F. N., & Patterson, J. (1986). A theory-based nursing assessment of the aged. *Topics in Clinical Nursing, 8*(1), 22-32.

Brauch, M. (1985). Self-care: Black perspectives. In J. Riehl-Sisca (Ed.), *The science and art of self-care* (pp. 181-188). Norwalk, CT: Appleton-Century-Crofts.

191

192 FOUNDATIONS OF NURSING THEORY

Brock, A. M., & O'Sullivan, P. (1985). A study to determine what variables predict institutionalization of the elderly. *Journal of Advanced Nursing, 10*, 533-537.

Bromley, B. (1980). Applying Orem's self-care theory in enterostomal therapy. *American Journal of Nursing, 80*, 245-249.

Campbell, J. C. (1986). Nursing assessment for risk of homicide with battered women. *Advances in Nursing Science, 8*(4) 36-51.

Campuzano, M. (1982). Self-care following coronary artery bypass surgery. *Focus on Critical Care, 9*(2), 55-56.

Chamorro, L. C. (1985). Self-care in the Puerto Rican community. In J. Riehl-Sisca (Ed.), *The science and art of self-care* (pp. 188-195). Norwalk, CT: Appleton-Century-Crofts.

Chang, B. (1980). Evaluation of health care professionals in facilitating self-care: Review of the literature and a conceptual model. *Advances in Nursing Science, 3*(1), 43-58.

Cleveland, S. A. (1989). Re: Perceived self-care agency: A LISREL factor analysis of Bickel and Hanson's Questionnaire [Letter to the editor]. *Nursing Research, 38*, 59.

Clinton, J. F., Denyes, M. J., Goodwin, J. O., & Koto, E. M. (1977). Developing criterion measures of nursing care: Case study of a process. *Journal of Nursing Administration, 7*(7), 41-45.

Davidhizar, R., & Cosgray, R. (1990). The use of Orem's model in psychiatric rehabilitation assessment. *Rehabilitation Nursing, 15*(1), 39-41.

Denyes, M. J. (1982). Measurement of self-care agency in adolescents [Abstract]. *Nursing Research, 31*, 63.

Denyes, M. J. (1988). Orem's model used for health promotion: Directions from research. *Advances in Nursing Science, 11*(1), 13-21.

Denyes, M. J., O'Connor, N. A., Oakley, D., & Ferguson, S. (1989). Integrating nursing theory, practice, and research through collaborative practice. *Journal of Advanced Nursing, 14*, 141-145.

Dodd, M. J. (1982). Assessing patient self-care for side effects of cancer therapy: Part I. *Cancer Nursing, 5*, 447-451.

Dodd, M. J. (1983). Self-care for side effects in cancer chemotherapy: An assessment of nursing interventions: Part II. *Cancer Nursing, 6*, 63-67.

Dodd, M. J. (1984a). Measuring informational intervention for chemotherapy knowledge and self-care behavior. *Research in Nursing and Health, 7*, 43-50.

Dodd, M. J. (1984b). Patterns of self-care in cancer patients receiving radiation therapy. *Oncology Nursing Forum, 11*, 23-27.

Dodd, M. J. (1984c, December). Self-care for patients with breast cancer to prevent side effects of chemotherapy: A concern for public health nursing. *Journal of Public Health Nursing*, pp. 202-209.

Dodd, M. J. (1987). Efficacy of proactive information on self-care of radiation therapy patients. *Patient Education, 16*(5), 538-544.

Dodd, M. J. (1988a). Efficacy of proactive information on self-care in chemotherapy patients. *Patient Education and Counseling, 11*, 215-225.

Dodd, M. J. (1988b). Patterns of self-care in patients with breast cancer. *Western Journal of Nursing Research, 10*, 7-24.

Dropkin, M. J. (1981). Development of a self-care teaching program for postoperative head and neck patients. *Cancer Nursing, 4*, 103-106.

Dunphy, J., & Jackson, E. (1985). Planning nursing care for the postpartum mother and her newborn. In J. Riehl-Sisca (Ed.), *The science of art of self-care* (pp. 63-90). Norwalk, CT: Appleton-Century-Crofts.

Eben, J. D., Gashti, N. N., Nation, M. J., Marriner-Tomey, A., & Nordmeyer, S. B. (1989). Dorothea E. Orem: Self-care deficit theory of nursing. In A. Marriner-Tomey (Ed.), *Nursing theorists and their work* (2nd ed., pp. 118-132). St. Louis: C. V. Mosby.

Eichelberger, K., Kaufman, D., Rundahl, M., & Schwartz, N. (1980). Self-care nursing plan: Helping children to help themselves. *Pediatric Nursing, 6*(3), 9-13.

Eliopoulos, C. (1984). A self-care model for gerontological nursing. *Geriatric Nursing, 5,* 366-370.

Ewing, G. (1989). The nursing preparation of stoma patients for self-care. *Journal of Advanced Nursing, 14*(5), 411-420.

Facteau, L. M. (1980). Self-care concepts and the care of the hospitalized child. *Nursing Clinics of North America, 15*(1), 145-155.

Faucett, J., Ellis, V., Underwood, P., Naqvi, A., & Wilson, D. (1990). The effect of Orem's self-care model on nursing care in a nursing home setting. *Journal of Advanced Nursing, 15* 659-666.

Fawcett, J. (1989). *Analysis and evaluation of conceptual models in nursing* (2nd ed.). Philadelphia: F. A. Davis.

Fawcett, J., Cariello, F. P., Davis, D. A., Farley, J., Zimmaro, D., & Watts, R. J. (1987). Conceptual models for nursing: Application to critical care nursing practice. *Dimensions of Critical Care Nursing, 6,* 202-213.

Fenner, K. (1979). Developing a conceptual framework. *Nursing Outlook, 27,* 122-126.

Fitzgerald, S. (1980). Utilizing Orem's self-care nursing model in designing an educational program for the diabetic. *Topics in Clinical Nursing, 2*(2), 57-65.

Frey, M. A., & Denyes, M. J. (1989). Health and illness self-care in adolescents with IDDM: A test of Orem's theory. *Advances in Nursing Science, 12*(1), 67-75.

Galli, M. (1984, March/April). Promoting self-care in hypertensive clients through patient education. *Home Healthcare Nurse,* pp. 43-45.

Garrett, A. P. (1985). A nursing system design for a patient with myocardial infarction. In J. Riehl-Sisca (Ed.), *The science and art of self-care* (pp. 142-160). Norwalk, CT: Appleton-Century-Crofts.

Gast, H. L., Denyes, M. J., Campbell, J. C., Hartweg, D. L., Schott-Baer, D., & Isenberg, M. (1989). Self-care agency: Conceptualizations and operationalizations. *Advances in Nursing Science, 12*(1), 26-38.

Gordon, M. (1982). *Manual of nursing diagnosis.* New York: McGraw-Hill.

Gulick, E. E. (1986). The self-assessment of health among the chronically ill. *Topics in Clinical Nursing, 8*(1), 74-72.

Gulick, E. E. (1987). Parsimony and model confirmation of the ADL self-care scale for multiple sclerosis persons. *Nursing Research, 36,* 278-283.

Hammonds, T. A. (1985). Self-care practices of Navajo Indians. In J. Riehl-Sisca (Ed.), *The science and art of self-care* (pp. 171-180). Norwalk, CT: Appleton-Century-Crofts.

Hanchett, E. S. (1988). Community assessment and intervention according to Orem's theory of self-care deficit. In E. S. Hanchett (Ed.), *Nursing frameworks and community as client: Bridging the gap* (pp. 25-39). Norwalk, CT: Appleton & Lange.

Hanchett, E. S. (1990). Nursing models and community as client. *Nursing Science Quarterly, 3*(2), 67-72.

Hankes, D. D. (1984). Self-care: Assessing the aged client's need for independence. *Journal of Gerontological Nursing, 10*(5), 27-31.

Hanson, B. R., & Bickel, L. (1985). Development and testing of the questionnaire on perception of self-care agency. In J. Riehl-Sisca (Ed.), *The science and art of self-care* (pp. 271-278). Norwalk, CT: Appleton-Century-Crofts.

Harper, D. C. (1984). Application of Orem's theoretical constructs to self-care medication behaviors of the elderly. *Advances in Nursing Science, 6*(3), 29-46.

Harris, J. (1980). Self-care is possible after cesarean delivery. *Nursing Clinics of North America, 15*(1), 191-204.

Harry S Truman Veterans' Administration. (1986). *Ideal sets of action for persons with laryngectomy and angina.* Unpublished manuscript, Columbia, MO.

Hartley, L. A. (1988). Congruence between teaching and learning self-care: A pilot study. *Nursing Science Quarterly, 1*(4), 161-167.

Hartweg, D. L. (1990). Health promotion self-care within Orem's general theory of nursing. *Journal of Advanced Nursing, 15*, 35-41.

Hartweg, D. L., & Metcalfe, S. A. (1986). Self-care attitude changes of nursing students enrolled in a self-care curriculum—A longitudinal study. *Research in Nursing and Health, 9*, 347-353.

Hautman, M. A. (1987). Self-care responses to respiratory illnesses among Vietnamese. *Western Journal of Nursing Research, 9*, 223-243.

Hedahl, K. (1983). Assisting the adolescent with physical disabilities through a college health program. *Nursing Clinics of North America, 18*, 257-274.

Helene Fuld Health Trust. (1988). *The nurse theorists: Portraits of excellence. Dorothea Orem* [Videocassette]. Oakland, CA: Studio III.

Henderson, V. (1966). *The nature of nursing: A definition and its implications for practice, research, and education.* New York: Macmillan.

Herrington, J. V., & Houston, S. (1984). Using Orem's theory: A plan for all seasons. *Nursing and Health Care, 5*(1), 45-47.

Hewes, C. J., & Hannigan, E. P. (1985). Self-care model and the geriatric patient. In J. Riehl-Sisca (Ed.), *The science and art of self-care* (pp. 161-167). Norwalk, CT: Appleton-Century-Crofts.

Horn, B. J., & Swain, M. A. (1977). *Development of criterion measures of nursing care* (Vols. 1-2, National Technical Information Service Nos. PB-267 004 & PB 267 005). Ann Arbor: University of Michigan Press.

Jirovec, M., & Kasno, J. (1990). Self-care agency as a function of patient-environmental factors among nursing home residents. *Research in Nursing and Health, 13*, 303-309.

Joseph, L. S. (1980). Self-care and the nursing process. *Nursing Clinics of North America, 15*, 131-143.

Kearney, B. Y., & Fleischer, B. J. (1979). Development of an instrument to measure the exercise of self-care agency. *Research in Nursing and Health, 2*, 25-34.

Kinlein, M. L. (1977a). *Independent nursing practice with clients.* Philadelphia: J. B. Lippincott.

Kinlein, M. L. (1977b). The self-care concept. *American Journal of Nursing, 77,* 598-601.

Koster, M. K. (1983). Self-care: Health behavior for the school-age child. *Topics in Clinical Nursing, 5,* 29-40.

Kotarbinski, T. (1965). *Praxiology: An introduction to the sciences of efficient action* (O. Wojtasiewicz, Trans.). New York: Pergamon.

Kubricht, D. W. (1984). Therapeutic self-care demands expressed by outpatients receiving external radiation therapy. *Cancer Nursing, 7,* 43-52.

Lonergan, B. J. F. (1958). *Insight: A study of human understanding.* New York: Philosophical Library.

MacBride, S. (1987). Validation of an instrument to measure exercise of self-care agency. *Research in Nursing and Health, 10,* 311-316.

Macmurray, J. (1957). *The self as agent.* London: Faber & Faber.

McCracken, M. J. (1985). A self-care approach to pediatric chronic illness. In J. Riehl-Sisca (Ed.), *The science and art of self-care* (pp. 91-104). Norwalk, CT: Appleton-Century-Crofts.

Meleis, A. I. (1985). *Theoretical nursing: Development and progress.* Philadelphia: J. B. Lippincott.

Michael, M., & Sewall, K. (1980). Use of the adolescent peer group to increase the self-care agency of adolescent alcohol abusers. *Nursing Clinics of North America, 15*(1), 157-176.

Michos, S. (1985). The application of Orem's conceptual framework to enhance self-care in a dialysis program. *American Nephrology Nurses Association Journal, 12*(1), 21-24.

Miller, J. F. (1980). The dynamic focus of nursing: A challenge to nursing administration. *Journal of Nursing Administration, 10*(1), 13-18.

Moore, J. B., & Gaffney, K. F. (1989). Development of an instrument to measure mothers' performance of self-care activities for children. *Advances in Nursing Science, 12*(1), 76-84.

Moscovitz, A. (1984). Orem's theory as applied to psychiatric nursing. *Perspectives in Psychiatric Care, 22*(1), 36-38.

Mullin, V. (1980). Implementing the self-care concept in the acute care setting. *Nursing Clinics of North America, 15*(1), 177-190.

Murphy, P. (1981). A hospice model and self-care theory. *Oncology Nursing Forum, 8*(2), 19-21.

Neufield, A., & Hobbs, H. (1985). Self-care in a high-rise for seniors. *Nursing Outlook, 33*(6), 298-301.

Nickel-Gallager, L. (1985). Structuring nursing practice based on Orem's general theory. A practitioner's perspective. In J. Riehl-Sisca (Ed.), *The science and art of self-care* (pp. 236-244). Norwalk, CT: Appleton-Century-Crofts.

NLN News. (1987). Newark Beth Israel Medical Center adopts Orem's self-care model. *Nursing & Health Care, 8*(10), 593-594.

Nowakowski, L. (1980). Health promotion/self-care programs for the community. *Topics in Clinical Nursing, 2*(2), 21-27.

Nursing Development Conference Group. (1973). *Concept formalization in nursing: Process and product.* Boston: Little, Brown.

Nursing Development Conference Group. (1979). *Concept formalization in nursing: Process and product* (2nd ed., D. E. Orem, Ed.). Boston: Little, Brown.

Orem, D. E. (1956, October). *Hospital nursing service: An analysis.* Indianapolis: Division of Hospital and Institutional Services, Indiana State Board of Health.

Orem, D. E. (1959). *Guides to developing curricula for the education of practical nurses.* Washington, DC: Government Printing Office.

Orem, D. E. (1971). *Nursing: Concepts of practice.* New York: McGraw-Hill.

Orem, D. E. (1980). *Nursing: Concepts of practice* (2nd ed.). New York: McGraw-Hill.

Orem, D. E. (1983a). Analysis and application of Orem's theory. In I. W. Clements & F. B. Roberts (Eds.), *Family health: A theoretical approach to nursing care* (pp. 205-217). New York: John Wiley.

Orem, D. E. (1983b). The family coping with a medical illness. Analysis and application of Orem's self-care theory. In I. W. Clements & F. B. Roberts (Eds.), *Family health: A theoretical approach to nursing care* (pp. 385-386). New York: John Wiley.

Orem, D. E. (1983c). The family experiencing emotional crisis. Analysis and application of Orem's self-care deficit theory. In I. W. Clements & F. B. Roberts (Eds.), *Family health: A theoretical approach to nursing care* (pp. 367-368). New York: John Wiley.

Orem, D. E. (1984). Orem's conceptual model and community health nursing. In M. K. Asay & C. C. Ossler (Eds.), *Conceptual models of nursing: Applications in community health nursing. Proceedings of the Eighth Annual Community Health Nursing Conference* (pp. 35-50). Chapel Hill: University of North Carolina, Department of Public Health Nursing, School of Public Health.

Orem, D. E. (1985a). A concept of self-care for the rehabilitation client. *Rehabilitation Nursing, 10,* 33-36.

Orem, D. E. (1985b). *Nursing: Concepts of practice* (3rd ed.). New York: McGraw-Hill.

Orem, D. E. (1987). Orem's general theory of nursing. In R. Parse (Ed.), *Nursing science: Major paradigms, theories, and critiques* (pp. 67-89). Philadelphia: W. B. Saunders.

Orem, D. E. (1988a). The form of nursing science. *Nursing Science Quarterly, 1*(2), 75-79.

Orem, D. E. (1988b, November). *A perspective on theory based nursing.* Paper presented at the Seventh Annual Self-Care Deficit Theory of Nursing Conference, St. Louis.

Orem, D. E. (1990, September). Discussions on issues in Self-Care Deficit Theory. Remarks presented at a conference on *Self-Care Deficit Theory: Contemporary Issues,* Veterans Administration Medical Center, Palo Alto, CA.

Orem, D. E. (1991). *Nursing: Concepts of practice* (4th ed.). St. Louis: Mosby-Year Book, Inc.

Orem, D. E., & Taylor, S. G. (1986). Orem's general theory of nursing. In P. Winstead-Fry (Ed.), *Case studies in nursing theory* (Publication No. 15-2152, pp. 37-71). New York: National League for Nursing.

Parsons, T., Bales, R., & Shils, W. (1953). *Working papers in the theory of action.* Glencoe, IL: Free Press.

Patterson, E. T., & Hale, E. S. (1985). Making sure: Integrating menstrual care practices into activities of daily living. *Advances in Nursing Science, 7*(3), 18-31.

Perras, S., & Zappacosta, A. (1982). The application of Orem's theory in promoting self-care in a peritoneal dialysis facility. *American Association of Nephrology Nurses and Technicians Journal, 9*(3), 37-39.

Perry, P., & Sutcliffe, S. (1982). Conceptual frameworks for clinical practice. *Journal of Neurosurgical Nursing, 14*(6), 318-321.

Piemme, J., & Trainor, M. (1977). A first-year nursing course in a baccalaureate program, *Nursing Outlook, 25,* 184-187.

Pridham, K. F. (1971). Instruction of a school-age child with chronic illness for increased self-care, using diabetes mellitus as an example. *International Journal of Nursing Studies, 8,* 237-246.

Riesch, S. K., & Hauck, M. R. (1988). The exercise of self-care agency: An analysis of construct and discriminant validity. *Research in Nursing & Health, 11,* 245-255.

Rosenbaum, J. N. (1989). Self-caring: Concept development for nursing. *Recent Advances in Nursing, 24,* 18-31.

Saucier, C. (1984). Self-concept and self-care management in school-age children with diabetes. *Pediatric Nursing, 10*(2), 135-138.

Scarborough General Hospital Nursing Department. (1987). *Self-care deficit theory case study guide.* Scarborough, Ontario: Author.

Silva, M. C. (1986). Research testing nursing theory: State of the art. *Advances in Nursing Science, 9*(1), 1-11.

Smith, M. C. (1987). A critique of Orem's theory. In R. R. Parse (Ed.), *Nursing science: Major paradigms, theories, and critiques* (pp. 91-105). Philadelphia: W. B. Sanders.

Smith, M. C. (1989). An application of Orem's theory in nursing practice. *Nursing Science Quarterly, 2*(4), 159-161.

Steiger, N. J., & Lipson, J. G. (1985). *Self-care nursing. Theory & practice.* Bowie, MD: Brady Communications.

Stollenwerk, R. (1985). An emphysema client: Self-care. *Home Healthcare Nurse, 3*(2), 36-40.

Sullivan, T. (1980). Self-care model for nursing. In *Directions for nursing in the 80s* (Publication No. G-147, pp. 57-68). Kansas City, MO: American Nurses' Association.

Sullivan, T., & Munroe, D. (1986). A self-care practice theory of nursing the elderly. *Educational Gerontology, 12,* 13-26.

Swindale, J. E. (1989). The nurse's role in giving pre-operative information to reduce anxiety in patients admitted to hospital for elective minor surgery. *Journal of Advanced Nursing, 14,* 899-905.

Tadych, R. (1985). Nursing in multiperson units: The family. In J. Riehl-Sisca (Ed.), *The science and art of self-care* (pp. 49-55). Norwalk, CT: Appleton-Century-Crofts.

Taylor, S. G. (1980). *Self-Care Deficit Theory curriculum network directory.* Columbia: University of Missouri School of Nursing.

Taylor, S. G. (Ed.). (1988, November). *Nursing agency and nursing systems.* Paper presented at the Sixth Annual Self-Care Deficit Theory Conference, November 11-13, 1987, St. Louis. Columbia: Curators of the University of Missouri.

Taylor, S. G. (1988). Nursing theory and nursing process: Orem's theory in practice. *Nursing Science Quarterly, 1,* 111-119.

Taylor, S. G. (1989). An interpretation of family within Orem's general theory of nursing. *Nursing Science Quarterly, 2*(3), 131-136.

Taylor, S. G. (1990, September). *Self-care deficit theory and research.* Paper presented at conference *Self-Care Deficit Theory: Contemporary Issues,* Veterans Administration Medical Center, Palo Alto, CA.

Taylor, S. G., & Geden, E. (1991). Construct and empirical validity of the self-as-carer inventory. *Nursing Research, 40*(1), 47-50.

Titus, S., & Porter, P. (1989). Orem's theory applied to pediatric residential treatment. *Pediatric Nursing, 15*(5), 465-468, 470-471, 556.

Wagnild, G., Rodriguez, W., & Pritchett, G. (1987). Orem's self-care theory: A tool for education and practice. *Journal of Nursing Education, 26*(8), 342-343.

Walborn, K. (1980). A nursing model for the hospice: Primary and self-care nursing. *Nursing Clinics of North America, 15,* 205-217.

Walker, L., & Avant, K. (1988). *Strategies for theory construction in nursing* (2nd ed.). Norwalk, CT: Appleton & Lange.

Wallace, W. A. (1979). Basic concepts: Natural and scientific. In *From a realist point of view: Essays in the philosophy of science.* Washington, DC: University Press of America.

Wallace, W. A. (1983). Being scientific in a practice discipline. In *From a realist point of view: Essays in the philosophy of science* (2nd ed., pp. 273-293). Washington, DC: University Press of America.

Weaver, M. T. (1987). Perceived self-care agency: A LISREL factor analysis of Bickel and Hanson's questionnaire. *Nursing Research, 36,* 381-387.

Weis, A. (1988). Cooperative care and an application of Orem's self-care theory. *Patient Education Counselor, 11*(2), 141-146.

Whetstone, W. R. (1987). Perceptions of self-care in East Germany: A cross-cultural empirical investigation. *Journal of Advanced Nursing, 12,* 167-176.

Whetstone, W. R., & Hansson, A. O. (1989). Perceptions of self-care in Sweden: A cross-cultural replication. *Journal of Advanced Nursing, 14,* 962-969.

Williams, A. (1979). The student and the alcoholic patient. *Nursing Outlook, 17,* 470-472.

Williams, P., Valderrama, D., Gloria, M., Pascoguin, L., Saavedra, L., De La Rama, D., Ferry, T., Abaguin, C., & Zaldivar, S. (1988). Effects of preparation for mastectomy/hysterectomy on women's post-operative self-care behaviors. *International Journal of Nursing Studies, 25*(3), 191-206.

Woods, N. F. (1985). Self-care practices among young adult married women. *Research in Nursing and Health, 8,* 21-31.

Woolery, L. F. (1983). Self-care for the obstetrical patient: A nursing framework. *Journal of Gynecological Nursing, 12,* 33-37.

Bibliography

Classic works, articles, and chapters by Orem; critiques; comparisons with other models; and some media are presented below. Many examples of application are presented in the References. The author recognizes the significant contribution of doctoral dissertations and proceedings of conferences to theory development; they are not included due to page constraints.

Classic Works

Nursing Development Conference Group. (1973). *Concept formalization: Process and product* (D. E. Orem, Ed.). Boston: Little, Brown.

Nursing Development Conference Group. (1979). *Concept formalization: Process and product* (2nd ed., D. E. Orem, Ed.). Boston: Little, Brown.

Orem, D. E. (1956, October). *Hospital nursing service: An analysis.* Indianapolis: Indiana State Board of Health, Division of Hospital and Institutional Services.

Orem, D. E. (1959) *Guides to developing curricula for the education of practical nurses* (Vocational Division No. 274, Trade and Industrial Education No. 68). Washington, DC: Government Printing Office.

Orem, D. E. (1971). *Nursing: Concepts of practice.* New York: McGraw-Hill.

Orem, D. E. (1980). *Nursing: Concepts of practice* (2nd ed.). New York: McGraw-Hill.

Orem, D. E. (1985). *Nursing: Concepts of practice* (3rd ed.). New York: McGraw-Hill.

Orem, D. E. (1991). *Nursing: Concepts of practice* (4th ed.). St. Louis: C. V. Mosby.

Articles and Book Chapters by Orem

Orem, D. E. (1981). Nursing: a triad of action systems. In G. Lasker (Ed.), *Applied systems and cybernetics: Vol. 4. Systems research in health care, biocybernetics and ecology.* New York: Pergamon.

Orem, D. E. (1983a). The self-care deficit theory of nursing: A general theory. In I. W. Clements & F. B. Roberts (Eds.), *Family health: A theoretical approach to nursing care* (pp. 205-217). New York: John Wiley.

Orem, D. E. (1983b). The family coping with a medical illness. Analysis and application of Orem's self-care theory. In I. W. Clements & F. B. Roberts (Eds.), *Family health: A theoretical approach to nursing care* (pp. 385-386). New York: John Wiley.

Orem, D. E. (1983c). The family experiencing emotional crisis. Analysis and application of Orem's self-care deficit theory. In I. W. Clements & F. B. Roberts (Eds.), *Family health: A theoretical approach to nursing care* (pp. 367-368). New York: John Wiley.

Orem, D. E. (1984). Orem's conceptual model and community health nursing. In M. K. Asay & C. C. Ossler (Eds.), *Conceptual models of nursing. Applications in community health nursing. Proceedings of the Eighth Annual Community Health Nursing Conference* (pp. 35-50). Chapel Hill: University of North Carolina, Department of Public Health Nursing, School of Public Health.

Orem, D. E. (1985). A concept of self-care for the rehabilitation client. *Rehabilitation Nursing, 10*(3), 33-36.

Orem, D. E. (1987). Orem's general theory of nursing. In R. Parse (Ed.), *Nursing science: Major paradigms, theories, and critiques* (pp. 67-89). Philadelphia: W. B. Saunders.

Orem, D. E. (1988). The form of nursing science. *Nursing Science Quarterly, 1*(2), 75-79.

Orem, D. E. (1989). Theories and hypotheses for nursing administration. In B. Henry, C. Arndt, M. Di Vincenti, & A. Marriner-Tomey (Eds.), *Dimensions of nursing administration.* Boston: Blackwell Scientific.

Orem, D. E., & Taylor, S. G. (1986). Orem's general theory of nursing. In P. Winstead-Fry (Ed.), *Case studies in nursing theory* (Publication No. 15-2152, pp. 37-71). New York: National League for Nursing.

Analyses and Critiques of Self-Care Deficit Theory of Nursing

Dashiff, C. J. (1988). Theory development in psychiatric-mental health nursing: An analysis of Orem's theory. *Archives of Psychiatric Nursing, 11,* 366-372.

Davidhizar, R. (1989). Critique of Orem's self-care model. *Nursing Management, 19*(11), 78-79.

Eben, J. D., Gashti, N. N., Nation, M. J., Marriner-Tomey, A., & Nordmeyer, S. B. (1989). Dorothea E. Orem: Self-care deficit theory of nursing. In A. Marriner-Tomey (Ed.), *Nursing theorists and their work* (2nd ed., pp. 118-132), St. Louis: C. V. Mosby.

Fawcett, J. (1989). *Analysis and evaluation of conceptual models in nursing* (2nd ed.). Philadelphia: F. A. Davis.

Johnston, R. L. (1989). Orem's self-care model of nursing. In J. Fitzpatrick & A. Whall (Eds.), *Conceptual models of nursing: Analysis and application* (2nd ed., pp. 165-184). Norwalk, CT: Appleton & Lange.

Foster, P. C., & Janssens, N. P. (1985). Dorothea E. Orem. In Nursing Theories Conference Group, *Nursing theories: The base for professional nursing practice* (2nd ed., pp. 124-139). Englewood Cliffs, NJ: Prentice Hall.

Meleis, A. I. (1985). *Theoretical nursing: Development and progress.* Philadelphia: J. B. Lippincott.

Meleis, A. I. (1991). *Theoretical nursing: Development and progress* (2nd ed.). Philadelphia: J. B. Lippincott.

Melynk, K. A. M. (1983). The process of theory analysis: An examination of the nursing theory of Dorothea E. Orem. *Nursing Research, 32,* 170-174. [Letters to the editor and responses by the author, *Nursing Research, 32,* 318, 381-383.]

Lundh, U., Soder, M., & Waerness, K. (1988). Nursing theories: A critical view. *Image: Journal of Nursing Scholarship, 20*(1), 36-40.

Smith, M. C. (1979). Proposed metaparadigm for nursing research and theory development. An analysis of Orem's self-care theory. *Image: Journal of Nursing Scholarship, 11,* 75-79.

Smith, M. J. (1987). A critique of Orem's theory. In R. R. Parse (Ed.), *Nursing science: Major paradigms, theories, and critiques* (pp. 91-105). Philadelphia: W. B. Saunders.

Stevens, B. J. (1984). *Nursing theory: Analysis, application, and evaluation. (2nd ed.).* Boston: Little, Brown.

Thibodeau, J. A. (1983). *Nursing models: Analysis and evaluation.* Monterey, CA: Wadsworth Health Science Division.

Whelan, E. G. (1984). Analysis and application of Dorothea Orem's self-care practice model. *Journal of Nursing Education, 23*(8), 342-345.

Media and Software

Helene Fuld Health Trust. (1988). *The nurse theorists: Portraits of excellence. Dorothea Orem* [Videocassette]. Oakland, CA: Studio III.

National League for Nursing. (1987). *Nursing theory: A circle of knowledge.* New York: Author.

Orem, D. E. (1978, December). *A general theory of nursing* [Audiocassette recording]. Paper presented at the Second Annual Nurse Educator Conference, New York.

Self-care deficit theory of nursing: Software for bedside care [Computer program]. Bordentown, NJ: Nursing Systems International.

Comparisons With Self-Care Models and Nursing Models

Butterfield, S. (1983). In search of commonalities: An analysis of two theoretical frameworks. *International Journal of Nursing Studies, 20,* 15-22.

Gantz, S. B. (1990). Self-care: Perspectives from six disciplines. *Holistic Nursing Practice, 4*(2), 1-12.

Hanucharurnkul, S. (1989). Comparative analysis of Orem's and King's theories. *Journal of Advanced Nursing, 14,* 365-372.

Rosenbaum, J. (1986). Comparison of two theorists: Orem and Leininger. *Journal of Advanced Nursing, 11,* 409-419.

Steiger, N. J., & Lipson, J. G. (1985). *Self-care nursing. Theory & practice.* Bowie, MD: Brady Communications.

Woods, N. F. (1989). Conceptualizations of self-care: Toward health-oriented models. *Advances in Nursing Science, 12*(1), 1-13.

PART V

Rosemarie Parse
Theory of Human Becoming

SHEILA McGUIRE BUNTING

Biographical Sketch of the Nurse Theorist
Rosemarie Rizzo Parse, PhD, RN, FAAN

Position: Professor and Coordinator of the Center for
   Nursing Research, Hunter College, New York
President of Discovery International, Inc.
Editor: *Nursing Science Quarterly*
BSN: Duquesne University, Pittsburgh
MS: University of Pittsburgh
PhD: University of Pittsburgh
Fellow: American Academy of Nursing

SOURCE: (Lee & Schumacher, 1989)

Foreword

There are those nursing leaders among us who call on us to question our traditions and stretch our boundaries beyond what *is* to what *is possible* for nursing's contribution to the health of humankind. Rosemarie Parse is one such leader. In her theory of human becoming she presents a conceptualization of nursing as a professional discipline—a basic science—focusing on the study of the human health experience. This science assigns nursing practice the goal of enhancing the quality of life as defined by our clients. Our clients become the experts on their health and their lives. They are not passive recipients of our care but instead are involved creators of their health. From this perspective, health cannot be assessed or diagnosed by the nurse. Health is a way of living according to personal values that reflects the unique process of becoming. Nursing practice, according to Parse, is being in relationship, in true loving presence, with clients while they describe the meaning of their lifeworld, struggle with the paradoxes inherent in health experiences, and discover and fulfill hopes and dreams.

This section provides an overview of Parse's foundational beliefs and theoretical constructs. Sheila McGuire Bunting may be congratulated for her summary and provocative presentation that continually invite students to explore the primary sources of the cited theory texts, practice examples, and research for deeper understandings. This work may be used as a springboard for study of the theory of human becoming. It introduces beginning students to the philosophical underpinnings, the assumptions about the nature of persons and health, the specific conceptual and propositional formulations of the theory, and the applications in practice and research. Also, Parse's particular practice and research methodologies are briefly described. Through her examples, Bunting seeks to lead students beyond the language and structure of the theory toward a grasp of its profound message and the uniqueness of the nursing practice that it generates.

Theories are not static entities "cast in stone," or in this case, "cast in print," in their original versions. Theories are dynamic; they change and grow as they are nurtured by the scholars who work with them in practice and in research. Since the first publication of *Man-Living-Health: A Theory of Nursing* in 1981, Parse has continued to modify and further develop the theory of human becoming. The theory has been adopted as a framework for practice by nurses throughout the world. Several evaluation studies have documented differences in client perceptions of quality of life, nurses' perceptions of their practice, and administrators' perceptions of morale and the quality of nursing practice following a 6- to 9-month implementation of Parse's theory in practice. The theory has been used as the philosophical and theoretical perspective of many master's theses and doctoral dissertations. Published research continues to contribute to the growth of the theory.

This section is a "snapshot" of Parse's theory. It is a glimpse into a distinctive world of nursing framed with respect for the mystery of health and the wonder of human becoming.

MARLAINE C. SMITH, RN, PHD
University of Colorado
School of Nursing

Acknowledgments

I would like to thank Dr. Marlaine Smith for her support and encouragement and for her patience and care in the reading and rereading of this manuscript. Dr. Louette Lutjens and editor Dr. Adele Webb, old friends and classmates, served as guides, offering long-distance counseling and advice at odd hours. I am grateful to Dr. Rosemarie Rizzo Parse for her past mentorship, for the assistance she has extended to me in my pursuit of this project, and, most particularly, for her theory, so grandly conceptualized and beautifully written, and for its potential to empower clients and enrich nursing.

23

Origins of the Theory

Historical Evolution of the Theory

Parse has pointed out that the discipline of nursing has traditionally been grounded in the natural sciences such as chemistry, physics, and physiology and that it has been guided by the medical model in its practice. She proposed the theory of human becoming (formerly called Man-Living-Health) as an alternative framework. This theory synthesized concepts from Rogers's conceptual system and major ideas from the existential-phenomenological philosophies of Heidegger, Sartre, Merleau-Ponty, and Marcel (Parse, 1981, p. 5).

Heidegger was a German philosopher who died in 1976. He was interested in analyzing the complexity of human existence, which he termed *Dasein*, meaning "being there" (Heidegger, 1962). The term *Dasein* signifies both the mystery and the randomness or chance associated with being in the world in a given time and place. Despite this view of the arbitrary nature of human existence, Heidegger focused on the freedom he believed each person possessed. This freedom included the choice to live authentically and to recognize the limits of one's human nature and confront the fact of one's nonbeing. This acceptance of one's finite existence and one's own death makes possible a life of conscience, care, and responsibility. Living authentically is discovering oneself in direct relation to the existing world. To live authentically, one must make the choice to do so, to reject the world of tasks, rules, and the urgency of external standards. "In choosing to make this choice, Dasein *makes possible* . . . its authentic potentiality-for-Being" (Heidegger, 1962, p. 313). An important part of existential-phenomenological philosophy is the view of time. The authentic present involves the dynamic interplay of the past and future; it is related to a past that one is reliving in the present and to a future anticipated as a present reality. The concepts of freedom, authenticity, and this multidimensional quality of time are important in Parse's theory. Other writers whose works presented the existential-phenomenological movement to the public included Jean-Paul Sartre (1956) and Maurice Merleau-Ponty (1962).

Parse believed that the medical model view of the person was that of a mechanistic being and that medicine traditionally treated the person in a fragmented manner. The particulate or *sum of parts* view is a logical extension of the view of the person as a collection of separate parts, called *Cartesian psychophysical dualism* (Lavine, 1984) after René Descartes. Descartes was a philosopher who believed in two separate kinds of reality. One was a physical substance that had no consciousness and took up space, and the other was a thinking, spiritual substance that, by definition, had no physical extension. In this view, the mind and spirit can be separated from the body.

The offering of an alternative to this *sum of parts* view of the person that had been maintained by many areas of medicine and nursing required a major change of perspective. Such a shift occurred when the work of Martha Rogers provided a unitary perspective of the human being and a new way to see the role of nursing (Rogers, 1970). Parse's theory is partially derived from this nursing framework.

Parse's ideas were influenced by her own nursing experiences involving teaching and persuading patients to do things that medical experts deemed "good for them." She concluded that the patients had their own reality and behaved accordingly (Parse, 1985a). The early premises of her theory appeared in her first book, *Nursing Fundamentals* (Parse, 1974). These premises included statements related to the focus and methods that should be the concern of nurses, the nature of the human being, and the important construct of the mutual, interactive manner in which the human and the environment evolve together (Parse, 1974; Smith & Hudepohl, 1988). During the early development of her theory in the 1970s, Parse was a member of the faculty at Duquesne University where there was an internationally recognized center in existential phenomenology. The study of and interactions with these philosophers formed a basis for the synthesis of the elements of these concepts within the assumptions of her theory (R. Parse, personal communication, April 1987; Smith & Hudepohl, 1988). The purpose of Parse's theory was to create a paradigm (or model guideline) of nursing rooted in the human sciences. She saw the human sciences as being directed toward uncovering the meaning of events in the lives of persons as these events were experienced by the persons themselves—the study of the human being's participative experience in a situation. In creating this theory, she synthesized Rogers's principles of helicy, complementarity (now called integrality), and resonancy and the building blocks of energy field, openness, pattern and organization, and four-dimensionality with the tenets and concepts of existential phenomenology (Parse, 1981, p. 13).

Martha Rogers's principle of integrality describes human beings and their environments as integrated and interacting energy fields that are continuously and mutually changing. These human and environmental fields are identified, according to Rogers's theory, by patterns and organizations of wave frequencies that are continuously changing "from lower-frequency, longer wave patterns to higher-frequency, shorter wave patterns" (Rogers, 1980, p. 333). Rogers termed this concept of changing waves and patterns *resonancy*. The direction of that change—Rogers's principle of *helicy*—is always new and always moving toward greater complexity, never going backwards or repeating its pattern. Rogers was very clear in specifying the open nature of the human and environmental fields: "Man and environment are continually exchanging matter and energy with one another" (Rogers, 1970, p. 54).

Parse's theory, then, has its base in Rogers's Science of Unitary Human Beings. Rogers's conceptual system, in turn, is rooted in humanistic and natural scientific thought. The basic statements of Parse's theory were written at a philosophical level from a combination of existential-phenomenological ideas (the tenets of subjectivity and intentionality and the concepts of coconstitution, coexistence, and situated freedom) synthesized with Rogers's principles and building blocks (Parse, 1987, p. 161).

The tenet of human *subjectivity* refers to the person as a conscious being who is capable of encountering the world, relating to it, and growing from the relationship. The human can and does give meaning to all of the things that occur between him or herself and the world, thereby taking an active part in creating and constituting the reality of both the self and the world. The tenet of *intentionality* means that the person is knowingly open to the world. To be human is to be intentionally involved with and present to the world (Parse, 1981). *Situated freedom* refers to the belief that one chooses the situations in which one finds oneself as well as one's attitude and response to the situations. The way in which a particular situation comes about and develops is related to the previous choices of that individual. The tenet of free choice for human beings has been synthesized by Parse from the work of Sartre (1956) and is an important element of her theory. *Coexistence* means that life as a person knows it is an experience of being with others. One is brought into the world by other beings and one's perceptions of self and the environment are formed with the input of others: "Without others one would not know that one is" or who one is (Parse, 1981, p. 20). *Coconstitution* signifies that the reality of any situation is related to all of the elements that make up that situation and the meaning assigned by the person. To say that humans coconstitute situations is to say that their perceptions together with the other elements of the situation create the reality. By being present in a situation and being in relationship to the multiple views of the world and others in the world, the individual influences these views and takes part in the *cocreation* of the situation and of the world.

The evolution of Parse's theory, synthesized from the elements of Rogers's framework and those of existential phenomenology, is illustrated in Figure 23.1.

Important differences between Rogers's and Parse's conceptualizations are the differing views of the human being and of health. Parse viewed the person as an open being who cocreates personal health rather than viewing the person as an energy field. She viewed health as a "process of becoming as experienced and described by the person" whereas Rogers viewed health as a value (Parse, 1992, p. 36). The human capacity to participate and shape the environment, to freely choose meaning in a situation, to take responsibility for choices and decisions, to mutually shape patterns of relating and existing, and to transcend beyond the present reality is central to Parse's theory and to her conceptualization of the person.

Parse continues to develop her theory through her own research and by working closely with other nursing scholars. This includes the mentoring of students, many of whom have used her theory to guide

Rogers		Existential Phenomenology	
Principles	Concepts	Concepts	Tenets
Helicy Complimentarity Resonancy	Energy Field Openness Pattern and Organization	Coconstitution Coexistence Situated Freedom	Intentionality Human Subjectivity

Assumptions

Human	Becoming
1. The human is coexisting while coconstituting rhythmical patterns with the universe.	5. Becoming is an open process experienced by the human.
2. The human is an open being, freely choosing meaning in situation, bearing responsibility for decisions.	6. Becoming is a rhythmically coconstituting process of human-universe interrelationship.
3. The human is a living unity continuously coconstituting patterns of relating.	7. Becoming is the human's pattern of relating value priorities.
4. The human is transcending multidimensionally with the possibles.	8. Becoming is an intersubjective process of transcending with the possibles.
	9. Becoming is human unfolding.

Principles

1. Structuring meaning multidimensionally is cocreating reality through the languaging of valuing and imaging.	2. Cocreating rhythmical patterns of relating is living the paradoxical unity of revealing-concealing and enabling-limiting while connecting-separating.	3. Cotranscending with the possibles is powering unique ways of originating in the process of transforming.

Figure 23.1. Evolution of the Theory of Human Becoming.
SOURCE: Adapted from Parse (1992).

their theses and doctoral dissertations (see listings in the bibliography). The primary texts of her work are *Man-Living-Health: A Theory of Nursing* (Parse, 1981) and the chapter titled "Man-Living-Health

Theory of Nursing" in her edited book, *Nursing Science: Major Paradigms, Theories and Critiques* (Parse, 1987). An excellent precis and update on the language of her theory appeared in a recent article in *Nursing Science Quarterly* (Parse, 1992).

24

Assumptions

Described in Parse's 1981 book and presented with updated language in 1992, the central conceptual units from Rogers's framework along with those from existential phenomenology are synthesized into nine assumptions (Parse, 1992, p. 38; see Figure 23.1). These assumptions state beliefs about human beings and health: Five address human beings, and four address health as human becoming.

Assumptions of a theory are statements that are accepted or assumed to be true without requiring proof. They are statements of foundational beliefs on which the theory is built. In selecting a theory to guide practice or research, an individual must first be sure that the assumptions of the theory are in agreement with his or her worldview. For instance, if one believes in absolute cause and effect, Parse's assumptions would not fit with one's worldview. Parse's theory is based on a belief that events and people mutually shape and influence one another. The idea of health as the person adapting to or coping with the environment is inconsistent with Parse's theory (Parse, 1987). In the theory of human becoming, the view that a person has a part in creating his or her own reality affects both the accepted assumptions and the basic principles of the theory. Parse stated that the most significant distinction of her theory from that of other nursing theorists is the belief that the human being, who is more than and different from the sum of the parts, "evolves mutually with the environment, participates in cocreating personal health by choosing meanings in situations, and conveys meanings that are personal values reflecting dreams and hopes" (Parse, 1987, p. 162).

In discussing the language used in her theory, originally called Man-Living-Health, Parse stated that the word *man* referred to *Homo sapiens*, or the human being in general, rather than to males only. She frequently uses participles and gerunds (verbs ending in "ing") to call attention to the fact that her theory deals with things that are in process (Parse, 1987); that is, they are happening as one thinks about them.

Assumption 1. "The human is coexisting while coconstituting rhythmical patterns with the universe" (Parse, 1992, p. 38). The meaning of the first assumption is that the individual exists with other persons, evolving as the universe is evolving. The patterns formed by the person exchanging energy with the universe are unique to that person. These particular patterns of relating distinguish an individual from the environmental pattern and from the patterns of all other persons in the universe. The person, then, "is a pattern of patterns of relating . . . the individual's unique way of being recognized" (Parse, 1981, p. 26). Important in Parse's theory is the active part taken by individuals in creating their own patterns and their own reality.

Assumption 2. "The human is an open being, freely choosing meaning in situation, bearing responsibility for decisions" (Parse, 1992, p. 38). This statement signifies that the human being *chooses* ways of being in a situation and is accountable for those choices. By choosing some meanings of the situations of his or her life and not choosing others, the individual opens many possibilities and closes others. These losses and gains, the "birthings and dyings . . . are the rhythmical happenings in day-to-day living" (Parse, 1981, p. 27). The events of a person's life and the meanings of those events are created as the individual, through the choices made, creates the possibilities that he or she can become. Even when people do not know the outcomes of the choices they make, they are responsible for those outcomes. Persons and the universe exchange energy to make the world. The individual chooses the meaning given to the situations he or she cocreates.

Assumption 3. "The human is a living unity continuously coconstituting patterns of relating" (Parse, 1992, p. 38). The idea of the human as a living unity means that he or she is more than and different from the sum of the parts, that is, the physiological, psychological, spiritual, sociological, and other classifications that are often assigned to dimensions of the person. Coconstitution is the individual's "active participation in creating meaning with others in the world" (Parse, 1981, p. 177). This meaning is created in the interactions that occur between individuals and their world. These coconstituted patterns of relating are the unitary person's ways of being. The patterns are expressed and identified "through gesture, movement, gaze, posture, touch, and speech" (Parse, 1981, p. 28). One can distinguish a person from all others in the universe by the patterns of appearance, mannerisms, voice, and other characteristics that make the person individual.

Assumption 4. "The human is transcending multidimensionally with the possibles" (Parse, 1992, p. 38). *Transcending* means "going beyond, exceeding" (Parse, 1981, p. 179). *Multidimensionality* "refers to human existence as beyond the temporo-spatial limits of a three-dimensional universe" (M. Smith, personal communication, October 1991). There are many levels of the universe experienced by a person simultaneously. Specifically, Parse (1987) refers to this concept as "explicit-tacit knowing" (p. 162). She pointed out that not all choices are made from the explicit level and that humans construct their meanings from a "whole sense of the situation" (Parse, 1987, p. 162). Cognitive logic and thought along with the intuitive "hunch" are experienced by the person as a unified impression all at once. The human being is capable of moving beyond the present reality, of growing and becoming something more and different from what the present limits may indicate. The choices to grow to new possible dimensions are decided from many types of knowledge, including a logical deductive reflection and a "prereflective" grasp of the situation.

Assumption 5. "Becoming is an open process, experienced by the human" (Parse, 1992, p. 38). The process of becoming is the human being's continuous growing through exchange of energy with the universe, and this process of becoming is health in Parse's theory. This process of health involves continuous change. The direction of change evolves toward more diversity and more complexity. As persons grow and develop they become more different from one another, more complicated, and more intricate. Part of the process of growing is choosing who one will be in a given situation (Parse, 1981). These choices are unique and personal, and they determine reality for a person: "An experience of a situation, while cocreated with others, belongs to one human being only" (Parse, 1981, p. 30). The person creates health by the choices made. Choosing some options automatically eliminates other options, so the person co-creates and experiences possibilities within a different perspective as he or she participates in the process of becoming, living health (Parse, 1981). Each time one makes a choice there are many things that are not chosen, some that one knows about and many that one does not or cannot know. Health, then, is cocreated by a person's choices.

Assumption 6. "Becoming is a rhythmically coconstituting process of the human-universe interrelationship" (Parse, 1992, p. 38). This assumption means that health, the process of becoming, is a continuous energy interchange created both by the human and the universe (cocreated) as they interrelate (Parse, 1981, pp. 30-31). Change occurs in this becoming and change involves an ongoing process of connecting with some things while separating from others. The human's health "is the rhythmic process of changing through the simultaneous connecting and separating" (Parse, 1987, p. 31) of the person with the environment. The people, beliefs, events, and other elements of the environment, which we connect with and separate from, change us and are changed by us in an ongoing rhythm. With all of these elements we coconstitute our health.

Assumption 7. "Becoming is the human's pattern of relating value priorities" (Parse, 1992, p. 38). This assumption means that health (human becoming) is the individual's way of living the particular ideals chosen and cherished by that person. Health is a synthesis of the values of an individual (Parse, 1987, p. 31). The choices the individual makes are an expression of cherished values and ways of relating and being. "These ways of being emerge in recognizable patterns" (Parse, 1981, p. 32). The way of being brings out emerging patterns that indicate the priorities and increasing complexity of each human being. These emerging patterns make up the individual's health.

Assumption 8. "Becoming is an intersubjective process of transcending with the possibles" (Parse, 1992, p. 38). This assumption, a statement about health as human becoming, "means that health is reaching beyond the actual to the possible through subject-to-subject energy interchange" (Parse, 1981, p. 32). Although *intersubjective* means between two separate conscious minds, in this assumption this interchange can and does occur between humans and other elements in the universe as well as between human beings. The genuine relating to another person is a risk, and it reflects individuals choosing ways of becoming more complex and more diverse. It means giving up the familiar to "struggle with the unfamiliar toward an imaged not-yet" (Parse, 1981, p. 32) as individuals reveal and conceal who they are and who they can become.

Assumption 9. "Becoming is human unfolding" (Parse, 1992, p. 38). This assumption means that health is the process of the human being "synergistically becoming more complex and more diverse in coexistence with others" (Parse, 1981, p. 33). Human becoming as an unfolding involves open systems exchanging energy and changing continuously, never going backwards or returning to a previous state. This idea of health proposes that health is "a nonspecific entity, continuously transforming" (Parse, 1981, p. 33) as the human being grows older. An important element in Parse's definition of health is that it is an ongoing process of the individual being with others. All humans and other elements of the universe are unfolding toward greater complexity.

Parse, in her 1987 book, further synthesized her nine assumptions into three assumptions:

1. Human becoming "is freely choosing personal meaning in situations in the intersubjective process of relating value priorities" (p. 161). In explaining this assumption, Parse stated that the human being, "through subject-to-subject-interchange in situation assigns meaning which reflects personal values" (p. 161). Because more than one meaning can always be given to any event or action, the

meaning that one chooses to give is determined by the individual's values and previous experiences. The person does not, however, assign these meanings in isolation. Meanings are always affected by communication with others in a person's life; that is, the meanings are created intersubjectively. An example of different meanings given to an event might be those assigned by persons taking a morning walk. To person A it is a chore she is forcing herself to do, to person B it is a gift of time for herself to be alone before she starts the day, and to person C it is the means of getting to a meeting with her lover. Because Parse's definition of health is that of a process, a personal choosing of meaning that cocreates reality with the universe, each of these persons can be seen as expressing cherished values and ways of relating and being. These emerging patterns make up the individual's health.

2. Human becoming "is cocreating rhythmical patterns of relating in open interchange with the environment" (p. 162). This means the person-universe interrelationship is reflected in the patterns created together. One can distinguish and recognize the human and the environment by their patterns. Parse stated that the human together with universe create the pattern of each. The human is distinguishable as human and environment as environment, "yet each is a coparticipant in the creation of the other" (p. 162). An example of this concept is a woman who lives in an intermediate care residence for the elderly. As she interrelates in her new setting, both she and the community of residents and attendants are mutually changing. Together they evolve patterns of being alone and together.

3. Human becoming "is cotranscending multidimensionally with the unfolding possibles" (p. 162). This means that human becoming is "moving beyond self at all levels of the universe as dreams become actualities" (p. 162). Cotranscending means "going beyond the actual in interrelationship with others" (p. 166). Multidimensionally refers to the various levels of the universe that are experienced simultaneously (p. 162). Or, it is all the ways that a person can "know" as a unified impression. An example might be a family working with a child with special health needs. As the family members work with the child and with one another, each moves beyond the self and the present reality to the possibles that unfold. This movement beyond is not a linear development but occurs on many levels at once (multidimensionally). The family's health is the movement toward and the expression of these possibles as they are chosen and lived.

25

Concepts, Principles,
and Theoretical Structures

According to Parse, the major themes emerging from the philosophical assumptions are meaning, rhythmicity, and cotranscendence (moving beyond with another). Each theme leads to the development of a principle of human becoming. The understanding of concepts unique to Parse's work is essential to comprehension of her theory.

Major Concepts

The principles of Parse's theory of human becoming contain nine major concepts, three from each of the principles. They are imaging, valuing, languaging, revealing-concealing, enabling-limiting, connecting-separating, powering, originating, and transforming. These are all processes in which individuals actively engage.

"What is real for each individual is structured by that individual" (Parse, 1992, p. 37). *Imaging* refers to knowing in the many ways a person can know something. It is the creating of perceptions (internal pictures, feelings, sounds) of events, ideas, and people—making them real. This creation of reality includes one's images of the past and the future as well as constructions of the present. In *languaging*, one communicates perceptions, beliefs, and priorities through verbal and nonverbal means—"Sharing valued images through symbols of words, gesture, gaze, touch, and posture" (Parse, 1981, p. 177). *Valuing* is "the process of living cherished beliefs while assimilating the new into a personal worldview. It emerges in the human-universe process and is the human being's confirming of cherished beliefs" (Parse, 1992, p. 37). By the life that one lives and the choices one makes, one expresses and testifies to one's beliefs and values.

Parse's paradoxical concepts concern the merging of seeming opposites in which the dialectical processes are occurring simultaneously. These processes can be thought of as background/foreground concepts. That is, one cannot think of one without implicitly summoning up the idea of the other, as the idea of noise is present in silence and the idea of white in thinking of the color black. *Connecting-separating,* according to Parse (1987), "is the rhythmical process of distancing and relating, that is, moving in one direction and away from others, yet always toward greater diversity" (p. 164). Each choice made brings a person closer to certain elements of the universe and farther from others. One meets different people and lives different experiences each year (or day) of one's life. This year is lived differently than last year, but the past experiences are now part of the living person, and he or she therefore has become more diverse and will continue to become more diverse. Connecting with some events and people and separating from others creates a rhythmic pattern because all connections and separations are related.

Connecting-separating with people and projects is *enabling-limiting* (Parse, 1987, p. 164) because each connection or separation choice contains a number of possibilities and also many limitations. Each road taken represents many roads one was unable to take. Each change that one makes in life enables one to envision new possibilities and limits one in the pursuit of other possibilities. As one relates to others, one is always *revealing-concealing* the personal self. One can never completely reveal the whole of the self to another, so the concealing is always there as a part of the revealing process. By choosing to reveal, one selects at the same time what one will conceal.

Parse's concept of *powering* is the energizing force behind creativity, the drive that provides the fuel to allow change and creativity to happen: "Powering is the pushing-resisting of interhuman encounters" (Parse, 1987, p. 165). *Originating* is creating and generating new and different ways of being in the world. Persons are originating when they initiate new patterns of interrelationships with their universes. Parse (1987) defines *transforming* as "the changing of change" (p. 165). Change itself is a continuous process of the human-universe interrelationship. It can be recognized by its ever increasing variety. The transcending, or moving beyond, which occurs through transforming, takes place through struggling. Transforming, or changing, "unfolds as the familiar is seen in a different light, thus shifting the view and illuminating new possibles" (Parse, 1987, p. 165).

Principles

Principle 1. "Structuring meaning multidimensionally is cocreating reality through the languaging of valuing and imaging" (Parse, 1987, p. 163). Principle 1 connects and relates Parse's concepts of imaging, valuing, and languaging. Structuring meaning multidimensionally signifies that individuals construct their meaning of situations from many levels of the universe, from an "explicit-tacit knowing" (Parse, 1987, p. 162). Not all choices are made from the explicit level; humans construct their meanings from a "whole sense of the situation" (Parse, 1987, p. 162; see Assumption 4). Individuals, by the choices they make between meanings, are active in cocreating (with their universe and the people around them) their personal reality. "Health is an expression of values at the moment, the meaning given to a situation" (Parse, 1987, p. 163).

Illustration: A young man who was recently diagnosed with AIDS feels devastated and helpless. He is confronting, on many levels, the meanings he has created from all that he knows from others' comments, what he has read, and from his own sense of the situation (structuring meaning multidimensionally). While talking to the nurse about his past life, his present, and his hopes for the future (languaging), he begins to see different meanings (cocreated reality). He is able to envision the past and present of his life and the different meanings he has constructed (imaging), realizing that he has been able and is presently able to live his cherished beliefs (valuing).

Principle 2. "Cocreating rhythmical patterns of relating is living the paradoxical unity of revealing-concealing, enabling-limiting, while connecting-separating" (Parse, 1987, p. 164). The human and the universe, including the people in one's life, cocreate a rhythmical interchange. As each person grows and changes, she or he forms bonds with some aspects of the universe, including people, places, and activities, and simultaneously breaks bonds with others. Other persons and elements in the universe are moving toward and away from one another as well, revealing aspects of themselves while concealing other aspects in an ongoing rhythmical pattern of interrelationships. Each pattern of the kaleidoscope is different, more complex, containing elements of all of the previous patterns.

Illustration: In order to be close by for her mother, whose dementia was becoming a safety factor, a woman made the decision to leave her valued and stimulating position in an office to do her work on consignment out of her home. She was conscious of separating from her former valued associates while connecting with new contacts and connecting in a new way with personal friends and family, particularly her daughters, who offered to help care for their grandmother. Her new work situation was enabling in that her time schedule was more open, but it was more limiting in its constrictions on her movements outside her home. She found herself relating differently to persons who had always known her as a person who worked outside the home. In her rhythmical interchanges with the persons who questioned her about her situation, she was aware of revealing some of the new meanings she had created while concealing others.

Principle 3. "Cotranscending with the possibles is powering unique ways of originating in the process of transforming" (Parse, 1987, p. 165). Parse's concepts of powering (energizing), originating (creating anew), and transforming (changing change) are related in this principle. Cotranscending is "going beyond the actual in interrelationship with others" (Parse, 1987, p. 166). The presence of others may help persons to move beyond the perceived limits of the present, though the person must do the moving herself or himself. This is an important concept because nurses can help clients move beyond. The actual impetus, or energy, for the moving beyond is termed *powering* by Parse. Moving beyond the present reality with other persons is energizing the creation of new realities in the process of making changes.

Illustration: A couple in a relationship involving spouse abuse expressed the desire to change their abusive pattern and to move beyond it together. The husband, a trainee in a very demanding executive development program for his new job, tended to cease interacting with his wife when he was panicked about his work. The wife valued intimacy and had a pattern of open communication of feelings. Faced with an unresponsive husband, her own anxiety led her to push him to talk about his feelings and resist his request to be left alone. He abused her verbally and struck her in the face.

Both parties valued the relationship and wanted to develop new ways of living together. They began to question the meanings of the connections and familiar patterns of their relating. As they talked about these meanings, they found themselves struggling with their past images and their expectations of one another in the present and future. The meanings began to transform, moving beyond the familiar to a new image of how they could be together.

Theoretical Structures

Parse's definition of a theoretical structure is "a statement interrelating concepts in a way that can be verified" (Parse, 1981, p. 68). Theoretical structures are "nondirectional propositions," that are "noncausal in nature and consistent with the assumptions and principles [of Parse's theory]" (Parse, 1987, p. 166). They are designed to guide practice and research. To make these operational in practice and research, "statements about nursing practice must be derived and lived experiences chosen for study" (Parse, 1987, p. 166). Parse suggested that it is appropriate to use one concept from each principle to derive a theoretical structure. The relationships between concepts, principles, and the three theoretical structures that have been derived and published are illustrated in Figure 25.1.

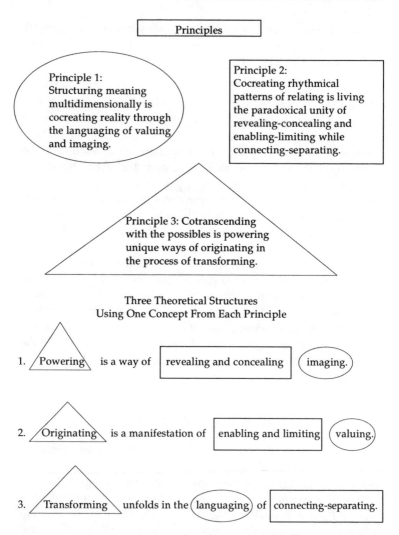

Figure 25.1. Derivation of theoretical structures from principles and concepts of the Theory of Human Becoming.

26

Major Nursing Concepts

The Simultaneity Paradigm

Four major concepts of concern to nursing are (a) the persons or groups who benefit from nursing services, (b) their environment, (c) their health, and (d) nursing. To describe the ways in which these concepts are viewed in Rogers's and Parse's nursing theories, Parse created the term *simultaneity paradigm,* which indicates different ways of looking at the human being, health, and the goals of nursing (Parse, 1987, pp. 136-137). The word *paradigm* indicates a way of thinking about concepts and their relationships, "a way of viewing a particular field of study" (Parse, 1981, p. 178). The condition of *simultaneity* is, according to the dictionary, the happening of two or more events at the same time. The term emphasizes that the concepts in Parse's theory are ever in process, always becoming. The naming of the simultaneity paradigm came from the consideration of the human being within this paradigm as "a synergistic being in open, mutual, simultaneous interchange with the environment" (Parse, 1985b, p. 1).

The person, as viewed in the simultaneity paradigm, is thought of as different from and more than the sum of parts. He or she is able to take part knowingly in the process of change, interacting continuously with the universe in a mutual, integral exchange of matter and energy. Health is seen as a process experienced by the person and unique to that person, not as a condition, a state, or an outcome. The goal of nursing in the simultaneity paradigm is service to persons (Rogers, 1987), focusing on the quality of life as the individual perceives it, regardless of society's designation of illness (Parse, 1987, pp. 136-137).

Human Becoming

Parse's man-living-health nursing theory has been renamed the *human becoming theory*. No changes have been made in the theory itself. The change in name reflects the change in the dictionary definition of *man*, which is now the male human (Parse, 1992). In 1980, when *Man-Living-Health: A Theory of Nursing* was being written, *man* was defined as the generic human. The putting together of *man, living*, and *health* into a hyphenated whole "creates a unity of meaning different from the individual words as they stand alone" (Parse, 1981, p. 39). The combined words make it clear that human health is the ongoing process of participation with the world. Man-Living-Health is a unitary phenomenon that refers to the person's becoming through cocreating rhythmical patterns of relating as energy is exchanged with the environment. Health, then, is a process of the human being relating to his or her universe, and it is created by the person and the universe together. Health in this theory is not thought of separately from the person and the environment:

> Health is Man's unfolding. It is Man's lived experiences, a nonlinear entity that cannot be qualified by terms such as good, bad, more, or less. It is not Man adapting or coping. Unitary Man's health is a synthesis of values, a way of living. It is not the opposite of disease or a state that man has, but rather is a continuously changing process that Man cocreates. (Parse, 1987, p. 160)

Nursing

Nursing as a process would not be included within the theoretical metaparadigm concepts in Parse's theory. *Nursing* is defined in Parse's theory as "a discipline focusing on the study of the health of persons in interrelationship with their environment" (M. Smith, per-

Dimensions	Processes
1. Illuminating meaning is shedding light through uncovering the what was, is, and will be, as it is appearing now. It happens in explicating what is.	1. Explicating is making clear what is appearing now through languaging.
2. Synchronizing rhythms happens in dwelling with the pitch, yaw, and roll of the interhuman cadence.	2. Dwelling with is giving self over to the flow of the struggle in connecting-separating.
3. Mobilizing transcendence happens in moving beyond the meaning moment to what is not yet.	3. Moving beyond is propelling toward the possibles in transforming.

Figure 26.1. The Theory of Human Becoming practice methodology.
SOURCE: Adapted from Parse (1992).

sonal communication, October 1991). Nursing practice was described by Parse as involving both science and art: "It is the utilization of nursing's abstract body of knowledge in the service to people" (Parse, 1981, p. 81). The reponsibility of nursing to society is to guide the choosing of possibilities in the changing health process. This guiding occurs through an intersubjective participation with persons and their families. The goal of nursing is to enhance the quality of life as perceived by the person and the family (Parse, 1987, p. 167).

Parse rejected the nursing process as not evolving from the science of nursing (Parse, 1987, p. 166). Dimensions of practice are illuminating meaning, synchronizing rhythms, and mobilizing transcendence. The processes Parse advocated for nursing practice are (a) explicating, defined as making clear what is appearing now through languaging; (b) dwelling with, which is giving self over to the flow of the struggle in connecting-separating; and (c) moving beyond, which is propelling toward the possibles in transforming (Parse, 1987, p. 169). The dimensions and processes of nurses practicing within the theory of human becoming are listed in Figure 26.1.

Parse stated that the person is an open being who freely chooses "meaning in situation and bears responsibility for the choices" (Parse, 1981, p. 39). Parse was very clear that the values of the individual must predominate and that the nurse serves in a supportive role rather than serving as the authority figure who knows and tells what is best for the person. Individuals are the experts on themselves and their health, and they are responsible and autonomous. Their judgments and their views are the significant ones.

27

Practice Methodologies

The methodology recommended for the theory of human becoming is a selection of dimensions and processes that are different from the nursing process (Mitchell & Santopinto, 1988). The practice methodology of human becoming is unlike the nursing process in which nurses, in assessing, ask specific questions of their clients and identify problems associated with isolated causal agents. The nurses then plan, carry out, and evaluate interventions. In nursing practice guided by the theory of human becoming, nurses do not "diagnose" or fit clients into preestablished categories, nor do they label any phenomena as "problems." There are no assumptions of linear cause and effect. The dimensions of the practice methodology for the theory of human becoming are related to Parse's three principles.

Illuminating Meaning

Principle 1, which is structuring meaning multidimensionally, gives rise to the dimension "Illuminating meaning through explicating" (Parse, 1987, p. 168): "Illuminating meaning involves shedding light through the uncovering" (Parse, 1987, p. 168) of the meaning of the past, the present, and the future from the client's/family's perspective. As clients talk about their meanings, the communicating of the impressions, thoughts, and feelings changes the meanings, making them more clear and explicit. This is accomplished by *languaging*, which is the sharing of their ideas and perceptions through words, gestures, facial expressions, touch, and body language (Parse, 1981, p. 177). The process related to this dimension is the nursing activity of explicating, which is "making clear what is appearing now through languaging" (Parse, 1987, p. 167). Thinking about and expressing to the nurse the thoughts and feelings connected with this moment in time can lead the client/family to a new way of viewing the familiar situation, allowing them to use new aspects of the universe in cocreating a different ongoing reality.

Synchronizing Rhythms

The dimension of "synchronizing rhythms through dwelling with the ebb and flow of human encounters" (Parse, 1987, p. 167) comes from Principle 2—cocreating rhythmical patterns. Parse observed that there are rhythms in the struggles and triumphs and the ups and downs of everyday living with others. Practicing within the theory of human becoming, the nurse does not try to change these rhythms or assist the family or individual to adapt but moves with the rhythm, guiding individuals and families to find their own harmony within the situation, leading them to find their own meaning. The process for the nurse: "Dwelling with is giving self over to the struggle in connecting-separating" (Parse, 1987, p. 167).

Mobilizing Transcendence

The dimension of "mobilizing transcendence through moving beyond" (Parse, 1987, p. 167) flows directly from Principle 3—cotranscending with the possibles. As the nurse dwells in true presence with clients/families as they struggle with the ever-changing situations, they move beyond (transcend) the present meaning of the events in their lives "to what is not yet . . . dreaming of the possibles and planning to reach for the dreams. The nurse guides individuals and families to plan for the changing of lived health patterns—these patterns uncovered in the illuminating of meaning, synchronizing of rhythms, and mobilizing of transcendence" (Parse, 1987, p. 169).

28

Clinical Example

An excellent example of the use of Parse's theory to guide clinical practice was described by Butler (1988) in the case of an elderly hospitalized father who was confused and frightened by treatment and who begged his family to take him home. The nurse, rather than attempting to orient the father or advise the family, guided them through the process of finding their own meaning in the situation (illuminating meaning through explicating). The nurse posed questions to the family and helped them clarify their thoughts and feelings and to share these with one another. The insights gained by the new meanings were explored and the family arrived at a new consensus and connectedness. Their altered view of the situation enabled them to support the father in his refusal to have physical therapy and led them to request that his tranquilizer be discontinued. In these decisions, the family elected to move with their father's reality. The nurse, in directing energy toward the planning for this different mode, was synchronizing the rhythms of the family (as well as those of the health care agency). The nurse asked questions, clarified perceptions, pointed out and explored options, and helped them to learn ways of taking care of the father in the daughter's home. The family, however, set their own rhythms, struggled with the responsibility of their choices, and came to live their own value priorities. The nurse neither advocated nor discredited the plan to remove the father from the hospital but went with the rhythm of the family.

Dramatic progress was evident in the father as soon as he began to live in his daughter's home, and, within 10 days, he requested to go to his own home. Again, the nurse dwelled with the family members in the revealing-concealing of their fears and concerns about the enabling-limiting possibilities of this proposed change. The second move represented a separating from a now familiar and safe environment while connecting with the cherished desire of living in his own home with his wife. The couple's home was altered to make it safer and easier for them to care for one another and the nurse arranged to make regular visits. The father, cotranscending with the new possibles, began to unfold a new pattern of health. His physicians were amazed at the progress of his medical condition. Leaving the doctors' offices with the nurse, the father, noting that it was raining, picked up his walker and ran to the car.

Butler (1988) stated that the dimension of mobilizing transcendence by moving beyond to new possibilities was evident in all facets of the nurse's practice (see appendix). This dimension was particularly evident when the nurse helped the family to image new possibilities and to move beyond in each of the connecting-separating instances when the father left the hospital and then his daughter's home.

Other published examples of clinical nursing practice guided by Parse's theory include the case of an elderly client who was actually in a hospital ward but whose coconstituted reality placed her in a park (Mitchell, 1986). Being present to the client's languaging, the nurse realized the client was multidimensionally experiencing her past (childhood and young adulthood), present, and future simultaneously. The nurse did not contradict the patient's reality but validated her feelings, guiding her to express her personal meanings and offering information and freedom to make choices. Another example of practice based on Parse's theory was an account of a nurse dwelling with a family that was cotranscending patterns of spouse abuse (Butler & Snodgrass, 1991).

29

Research Methodologies in the Theory of Human Becoming

Research Topics

The worldview and the assumptions of Parse's theory of human becoming lead the nurse to choose as the major focus for study the commonly lived experiences of human beings. Such health-related experiences include those which reflect the concepts of Parse's theory: being-becoming, value priorities, negentropic unfolding, and others relating to the quality of life for the person/family (Parse, 1987, p. 174). Examples of topics that have been studied are: *Persisting in Change Even Though It Is Difficult: The Lived Experience of Health* (Parse, 1985b) and *Struggling Through a Difficult Time for Unemployed Persons* (Smith, 1990).

Research Processes

Parse's is one of the few nursing theories for which a research methodology specific to the theory has been developed. The processes used to study the topics listed above connect with and are consistent with the theory. *Dialogical engagement* is the term for the discussion between participant and researcher (Parse, 1987). The researcher dwells with the ideas of the meaning of the experience and brings some questions and direction to begin the dialogue. These are not precise and predefined as in a printed questionnaire but a sharing of the sense of the question as it has originated. The genuine direction of the dialogue emerges from the lived experience and the recounting by the participant. *Extraction-synthesis* is the process by which the researcher dwells with the transcribed dialogue, moving to higher levels of abstraction to the structure of the evolved answers to the research question, which is "What is the structure of this lived experience?" (Parse, 1987, p. 177). The major processes used by the researcher are (a) extracting essences, (b) synthesizing essences, (c) formulating propositions, (d) extracting concepts, and (e) synthesizing a structure of the lived experience from the extracted concepts.

Heuristic interpretation consists of *structural integration* in which the propositions and structures are connected to the theory, and *conceptual interpretation* that interprets the essences synthesized from the lived experiences in light of the concepts of Parse's theory. These processes lead to the formulation of specific theoretical structures derived from the theory (see "Theoretical Structures," described above). "The heuristic interpretation weaves the ideas of the structure as lived into the theory and propels it beyond to posit ideas for research studies and possible practice activities" (Parse, 1987, p. 177).

Example of Research Methodology

Kelley (1991) used Parse's methodology to generate a study of the lived experience of "struggling with going along in a situation you do not believe in." Following Parse's guidelines, the researcher centered on the meaning of the phenomenon and then made herself authentically present to the study participants in dialogical engagement, allowing their experiences to emerge in the open interviews. The researcher then spent time listening intensively to the tapes and reading the transcripts, dwelling with the data to extract essences, or core ideas, and synthesizing these essences at a higher level of abstraction. Propositions were formulated for each participant, and core concepts for the group were extracted. The concepts were then synthesized into a structure of the lived experience. Core concepts identified by Kelley were (a) justifiable yielding, (b) opposing views intensifying personal convictions, and (c) compelled disclosure while suffering consequences (Kelley, 1991, p. 127). *Structural integration,* defined as connecting the structure of the lived experience with the theory, raised the abstraction of the concepts to (a) choosing priorities, (b) pushing-resisting, and (c) disclosing-not disclosing. The conceptual interpretation of these within Parse's theory was (a) valuing, (b) powering, and (c) revealing-concealing, or "struggling with going along in a situation you do not believe in is valuing the powering of revealing-concealing" (Kelley, 1991, p. 128).

The emerging methodology briefly described here differs from other methods used in nursing research. Because it focuses on the lived experiences of human beings, Parse presented it as an appropriate methodology to study the phenomena of interest to nurses.

30

Conclusion

Parse's theory of human becoming is important in its position among nursing theories that strive to provide the profession with guidelines for nursing practice, research, and education in a new age. It offers assumptions that provide a new and different view of health and an insight into the participation of persons in creating their own reality, a factor that nurses have always recognized. This theory provides concepts and tools for nurses to think about and to help them work with these client realities. Firmly rooted in the human sciences, Parse's theory fits with the intuitive search for frameworks that describe what some nurses have come to believe about their discipline and profession as well as what nurses actually do in their interaction with clients. It provides a map for many of the entities that nurses are dealing with: meanings, feelings, alternate interpretations of reality, communications, and values. It is also a very useful theory in that it addresses the struggles of clients, nurses, and families to assimilate and integrate change.

Appendix:
Clinical Example

Dimension	Processes of Nurse	Processes of Family
Illuminating meaning	Assisting family members in clarifying their ideas, sharing their thoughts	Exploring meaning of father's reality with him
	Posing questions	Expressing feelings including guilt, loneliness, and frustration
	Guiding the family in explicating the meaning of their current situation	Sharing feelings, values, and dreams
		Developing a consensus on new insights into the father's and family's situation (a cocreated different view)
Synchronizing rhythms	Directing family's energy toward planning for the new possibility	Family makes a choice to go with the rhythm set by the father
		Begin to discuss how a reuniting of the family might be brought about

(continued)

Dimension	Processes of Nurse	Processes of Family
	Helping the family explore the merits and drawbacks of all suggested possibilities	Exploring the possibilities of taking the father home
	Questioning, clarifying answers	Struggling with responsibilities and options
	Suggesting and exploring options	Devising a plan
	Neither advocating nor discrediting any plan proposed by family	Learning to perform some tasks for the father
	Going with the flow of the family's struggle to get the father home	Setting their own rhythm in devising their plan. Becoming more aware of their own and one another's values in self- disclosure (revealing-concealing)
		Coconstituting desired ways of being in the world
		Living their value priorities
Mobilizing transcendence	Preparing family to take father home	Family members move toward a clear understanding of the situation and one another
	Moving beyond at each level with the family	
	Being with the family as they struggle with familiar and unfamiliar patterns in finding new ways of being	Each member changes and the family struggles to find new ways of being together
		They achieve their goal of making their father comfortable in his own home

(continued)

Dimension	Processes of Nurse	Processes of Family
	Helping the family to be with the cherished familiar in new ways by exploring options, listening to ideas, analyzing viewpoints	They create a new emergence by inventing different ways of living their values

SOURCE: Butler (1988).

Glossary

Coconstitution
The human being's "active participation in creating meaning with others and the world" (Parse, 1981, p. 177).

Cocreate
"Initiate anew with another; coconstitute" (Parse, 1981, p. 177).

Cotranscending
"Going beyond the actual in interrelationship with others" (Parse, 1987, p. 166).

Health
"Process of becoming as experienced and described by the person" (Parse, 1992, p. 36). "Health is man's patterns of relating value priorities . . . an intersubjective process of transcending with the possibles" (Parse, 1981, p. 33). "Health is Man's unfolding. It is Man's lived experiences, a nonlinear entity that is not qualified or quantified by terms such as good, bad, more, or less. It is not Man adapting or coping. Unitary Man's health is a synthesis of values, a way of living. It is not the opposite of disease or a state that man has, but rather is a continuously changing process that Man cocreates" (Parse, 1987, p. 160). "Health is an expression of values at the moment, the meaning given to a situation" (Parse, 1987, p. 163). "It is just the way the human is! Health is cocreated through the human-environment interrelation-

ship, and it is lived in rhythmical patterns of relating that incarnate the meaning that the human being gives to situations" (Parse, 1990, p. 137).

Helicy

"Continuous, innovative, unpredictable, increasing diversity of human and environmental field patterns" (Rogers, 1990, p. 8).

Imaging

"Symbolizing or picturing" (Parse, 1981, p. 177). "Imaging refers to knowing; exists at the explicit and tacit realms" (Parse, 1992, p. 37).

Integrality

"Continuous mutual human field and environmental field process" (Rogers, 1990, p. 8). Formerly termed *complementary.*

Intersubjectivity

Subject-to-subject relationship involving true presence (Parse, 1981, p. 177).

Knowing

"Personal knowledge is shaped through prereflective-reflective imaging, explicitly and tacitly all at once. Explicit knowing is reflected upon critically; tacit knowing is prearticulate and acritical" (Parse, 1992, p. 37).

Languaging

"Sharing valued images through symbols of words, gesture, gaze, touch, and posture" (Parse, 1981, p. 177). It "is the way human beings represent personal structures of reality" (Parse, 1992, p. 37).

Man

"Refers to *Homo sapiens*" (Parse, 1981, p. xiii). "Man is an open being, more than and different from the sum of parts in mutual simultaneous interchange with the environment who chooses from options and bears responsibility for choices. Man cocreates patterns of relating with the environment and is recognized by these patterns" (Parse, 1987, p. 160). "Man is coexisting while coconstituting rhythmical patterns with the environment. . . . Man is transcending multidimensionally with the possibles" (Parse, 1981, p. 33).

Man-living-health

"A unitary phenomenon that refers to man's becoming through cocreating rhythmical patterns of relating in open energy interchange with the environment" (Parse, 1981, p. 39). This combination of words with their hyphens indicates one concept with a meaning different from the separate words. The phrase *man-living-health* indicates "health as ongoing participation with the world" (Parse, 1981, p. 39).

Multidimensionally

"Refers to the various levels of the universe that Man experiences all at once. Specifically the term refers to explicit-tacit knowing. Not all choices are made from the explicit level. Man chooses possibilities from the whole sense of the situation. With each situation there are multiple possibles unfolding. What unfolds surfaces in relationship to others and the environment as dreams of what can be become actualities" (Parse, 1987, pp. 161-162).

Originating

"Creating anew, generating unique ways of living which surface through interconnections with people and projects" (Parse, 1992, p. 38).

Paradigm

"A way of viewing a particular field of study" (Parse, 1981, p. 178).

Paradox

"Refers to apparent opposites. These rhythmical patterns are not opposites; they are two sides of the same rhythm that coexist all at once" (Parse, 1992, p. 38).

Pattern

"A configuration of man-environment interrelationship" (Parse, 1981, p. 178).

Phenomenology

"The study of phenomena as they unfold" (Parse, 1981, p. 178).

Possibles

"The imaginables toward which one reaches" (Parse, 1981, p. 178).

Powering

"Is the pushing-resisting rhythm in all and human-universe interrelationships. It is the back and forth experienced by humans in all life situations, an energizing force which sparks moving beyond the moment" (Parse, 1992, p. 38).

Theoretical structures

"A statement interrelating concepts in a way that can be verified" (Parse, 1981, p. 179). "Nondirectional propositions," statements that are "noncausal in nature and consistent with the assumptions and principles [of Parse's theory]." "They are designed to guide practice and research" (Parse, 1987, p. 166). "To make these usable in practice and research, statements about nursing practice must be derived and lived experiences chosen for study" (Parse, 1987, p. 166).

Transcending

"Going beyond; exceeding" (Parse, 1981, p. 179).

Transforming

"The shifting of views of the familiar as different light is shed on what is known. Change itself is a continuous ongoing process in the human-universe process which is recognized by increasing diversity" (Parse, 1992, p. 39).

Valuing

"The process of living cherished beliefs while assimilating the new into a personal worldview. It emerges in the human-universe process and is the human being's confirming of cherished beliefs" (Parse, 1992, p. 37).

Wholeness

"More than and different from the sum of parts" (Parse, 1981, p. 179).

References

Butler, M. J. (1988). Family transformation: Parse's theory in practice. *Nursing Science Quarterly, 1*, 68-74.

Butler, M. J., & Snodgrass, F. G. (1991). Beyond abuse: Parse's theory in practice. *Nursing Science Quarterly, 4*, 76-82.

Heidegger, M. (1962). *Being and time.* New York: Harper & Row.

Kelley, L. S. (1991). Struggling with going along when you do not believe. *Nursing Science Quarterly, 4*(3), 123-129.

Lavine, T. Z. (1984). *From Socrates to Sartre: The philosophic quest.* New York: Bantam.

Lee, R. E., & Schumacher, L. P. (1989). Rosemarie Rizzo Parse. In A. Marriner-Tomey (Ed.), *Nursing theorists and their work* (2nd ed., pp. 174-186). St. Louis: C. V. Mosby.

Merleau-Ponty, M. (1962). *Phenomenology of perception.* New York: Humanities Press.

Mitchell, G. J. (1986). Utilizing Parse's theory of Man-Living-Health in Mrs. M's neighborhood. *Perspectives, 10*(4), 5-7.

Mitchell, G. J., & Santopinto, M. (1988). An alternative to nursing diagnosis. *The Canadian Nurse, 84*(10), 25-28.

Parse, R. R. (1974). *Nursing fundamentals.* Flushing, NY: Medical Examination.

Parse, R. R. (1981). *Man-Living-Health: A theory of nursing.* New York: John Wiley.

Parse, R. R. (Speaker). (1985a). *Presentation at nurse theorist conference* (Cassette Recording No. DII-105). Louisville, KY: Meetings Internationale.

Parse, R. R. (1985b). Nursing research traditions quantitative and qualitative approaches. In R. R. Parse, A. B. Coyne, & M. J. Smith (Eds.), *Nursing research qualitative methods* (pp. 1-8). Bowie, MD: Brady Communications.

Parse, R. R. (1987). Man-Living-Health theory of nursing. In R. R. Parse (Ed.), *Nursing science: Major paradigms, theories and critiques* (pp. 159-180). Philadelphia: W. B. Saunders.

Parse, R. R. (1990). Health: A personal commitment. *Nursing Science Quarterly, 3*(3), 136-140.

Parse, R. R. (1992). Human becoming: Parse's theory of nursing. *Nursing Science Quarterly, 5*(1), 35-42.

Rogers, M. E. (1970). *An introduction to the theoretical basis of nursing.* Philadelphia: F. A. Davis.

Rogers, M. E. (1980). Nursing: A science of unitary man. In J. P. Riehl & C. Roy (Eds.), *Conceptual models for nursing practice* (2nd ed., pp. 329-337). New York: Appleton-Century-Crofts.

Rogers, M. E. (1987). Rogers's science of unitary human beings. In R. R. Parse (Ed.), *Nursing science: Major paradigms, theories, and critiques* (pp. 139-146). Philadelphia: W. B. Saunders.

Rogers, M. E. (1990). Nursing: Science of unitary, irreducible, human beings: Update 1990. In E. A. M. Barrett (Ed.), *Visions of Rogers's science-based nursing* (pp. 5-11). New York: National League for Nursing.

Sartre, J.-P. (1956). *Being and nothingness.* New York: Washington Square Press.

Smith, M. C. (1990). Struggling through a difficult time for unemployed persons. *Nursing Science Quarterly, 3,* 18-28.

Smith, M. C., & Hudepohl, J. H. (1988). Analysis and evaluation of Parse's theory of Man-Living-Health. *Canadian Journal of Nursing Research, 20*(4), 43-58.

Bibliography:
References Related to Parse's Work

Primary Sources

Books

Parse, R. R. (1974). *Nursing fundamentals.* Flushing, NY: Medical Examination.

Parse, R. R. (1981). *Man-living-health: A theory of nursing.* New York: John Wiley.

Parse, R. R. (1987). *Nursing science: Major paradigms, theories, and critiques.* Philadelphia: W. B. Saunders.

Parse, R. R., Coyne, A. B., & Smith, M. J. (1985). *Nursing research: Qualitative methods.* Bowie, MD: Brady.

Doctoral Dissertation

Parse, R. R. (1969). An instructional model for the teaching of nursing, interrelating objectives and media (Doctoral dissertation, University of Pittsburgh). *Dissertation Abstracts International, 31,* 180A.

Book Chapters, Articles, and Editorials

Parse, R. R. (1967, August). The advantages of the ADN program. *Journal of Nursing Education, 6*(15).

Parse, R. R. (1978). Rights of medical patients. In C. Fisher (Ed.), *Client participation in human services.* New Brunswick, NJ: Transaction.

Parse, R. R. (1980). Caring from a human science perspective. In M. M. Leininger (Ed.), *Caring: A human helping process*. Salt Lake City, UT.

Parse, R. R. (1981). Caring from a human science perspective. In M. M. Leininger (Ed.), *Caring: An essential human need*. Thorofare, NJ: Charles B. Slack.

Parse, R. R. (1988). Beginnings. *Nursing Science Quarterly, 1*, 1.

Parse, R. R. (1988). Creating traditions: The art of putting it together. *Nursing Science Quarterly 1*, 45.

Parse, R. R. (1988). Scholarly dialogue: The fire of refinement. *Nursing Science Quarterly, 1*, 141.

Parse, R. R. (1988). The mainstream of science: Framing the issue. *Nursing Science Quarterly, 1*, 93.

Parse, R. R. (1989). Essentials for practicing the art of nursing. *Nursing Science Quarterly, 2*, 111.

Parse, R. R. (1989). Making more out of less. *Nursing Science Quarterly, 2*, 155.

Parse, R. R. (1989). Man-living-health: A theory of nursing. In J. Riehl-Sisca (Ed.), *Conceptual models for nursing practice* (3rd ed.). Norwalk, CT: Appleton & Lange.

Parse, R. R. (1989). Martha E. Rogers: A birthday celebration. *Nursing Science Quarterly, 2*, 55.

Parse, R. R. (1989). Parse's man-living-health model and administration of nursing services. In B. Henry, C. Arndt, M. Di Vincenti, & A. Marriner-Tomey (Eds.), *Dimensions of nursing administration: Theory, research, education, and practice*. Cambridge, MA: Blackwell Scientific.

Parse, R. R. (1989). Qualitative research: Publishing and funding. *Nursing Science Quarterly, 2*, 1.

Parse, R. R. (1989). The phenomenological research method: Its value for management science. In B. Henry, C. Arndt, M. Di Vincenti, & A. Marriner Tomey (Eds.), *Dimensions of nursing administration: Theory, research, education, and practice*. Cambridge, MA: Blackwell Scientific.

Parse, R. R. (1990). A time for reflection and projection. *Nursing Science Quarterly, 3*, 141-143.

Parse, R. R. (1990). Health: A personal commitment. *Nursing Science Quarterly, 3*, 136-140.

Parse, R. R. (1990). Nurse theorist conference comes to Japan. *Japanese Journal of Nursing Research, 23*(3).

Parse, R. R. (1990). Nursing theory-based practice: A challenge for the 90s. *Nursing Science Quarterly, 3*, 53.

Parse, R. R. (1990). Parse's research methodology with an illustration of the lived experience of hope. *Nursing Science Quarterly, 3*, 9-17.

Parse, R. R. (1990). Promotion and prevention: Two distinct cosmologies. *Nursing Science Quarterly, 3*, 101.

Parse, R. R. (1991). Electronic publishing: Beyond browsing. *Nursing Science Quarterly, 4*, 1.

Parse, R. R. (1991). Growing: The discipline of nursing. *Nursing Science Quarterly, 4*, 139.

Parse, R. R. (1991). Mysteries of health and healing: Two perspectives. *Nursing Science Quarterly, 4*, 93.

Parse, R. R. (1991). Phenomenology and nursing. *Japanese Journal of Nursing, 17*(2), 261-269.

Parse, R. R. (1991). The right soil, the right stuff. *Nursing Science Quarterly, 4,* 47.

Parse, R. R. (in press). Man-living-health: A theory of nursing. In M. Mischo-Kelling & K. Wittneben (Eds.), *Auffassungen von Pflege in theorie und praxis.*

Unpublished Manuscripts (past 4 years)

Parse, R. R. (1987). *Man-living-health and the meaning of aging.* Paper presented at the annual meeting of the Gerontological Society, Washington, DC.

Parse, R. R. (1988). *Nursing science: The development and testing of theory.* Keynote address given at the Southern Council on Collegiate Education for Nursing Research conference, Atlanta.

Parse, R. R. (1988). *Parse's theory, research and practice.* Paper presented at the Annual Doctoral Students Research Conference, Wayne State University, School of Nursing, Detroit.

Parse, R. R. (1988). *Parse's theory in practice: An evaluation study.* Paper presented at the National Symposium of Nursing Research, San Francisco.

Parse, R. R. (1989). *Nursing as a discipline: Its theories and methods of inquiry.* State University of New York, Downstate.

Parse, R. R. (1989). *Parse's theory of nursing.* Cedars Medical Center Nursing Theory Conference, Miami, FL.

Parse, R. R. (1989). *Publications in scholarly journals.* ANA Council of Nurse Researchers, Chicago.

Parse, R. R. (1989). *Qualitative research: The new story in sciencing.* Keynote address given at Barry University, University of Miami, and South Florida Nursing Research Society, Miami.

Parse, R. R. (1989). Symposium for doctoral students and faculty on research and theory development, simultaneity paradigm, Medical College of Georgia, Augusta.

Parse, R. R. (1989). *The quest for knowledge: Imagining, enlightening, enlivening.* Paper presented at the Barry University 50th Jubilee, Miami Shores, FL.

Parse, R. R. (1989). *Using nursing knowledge in practice.* Keynote address given at the Cedars Medical Center Nursing Theory Conference, Miami, FL.

Parse, R. R. (1990). *Research methods unique to nursing.* Keynote address given at the Barry University, University of Miami, and South Florida Nursing Research Society, Miami.

Parse, R. R. (1990). *A dialogue with nurse theorists: A basis for differentiating nursing practice.* Paper presented at the annual meeting of the American Academy of Nursing, Charleston, SC.

Parse, R. R. (1990). *Advancing nursing science through qualitative research.* Paper presented at the annual meeting of the Eastern Nursing Research Society, New York.

Parse, R. R. (1990). *Man-living-health: Theory, research and practice.* Paper presented at the College of Nursing, University of South Carolina, Columbia.

Parse, R. R. (1990). *Man-living-health theory and the meaning of health and cultural values in elders.* Paper presented at the 43rd Annual Scientific Session of the Gerontological Society of America, Boston.

Parse, R. R. (1990). *Parse's research and practice methodologies.* Paper presented at the Discovery International, Inc. Nursing Science Seminar, Vernon Manor Hotel, Cincinnati, OH.

Parse, R. R. (1990). *Parse's theory: A way of living nursing.* Paper presented to the Nursing Division, Queen Elizabeth Hospital, Toronto, Ontario, Canada.

Parse, R. R. (1990). *Parse's theory in practice: A workshop.* Paper presented at the North Shore Medical Center, Miami, FL.

Parse, R. R. (1990). *Parse's theory in practice and research.* Paper presented at Sigma Theta Tau, Alpha Phi Chapter, Annual Research Day, Hunter-Bellevue School of Nursing, New York.

Parse, R. R. (1990). *Parse's theory in research and practice.* Paper presented at the UCLA Neuro-Psychiatric Institute and Hospital, Nursing Department, Los Angeles.

Parse, R. R. (1990). *Qualitative research.* Paper presented at the College of Nursing, University of South Carolina, Columbia.

Parse, R. R. (1990). *Reporting research: From article to abstract.* Paper presented at Teachers College, Columbia University, New York.

Parse, R. R. (1990). *Simultaneity paradigm and Parse's theory.* Paper presented at the University of Pittsburgh, Pittsburgh.

Parse, R. R. (1990). *The meaning of choosing health.* Paper presented at the Harmarville Rehabilitation Center, Harmarville, PA.

Parse, R. R. (1991). *Man-living health, theory, research and practice.* Paper presented at Kyoto, Japan.

Parse, R. R. (1991). *Nursing knowledge for the 21st century: An international commitment.* Keynote address given at the Discovery International, Inc. Biennial Nurse Theorist Conference, Tokyo, Japan.

Parse, R. R. (1991). *Nursing theory-based practice: Does it make a difference?* Paper presented at the Battle Creek Veterans Administration Medical Center Conference, Kalamazoo, MI.

Parse, R. R. (1991). *Parse in question and answer.* Paper presented at the Discovery International, Inc. Biennial Nurse Theorist Conference, Tokyo, Japan.

Parse, R. R. (1991). *Parse's human becoming theory of nursing.* Paper presented at the Battle Creek Veterans Administration Medical Center Conference, Kalamazoo, MI.

Parse, R. R. (1991). *Parse's theory.* Paper presented at the Discovery International, Inc. Biennial Nurse Theorist Conference, Tokyo, Japan.

Parse, R. R. (1991). *Phenomenology as a way of living.* Paper presented at the annual meeting of the Interpersonal Relationships Society, Tokyo, Japan.

Parse, R. R. (1991). *Theory and research as tools for practice.* Paper presented at the University of Michigan School of Nursing Centennial Celebration, Ann Arbor.

Cassette Recordings

Parse, R. R. (Speaker). (1985). *Nursing education in the 21st century* (Cassette Recording No. DII-113). Louisville, KY: Meetings Internationale.

Parse, R. R. (Speaker). (1985). *Presentation at nurse theorist conference* (Cassette Recording No. DII-105). Louisville, KY: Meetings Internationale.

Parse, R. R., Orem, D. E., Roy, D., King, I. M., Rogers, M. E., & Peplau, H. E. (Speakers). (1985). *Panel discussion with nurse theorists* (Cassette Recording No. DII-112). Louisville, KY: Meetings Internationale.

Parse, R. R., & Phillips, J. R. (Speakers). (1985). *Parse's man-living-health theory of nursing* (Cassette Recording No. DII-109). Louisville, KY: Meetings Internationale.

Parse, R. R. (Speaker). (1986). *An emerging research methodology unique to nursing* (Cassette Recording No. DII-303). Louisville, KY: Meetings Internationale.

Parse, R. R. (Speaker). (1986). *Panel discussion* (Cassette Recording No. DII-305). Louisville, KY: Meetings Internationale.

Parse, R. R. (Speaker). (1986). *Quantitative and qualitative methods in nursing research* (Cassette Recording No. DII-201). Louisville, KY: Meetings Internationale.

Parse, R. R. (Speaker). (1986). *The ethnographic method* (Cassette Recording No. DII-204). Louisville, KY: Meetings Internationale.

Parse, R. R. (Speaker). (1986). *The phenomenological method* (Cassette Recording No. DII-202[A&B]). Louisville, KY: Meetings Internationale.

Parse, R. R. (Speaker). (1987). *Panel discussion with theorists* (Cassette Recording No. DII-408). Louisville, KY: Meetings Internationale.

Parse, R. R. (Speaker). (1987). *Parse's theory* (Cassette Recording No. DII-403). Louisville, KY: Meetings Internationale.

Parse, R. R. (Speaker). (1987). *Small group C* (Cassette Recording No. DII-411). Louisville, KY: Meetings Internationale.

Parse, R. R. (Speaker). (1989). *Health as a personal commitment in Parse's theory* (Cassette Recording No. DII-503). Louisville, KY: Meetings Internationale.

Parse, R. R. (Speaker). (1989). *Panel discussion with theorists* (Cassette Recording No. DII-507). Louisville, KY: Meetings Internationale.

Parse, R. R. (Speaker). (1990). *Panel discussion/retrospective and evaluation* (Cassette Recording No. DII-605). Louisville, KY: Meetings Internationale.

Parse, R. R. (Speaker). (1990). *Parse's research and practice methodologies* (Cassette Recording No. DII-601). Louisville, KY: Meetings Internationale.

Videotape Recordings

Parse, R. R., Orem, D. E., Roy, C., King, I. M., Rogers, M. E., & Peplau, H. E. (Speakers). (1985). *Panel discussion with theorists* (Videotape Recording No. DII-V-112). Louisville, KY: Meetings Internationale.

Parse, R. R. (Speaker). (1987). *Parse's theory* (Videotape Recording No. DII-V-403). Louisville, KY: Meetings Internationale.

Parse, R. R., Peplau, H. E., King, I. M., Roy, C., Rogers, M. E., Watson, J., & Leininger, M. (Speakers). (1987). *Panel discussion with theorists* (Videotape Recording No. DII-V-408). Louisville, KY: Meetings Internationale.

Parse, R. R. (Speaker). (1989). *Health as a personal commitment in Parse's theory* (Videotape Recording No. DII-V-503). Louisville, KY: Meetings Internationale.

Parse, R. R., Meleis, A. I., Neuman, B. M., Rogers, M. E., Pender, N. J., & King., I. M. (Speakers). (1989). *Panel discussion with theorists* (Videotape Recording No. DII-V-507). Louisville, KY: Meetings Internationale.

Parse, R. R. (Speaker). (1990). *A portrait in excellence* [Videotape]. Helene Fuld Health Trust. Oakland, CA: Studio Three Production.

Secondary Sources

Book Reviews on Parse's Books

Parse, R. R. (1975). *Nursing fundamentals.* In *Australian Nurses Journal, 5*(37).

Parse, R. R. (1981). *Man-living-health: A theory of nursing.* In *International Journal of Rehabilitation Research, 4,* 449, and in *Western Journal of Nursing Research, 5,* 105-106, Winter 1982.

Parse, R. R., Coyne, A. B., & Smith, M. J. (1986). *Nursing research: Qualitative methods.* In E. R. Lenz (Reviewer), Review of four general nursing research methods tests. In *Nursing Science Quarterly, 1,* 86-90.

Parse, R. R. (1988). *Nursing science: Major paradigms, theories, and critiques.* In M. K. Jacobs-Kramer, M. E. Levine, & E. M. Menke (Reviewers), Three perspectives on a scholarly work. In *Nursing Science Quarterly, 1,* 182-186.

Books and Articles Mentioning Parse's Theory

Chinn, P. L., & Jacobs, M. K. (1987). *Theory and nursing: A systematic approach* (2nd ed.). St. Louis: C. V. Mosby.

Fitzpatrick, J. J., & Whall, A. L. (1989). *Conceptual models of nursing: Analysis and application* (2nd ed.). Norwalk, CT: Appleton & Lange.

George, J. (1990). *Nursing theories: The base for professional nursing practice* (3rd ed.). New York: Prentice Hall.

Kleffel, D. (1991). Rethinking the environment as a domain of nursing knowledge. *Advances in Nursing Science, 14,* 10-51.

Marriner-Tomey, A. (1989). *Nursing theorists and their work* (2nd ed.). St. Louis: C. V. Mosby.

Meleis, A. I. (1985). *Theoretical nursing: Development and progress.* Philadelphia: J. B. Lippincott.

Mitchell, G. J. (1991). Nursing diagnosis: An ethical analysis. *Image: Journal of Nursing Scholarship, 23,* 99-103.

Nagle, L. M., & Mitchell, G. J. (1991). Theoretic diversity: Evolving paradigmatic issues in research and practice. *Advances in Nursing Science, 14,* 17-25.

Newman, M. A., Sime, A. M., & Corcoran-Perry, S. A. (1991). The focus of the discipline of nursing. *Advances in Nursing Science, 14,* 1-6.

Book Chapters and Articles by Others on Parse

Cowling, W. R. (1989). Parse's theory of nursing. In J. J. Fitzpatrick & A. L. Whall (Eds.), *Conceptual models of nursing: Analysis and application* (2nd ed., pp. 385-399). Norwalk, CT: Appleton & Lange.

Hickman, J. S. (1990). Rosemarie Rizzo Parse. In J. B. George (Ed.), *Nursing theories: The base for professional nursing practice* (3rd ed., pp. 311-332). Norwalk, CT: Appleton & Lange.

Lee, R. E., & Schumacher, L. P. (1989). Rosemarie Rizzo Parse: Man-living-health. In A. Marriner-Tomey (Ed.), *Nurse theorists and their work* (2nd ed., pp. 174-186). St. Louis: C. V. Mosby.

Phillips, J. (1987). A critique of Parse's man-living-health theory. In R. R. Parse, *Nursing science: Major paradigms, theories and critiques* (pp. 181-204). Philadelphia: W. B. Saunders.

Pugliese, L. (1989). The theory of man-living-health: An analysis. In J. Riehl-Sisca (Ed.), *Conceptual models for nursing practice* (3rd ed., pp. 259-265). Norwalk, CT: Appleton & Lange.

Smith, M. C., & Hudepohl, J. H. (1988). Analysis and evaluation of Parse's theory of man-living-health. *Canadian Journal of Nursing Research: Nursing Papers, 20*(4), 43-58.

Winkler, S. J. (1983). Parse's theory of nursing. In J. J. Fitzpatrick & A. L. Whall (Eds.), *Conceptual models of nursing: Analysis and application* (pp. 275-294). Bowie, MD: Brady.

Directories and Biographical Sources

Fellow in the American Academy of Nursing. (1989). *Directory of Fellows in AAN.*

Sigma Theta Tau. (1987). *Directory of nurse researchers* (2nd ed.). Indianapolis, IN: Author.

Articles About Parse's Theory

Banonis, B. C. (1989). The lived experience of recovering from addiction: A phenomenological study. *Nursing Science Quarterly, 2*, 37-43.

Butler, M. J. (1988). Family transformation: Parse's theory in practice. *Nursing Science Quarterly, 1*, 68-74.

Butler, M. J., & Snodgrass, F. G. (1991). Beyond abuse: Parse's theory in practice. *Nursing Science Quarterly, 4*, 76-82.

Cody, W. K. (in press). Grieving a personal loss. *Nursing Science Quarterly, 4*, 61-68.

Heine, C. (1991). Development of gerontological nursing theory: Applying man-living-health theory of nursing. *Nursing & Health Care, 12*, 184-188.

Kelley, L. M. (1991). Struggling with going along when you do not believe. *Nursing Science Quarterly, 4*, 123-129.

Liehr, P. R. (1989). The core of true presence: A loving center. *Nursing Science Quarterly, 2*, 7-8.

Mattice, M. (1991). Parse's theory of nursing in practice: A manager's perspective. *Canadian Journal of Nursing Administration, 23,* 11-13.

Mattice, M., & Mitchell, G. J. (1991). Caring for confused elders. *The Canadian Nurse, 86*(11), 16-17.

Mitchell, G. J. (1986). Utilizing Parse's theory of man-living-health in Mrs. M's neighborhood. *Perspectives, 10*(4), 5-7.

Mitchell, G. J. (1988). Man-living-health: The theory in practice. *Nursing Science Quarterly, 1,* 120-127.

Mitchell G. J. (1990). Struggling in change: From the traditional approach to Parse's theory-based practice. *Nursing Science Quarterly, 3,* 170-176.

Mitchell, G. J. (1990). The lived experience of taking life day-by-day in later life: Research guided by Parse's emergent method. *Nursing Science Quarterly, 3,* 29-36.

Mitchell, G. J. (1991). Diagnosis: Clarifying or obscuring the nature of nursing. *Nursing Science Quarterly, 4,* 52-53.

Mitchell, G. J. (1991). Nursing diagnosis: An ethical analysis. *Image: Journal of Nursing Scholarship.*

Mitchell, G. J., & Copplestone, C. (1990). Applying Parse's theory to perioperative nursing: A nontraditional approach. *AORN Journal, 51*(3), 787-798.

Mitchell, G. J., & Pilkington, B. (1990). Theoretical approaches in nursing practice: A comparison of Roy and Parse. *Nursing Science Quarterly, 3,* 81-87.

Mitchell, G. J., & Santopinto, M. D. A. (1988). An alternative to nursing diagnosis. *The Canadian Nurse, 84*(10), 25-28.

Mitchell, G. J., & Santopinto, M. D. A. (1988). The expanded role nurse: A dissenting viewpoint. *Canadian Journal of Nursing Administration, 4*(1), 8-14.

Nokes, K. M., & Carver, K. (1991). The meaning of living with AIDS: A study of using Parse's theory of man-living-health. *Nursing Science Quarterly, 4,* 174-179.

Quiquero, A., Knights, D., & Meo, C. O. (1991). Theory as a guide to practice: Staff nurses choose Parse's theory. *Canadian Journal for Nursing Administration, 23,* 14-16.

Rasmusson, D., Jonas, C. M., & Mitchell, G. J. (in press). The eye of the beholder: Applying Parse's theory with homeless individuals. *Clinical Nurse Specialist Journal.*

Santopinto, M. D. A. (1989). The relentless drive to be ever thinner: A study using the phenomenological method. *Nursing Science Quarterly, 2,* 29-36.

Smith, M. C. (1990). Struggling through a difficult time for unemployed persons. *Nursing Science Quarterly, 2,* 29-36.

Smith, M. J. (1989). Research and practice application related to man-living-health. In J. Riehl-Sisca (Ed.), *Conceptual models for nursing practice* (3rd ed., pp. 267-276). Norwalk, CT: Appleton & Lange.

Wondolowski, C., & Davis, D. K. (1988). The lived experience of aging in the oldest old: A phenomenological study. *American Journal of Psychoanalysis, 48,* 261-270.

Wondolowski, C., & Davis, D. K. (1991). The lived experience of health in the oldest old: A phenomenological study. *Nursing Science Quarterly, 4,* 113-118.

Unpublished Manuscripts

Banonis, B. (1989). *The lived experience of recovering from addiction: A phenomenological study*. Paper presented at the UCLA National Nursing Theory Conference, Los Angeles.

Beauchamp, C. J. (1990). *The lived experience of struggling with making a decision in a critical life situation*. Paper presented at the Discovery International, Inc. Nursing Science Seminar on Research and Practice Related to Parse's Theory of Nursing, Cincinnati, OH.

Cody, W. K. (1990). *Parse's theory in practice with a grieving family*. Paper presented at the Sigma Theta Tau, Alpha Phi Chapter, Annual Research Day, Hunter-Bellevue School of Nursing, New York.

Cody, W. K. (1990). *The lived experience of grieving a personal loss*. Paper presented at the Discovery International, Inc. Nursing Science Seminar on Research and Practice Related to Parse's Theory of Nursing, Cincinnati, OH.

Cody, W. K. (1990). *The lived experience of grieving a personal loss*. Paper presented at the UCLA National Nursing Theory Conference, Los Angeles.

Jonas, C. (1989). *Parse's theory: Research and practice*. Paper presented at the School of Nursing, University of Toronto, Ontario, Canada.

Jonas, C. (1989). *Parse's theory in practice with older people*. Paper presented at St. Michael's Hospital, Toronto, Ontario.

Jonas, C. (1989). *The lived experience of being an elder in Nepal*. Research study presented at the World Congress on Gerontology, Acapulco, Mexico.

Jonas, C. (1990). *Practicing Parse's theory with groups of individuals in the community*. Paper presented at Queen Elizabeth Hospital, Toronto, Ontario, Canada.

Kelley, L. S. (1989). *The lived experience of "struggling with going along in a situation you do not believe in": Using the man-living-health methodology*. Paper presented at the conference sponsored by Barry University, School of Nursing, Honor Society, Sigma Theta Tau, Beta Tau Chapter, University of Miami, and South Florida Nursing Research Society, Miami.

Kelley, L. S. (1990). *The lived experience of "struggling with going along in a situation you do not believe in": Using the man-living-health methodology*. Paper presented at the UCLA National Nursing Theory Conference, Los Angeles.

Liehr, P. R. (1988, December). *A study of the experience of "living on the edge."* Research study presented at the Southern Council on Collegiate Education for Nursing, Atlanta.

Mattice, M. (1990). *Evaluating Parse's theory in practice*. Paper presented at Queen Elizabeth Hospital, Toronto, Ontario, Canada.

Menke, E. M. (1990). *Critique of the research studies and the research methodology*. Paper presented at the Discovery International, Inc. Nursing Science Seminar on Research and Practice Related to Parse's Theory of Nursing, Cincinnati, OH.

Misselwitz, S. K. (1989). *A phenomenological study of getting through the day for women who are homeless*. Research study presented at the conference sponsored by Barry University, School of Nursing, Honor Society, Sigma Theta Tau, Beta Tau Chapter, University of Miami, and South Florida Nursing Research Society, Miami.

Mitchell, G. J. (1987). *Man-living-health in practice with the elderly*. Paper presented at the annual meeting of the Gerontological Society, Washington, DC.

Mitchell, G. J. (1988). *Man-living-health in practice.* Paper presented at the Wayne State University Summer Research Symposium, Detroit.

Mitchell, G. J. (1990). *A dialogue with nurse theorists: A basis for differentiating nursing practice—Parse in practice.* Paper presented at the annual meeting of the American Academy of Nursing, Charleston, SC.

Mitchell, G. J. (1990). *An evaluation study of Parse's theory of nursing in an acute care setting.* Conducted and presented study at St. Michael's Hospital, Nursing Department, Toronto, Ontario, Canada.

Mitchell, G. J. (1990). *From traditional nursing to Parse's theory.* Paper presented at Queen Elizabeth Hospital, Toronto, Ontario, Canada.

Mitchell, G. J. (1990). *Nursing practice guided by Parse's theory.* Paper presented at the North Shore Medical Center, Miami, FL.

Mitchell, G. J. (1990). *Parse in practice.* Paper presented at the UCLA National Nursing Theory Conference, Los Angeles.

Mitchell, G. J. (1990). *Parse's theory as a guide to practice.* Paper presented at the Discovery International, Inc. Nursing Science Seminar on Research and Practice Related to Parse's Theory of Nursing, Cincinnati, OH.

Pilkington, B. (1990). *Research guided by Parse's theory.* Paper presented at Queen Elizabeth Hospital, Toronto, Ontario, Canada.

Santopinto, M. D. A. (1987). *Parse's theory of nursing as a base for innovative practice.* Paper presented at Hamilton psychiatric Hospital, Hamilton, Ontario.

Santopinto, M. D. A. (1988). *A qualitative evaluation study of Parse's theory in practice: What happens when theory is implemented?* Research study presented at the Eighth Annual SCCEN Research Conference, Emory University, Atlanta.

Santopinto, M. D. A. (1988). *A test of Parse's theory in a gerontological setting: An evaluation study.* Research study presented at the Ryerson Theory Congress, Toronto, Ontario, Canada.

Santopinto, M. D. A. (1988). *Close encounters of the theoretical kind: Three theory-based approaches.* Paper presented at the Tenth Southeastern Conference of Specialists in Psychiatric-Mental Health Nursing, Asheville, NC.

Santopinto, M. D. A. (1989). *An emergent methodology study of caring about self for individuals who exercise relentlessly.* Research study presented at the Scientific Sessions of the Sigma Theta Tau Research Conference, Taipei, Taiwan.

Santopinto, M. D. A. (1989). *An evaluation study of Parse's practice methodology in a chronic care setting.* Research study presented at the 19th Quadrennial Congress of the International Council of Nurses, Seoul, Korea.

Santopinto, M. D. A. (1990). *An evaluation of Parse's theory.* Paper presented at the UCLA National Nursing Theory Conference, Los Angeles.

Santopinto, M. D. A. (1990). *An evaluation study of Parse's theory in practice.* Paper presented at the Discovery International, Inc. Nursing Science Seminar on Research and Practice Related to Parse's Theory of Nursing, Cincinnati, OH.

Santopinto, M. D. A. (1990). *An evaluation study of Parse's theory in practice in a chronic long-term setting.* Paper presented at the Battle Creek Veterans Administration Medical Center Conference, Kalamazoo, MI.

Smith, M. C. (1990). *Speculation on Parse in nursing education.* Paper presented at Queen Elizabeth Hospital, Toronto, Ontario, Canada.

Smith, M. C. (1990). *The lived experience of hope in families of critically ill persons.* Paper presented at the UCLA National Nursing Theory Conference, Los Angeles.

Cassette Recordings

Beauchamp, C. J. (Speaker). (1990). *The lived experience of struggling with making a decision in a critical life situation* (Cassette Recording No. DII-602). Louisville, KY: Meetings Internationale.

Cody, W. K. (Speaker). (1990). *The lived experience of grieving a personal loss* (Cassette Recording No. DII-602). Louisville, KY: Meetings Internationale.

Menke, E. M. (Moderator). (1990). *Panel discussion/retrospective and evaluation* (Cassette Recording No. DII-605). Louisville, KY: Meetings Internationale.

Menke, E. M. (Speaker). (1990). *Critique of the research studies and the research methodology* (Cassette Recording No. DII-603). Louisville, KY: Meetings Internationale.

Mitchell, G. J. (Speaker). (1990). *Parse's theory as a guide to practice* (Cassette Recording No. DII-604). Louisville, KY: Meetings Internationale.

Santopinto, M. D. A. (Speaker). (1990). *An evaluation study of Parse's theory in practice* (Cassette Recording No. DII-604). Louisville, KY: Meetings Internationale.

Sklar, M. (Speaker). (1986). *The experience of living in a three generational family constellation: A case study* (Cassette Recording No. DII-302). Louisville, KY: Meetings Internationale.

Smith, M. J. (Moderator). (1986). *Panel discussion of research related to Man-Living-Health: Evaluation* (Cassette Recording No. DII-305). Louisville, KY: Meetings Internationale.

Smith, M. J. (Speaker). (1986). *The experience of being confined: A study using the emerging method* (Cassette Recording No. DII-304). Louisville, KY: Meetings Internationale.

Smith, M. C. (Speaker). (1990). *The lived experience of struggling through difficult times* (Cassette Recording No. DII-603). Louisville, KY: Meetings Internationale.

Theses and Dissertations Using Parse's Theory

Beauchamp, C. (1990). *The lived experience of struggling with making a decision in a critical life situation.* Unpublished doctoral dissertation, University of Miami, FL.

Brunsman, C. S. (1988). *A phenomenological study of the lived experience of hope in families with chronically ill children.* Unpublished master's thesis, Michigan State University, Lansing.

Cody, W. K. (1989). *Grieving a personal loss: A preliminary investigation of Parse's man-living-health methodology.* Unpublished master's thesis, Hunter College, City University of New York.

Dowling, T. C. (1987). *Sharing who you really are with another: A phenomenological inquiry.* Unpublished master's thesis, Hunter College, City University of New York.

Huckshorn, K. A. (1988). *The lived experience of creating a new way of being.* Unpublished master's thesis, Florida State University, Tallahassee.

Nickitas, D. M. (1989). *The lived experience of choosing among life goals: A phenomenological study.* Unpublished doctoral dissertation, Adelphi University, Garden City, NY.

Petras, E. M. (1986). *The lived experience of sharing a painful moment with someone close: A phenomenological study.* Unpublished master's thesis, Hunter College, City University of New York.

Santopinto, M. D. A. (1987). *The relentless drive to be ever thinner: A phenomenological study.* Unpublished master's thesis, University of Western Ontario, London, Ontario, Canada.

Sklar, M. B. (1985). *Qualitative investigation of the health patterns lived in an intergenerational family lifestyle.* Unpublished master's thesis, Hunter College, City University of New York.

Authors Citing Parse's Works

Batra, C. (1987). Nursing theory for undergraduates. *Nursing Outlook, 35*(4), 189-192.

Boyd, C. O. (1989). Dialogue on a research issue: Phenomenological research in nursing—response. *Nursing Science Quarterly, 2,* 16-19.

Boyd, C. O. (1990). Critical appraisal of developing nursing research methods. *Nursing Science Quarterly, 3,* 42-43.

Campbell, J. (1986). A survivor group for battered women. *Advances in Nursing Science, 8*(2), 13-20.

Cohen, M. Z. (1987). A historical overview of the phenomenological movement. *Image, 19*(1), 31-34.

Counts, M. M., & Boyle, J. S. (1987). Nursing, health, and policy within a community context. *Advances in Nursing Science, 9*(3), 12-23.

Cull-Willby, B. L., & Pepin, J. I. (1987). Toward a co-existence of paradigms in nursing knowledge development. *Journal of Advanced Nursing, 12*(4), 515-521.

DeFeo, D. J. (1990). Change: A central concern in nursing. *Nursing Science Quarterly, 3,* 88-94.

Duffy, M. E. (1986). Qualitative research: An approach whose time has come. *Nursing and Health Care, 7*(5), 237-239.

Gortner, S. R., & Schultz, P. R. (1988). Approaches to nursing science methods. *Image, 20*(1), 22-24.

Haase, J. E. (1987). Components of courage in chronically ill adolescents: A phenomenological study. *Advances in Nursing Science, 9*(2), 64-80.

Kidd, P., & Morrison, E. F. (1988). The progression of knowledge in nursing: A search for meaning. *Image: Journal of Nursing Scholarship, 20.*

Limandri, B. J. (1982). Book reviews. *Western Journal of Nursing Research, 4*(1), 105-106.

Malinski, V. M. (1990). Three perspectives on a scholarly issue. *Nursing Science Quarterly, 3,* 49-50.

Moch, S. D., & Diemert, C. A. (1987). Health promotion within the nursing environment. *Nursing Administration Quarterly, 11*(3), 9-12.

Moody, L. (1990). *Advancing nursing science through research* (Vols. 1-2). Newbury Park, CA: Sage.

Pearson, B. D. (1987). Pain control: An experiment with imagery. *Geriatric Nursing, 8*(1), 28-30.

Perry, J. (1985). Has the discipline of nursing developed to the stage where nurses do think nursing? *Journal of Advanced Nursing, 10*(1), 31-37.

Phillips, J. R. (1990). Guest editorial: New methods of research: Beyond the shadows of nursing science. *Nursing Science Quarterly, 3*, 1-2.

Ray, M. A. (1987). Technological caring: A new model in critical care. *Dimensions of Critical Care Nursing, 6*(3), 166-173.

Ray, M. A. (1990). Critical reflective analysis of Parse's and Newman's research methodologies. *Nursing Science Quarterly, 3*, 44-46.

Reed, P. G. (1986). Religiousness among terminally ill and healthy adults. *Research in Nursing and Health, 9*(1), 35-41.

Reed, P. G. (1987). Constructing a conceptual framework for psychosocial nursing. *Journal of Psychosocial Nursing and Mental Health Services, 25*(2), 24-28.

Ruffingrahal, M. A. (1985). Qualitative methods in community analysis. *Public Health Nursing, 2*, 130-137.

Sarter, B. (1987). Evolutionary idealism: A philosophical foundation for holistic nursing theory. *Advances in Nursing Science, 9*, 1-9.

Sarter, B. (1988). Philosophical sources of nursing theory. *Nursing Science Quarterly, 1*, 52-59.

Smith, M. J. (1984). Transformation: A key to shaping nursing. *Image, 16*(1), 28-30.

Smith, M. C. (1990). Nursing's unique focus on health promotion. *Nursing Science Quarterly, 3*, 105-106.

Smith, M. C. (1990). Pattern in nursing practice. *Nursing Science Quarterly, 3*, 57-59.

Thompson, J. L. (1985). Practical discourse in nursing: Going beyond empiricism and historicism. *Advances in Nursing Science, 7*(4), 59-71.

Uys, L. R. (1987). Foundational studies in nursing. *Journal of Advanced Nursing, 12*(3), 275-280.

PART VI

Margaret Newman

Health as Expanding Consciousness

JOANNE MARCHIONE

Biographical Sketch of the Nurse Theorist: Margaret Newman, RN, PhD, FAAN

Born: 1933

Current Position: Professor, School of Nursing, University of Minnesota; Nurse theorist

Education: BSHE, Home Economics and English, Baylor University, Texas; BSN, University of Tennessee, Memphis; M.S., University of California, San Francisco; PhD, New York University

Service on editorial boards: *Advances in Nursing Science, Nursing Science Quarterly, Journal of Professional Nursing, Nursing Research* (Past), *Nursing and Health Care* (Past), *Western Journal of Nursing Research* (Past)

Previous Faculty Positions: University of Tennessee, New York University, Pennsylvania State University

Honors: Fellow, American Academy of Nursing, admitted 1976; *Who's Who in American Women;* Latin American Teaching Fellow; University of Tennessee, College of Nursing, Outstanding Alumnus Award; New York University, Division of Nursing, Distinguished Alumnus Award

Foreword

I believe Margaret Newman's theory of health is the latest turn in nursing theory and represents some of the most astute thinking in contemporary nursing. In 1987, I was honored to review her book *Health as Expanding Consciousness* (Watson, 1987), which laid out her evolving theory. Now I am equally honored to do the foreword to Joanne Marchione's fine section on Newman's work.

As Newman continues to take nursing significant steps forward in transforming the old paradigm of science, nursing, and health into the new world of science, nursing, and health, Marchione's clear application of the theory to individual, family, and community health praxis helps us reach yet another level of evolution and "expanding consciousness" with respect to Newman's work.

Marchione's work reflects several years of continuous experimentation and application of Newman's theory whereby she has had the opportunity to change as the theory has changed. Thus this section comes after Marchione's sustained theoretical and experiential inquiry and dialogue with the nurse theorist. As such, it represents the latest thinking and translation of Newman's concepts of consciousness, time-space, movement, pattern recognition, pattern, and health as expanding consciousness, to praxis.

Marchione's lucid and succinct overview of Newman's theory provides both a summary and an intepretation of the theory as well as a conceptual translation that allows one to apply all of the theoretical assumptions and key concepts. She makes the theory live and breath through her straightforward presentation of case studies that transfer theoretical concepts of "pattern of the whole" to concrete application to individual and family health.

The discussion on praxis research provides an informed, contemporary perspective on the nature of appropriate, productive, and congruent research and methods of inquiry related to Newman's (and others) evolving theory. Marchione's experience and examples invite dialogue with the reader; this, in turn, has the effect of modeling both theory and method through the author-reader exchange that compiles the narrative for the text. This very process thereby mirrors the theory and praxis method being presented. Thus, in an indirect way, engaging with the ideas in the book becomes an exemplar of the very theory of expanding consciousness, which in turn has the effect of verifying and experientially validating the theory.

This work offers a special invitation for nurses and nursing to come into a new unitary relationship with theory, research, and clinical practice—a form of praxis and process that is dialogic, narrative, and evolving. To come into a new expanding health consciousness—consciousness that is evolving and whole. To come into a new form of holographic science that is pattern laden and unfolding. To come into a new form of nursing that is informed by consciousness, by process, by health and wholeness—a new form of nursing that is overtly value laden and continuous in time and space, yet transcendent of time and space. To come into a new convergence of nursing theory and nursing assessment and praxis that is choosing, communicating, exchanging, feeling, knowing, moving, perceiving, relating, and valuing of process, pattern, and expanding health consciousness. All of these "coming togethers" in Marchione's section help one to see the importance of Margaret Newman's contribution to nursing and the spin-offs her work is bringing to the nursing profession and to the broader health sciences.

The intellectual and praxis excitement of Newman's and Marchione's work is that they are open, in process, and ready to discover new patterns; they are receptive to exchange to allow emergence of the whole to unfold as this theory continues to evolve. We are all invited to participate in this excitement of unfolding, evolution, and discovery in our unitary transformative praxis of health as expanding consciousness.

JEAN WATSON, RN, PHD, FAAN
Professor of Nursing and Director of the Center for Human Caring
University of Colorado, Health Sciences Center
Denver, Colorado

Preface

Theory development in nursing is the process by which the discipline of nursing is respected as a science and is recognized for its special focus on health and human caring.

In recent times, several nurse theorists have developed diverse and respected models and theories for nursing, thus contributing to the advancement of nursing science.

Margaret Newman is one of several internationally renowned nursing theorists who have led the way in the development of nursing science. A current description of Newman's theory of health is set forth in this section. The concepts, propositions, assumptions, and practice/research applications of the theory are summarized and presented, with the advice that this section is to be viewed as a supplement to Newman's (1979, 1986) primary texts. Primary and recent writings that explicate her theory can be found in the bibliography. The references and sources cited there serve as means to encourage additional reading.

The intent of this section is to assist students in nursing to clarify concepts, identify assumptions, relate propositions, and understand practice/research applications of Newman's theory. Nursing faculty may also find the text useful for a succinct and current review of Newman's theory of health.

My sincere thanks are extended to Margaret Newman, who so generously consented to review and critique a draft of this section prior to its publication. I am especially grateful to Newman for encouraging me to engage in an independent study with her at Pennsylvania State University in 1983 and for her continued support and encouragement over the past several years.

A special thank-you is extended to Associate Professor Susan Stearns, M.S.N., of the College of Nursing, University of Akron. Her gentle advice and sensitive critiques have been vital to the completion of this project.

JOANNE MARCHIONE

Acknowledgments

For my family and friends.

In honor of the memories of my father, my Uncle Tony, and Alfalfa. The spirit and essence of each of these three special relatives were with me as I moved, in an ever-expanding consciousness, to complete this project.

In gratitude for their unconditional love, loyal friendship, and energizing encouragement, I dedicate this section to my mother, to Tony III, Anthony, Dean, Gloria, Ruby, Pauline, Adam, Angie, Camille, Gregory, Cindy, Sally, Dianne, Lori, Pam, Terri, Bradley, Mark, Ben, Echo, Sandie, Dustin, Erin, Susan, June, Mary, Bob, Gharith, and there are many others.

31

Origin of the Theory

Margaret Newman traced the origin of her theorizing on health to her prenursing days. As a young woman, Newman was influenced intuitively by her mother, who was diagnosed with amyotrophic lateral sclerosis. Newman (1986) noted while caring for her mother that although her mother was physically incapacitated she was a whole person, viewed herself like any other person, and did not consider herself ill. Later, Newman formulated the premise that illness was part of health and reflected the life pattern of a person. She arrived at this formulation through a synthesis of the knowledge gained in graduate study and her experiences with her mother. Newman claimed that nurses should recognize a person's life pattern and accept the pattern for what it means to that person. Newman first presented her theory at a nurse theorist conference in 1978. Newman (1979) first published her theory of health in a text titled *Theory Development in Nursing*. Her ideas were set forth in a chapter titled "Toward a Theory of Health."

Newman credits nurse theorists, philosophers, and scholars with influencing her work. She was stimulated by discussions with Martha Rogers, who was one of her professors when she was a graduate student in nursing at New York University. Newman (1986) claims she was "intrigued and plagued" by Rogers's statement that "health and illness are simply expressions of the life process—one no more important than the other" (p. 4). She debated with Rogers about this idea. After considerable thought, Newman (1986) came to the realization that health and illness are a single process. She likened this process to rhythmic phenomena, "manifest in ups and downs, peaks and troughs, moving through varying degrees of organization and disorganization, but all as one unitary process" (p. 4). Newman (1986) formulated this unitary process of health and illness into a concept that she called "pattern of the whole" (p. 12). She referred to this pattern of the whole as expanding consciousness. Newman (1990a) claims that her theory of health as expanding consciousness stems from Rogers's (1970) theory of unitary human beings. Rogers's assumption regarding the patterning of persons in interaction with the environment is basic to Newman's view that consciousness is a manifestation of an evolving pattern of person-environment interaction.

Other scholars who influenced Newman in the development of her theory of health were biomedical engineer Itzhak Bentov (1978), philosopher Teilhard de Chardin (1959), physicist David Bohm (1980), mathematician Arthur Young (1976a, 1976b), and physician Richard Moss (1981). Bentov's (1978) writing on the evolution of consciousness provided Newman with logical explanations for her earlier intuitive formulations. Teilhard de Chardin's (1959) proposition that a person's consciousness continues to develop beyond the physical life and becomes a part of a universal consciousness was congruent with Newman's view of health as expanding consciousness. Bohm's (1980) theory of implicate order helped Newman to frame her theory of health into a perspective of an underlying unseen pattern that manifests itself in varying forms, including disease, and in the interconnectedness and omnipresence of all that there is in life. Young's (1976a, 1976b) theory of human evolution illuminated the critical importance of pattern recognition or insight in the process of expanding consciousness (health). Young's theory provided Newman with the impetus for the integration of her basic concepts of movement, space, time, and consciousness into a dynamic portrayal of health and life. Last, the description by Moss (1981) of love as the highest level of consciousness provided Newman with an "affirmation and elaboration" of her "intuitions regarding the nature of health" (Newman, 1986, pp. 5-6).

32

Assumptions of the Theory

Assumptions are statements accepted as given truths without proof. In order to use a theory, the assumptions must be accepted by the user. Assumptions set the foundation for the application of a particular theory.

Explicit Assumptions

An explicit assumption is a statement of truth that is fully and clearly expressed. The explicit assumptions of Newman's theory flow from her proposition that health is a synthesis of disease and non-disease. According to Newman (1979), the following assumptions are considered basic to her theory:

1. Health encompasses conditions heretofore described as illness, or in medical terms, pathology.
2. These pathological conditions can be considered a manifestation of the total pattern of the individual.
3. The pattern of the individual that eventually manifests itself as pathology is primary and exists prior to structural or functional changes.
4. Removal of the pathology in itself will not change the pattern of the individual.

5. If becoming "ill" is the only way an individual's pattern can manifest itself, then that is health for that person.
6. Health is the expansion of consciousness. (pp. 56-58)

Newman (1986) later regarded the sixth assumption as *the* theory,
that is, *the* explanatory idea. It is this theory, the idea of health as
expanding consciousness, that is elaborated by Newman.

Newman assumes that pattern is "an identification of the wholeness of the person" (Newman, 1990b, p. 132). Whatever manifests
itself in a person's life is "an explication of the underlying pattern for
that person" (Newman, 1990a, p. 38). Another assumption is that
one's personal pattern is "part of a larger, undivided pattern of an
expanding universe" (Newman, 1990a, pp. 38, 40). Basic to the understanding of Newman's theory of health is the assumption that one's
personal "pattern is evolving unidirectionally . . . toward a higher
consciousness" (Newman, 1990b, p. 132).

Implicit Assumptions

Implicit assumptions are implied, rather than expressly stated,
truths and are potentially contained or suggested in the descriptions
of a theory. Implicit in Newman's theory are the two assumptions that
humans are open energy systems and that humans are in continual
interconnectedness with a universe of open systems, frequently referred to as the environment. Another implicit assumption is that
humans are continuously active in evolving their own pattern of the
whole (health). A fourth implicit assumption is that humans are
intuitive as well as cognitive and affective beings. This assumption is
in tandem with the assumption that humans are capable of abstract
thinking as well as sensation. There is also the implicit assumption
that humans are more than the sum of their parts. Many of these
assumptions were derived from Rogers's (1970) theory of unitary
human beings.

33

Concepts of the Theory

Concepts are abstract ideas that provide a focus for thinking in a particular way. All theories have their own specific set of concepts that assist the student in understanding the meaning of the particular theory and its potential applications.

The basic concepts of Newman's theory of health are *consciousness, movement, space,* and *time.* Newman (1979) postulated that these concepts are interrelated in the following way:

1. Time and space have a complementary relationship.
2. Movement is a means by which space and time become a reality.
3. Movement is a reflection of consciousness.
4. Time is a function of movement.
5. Time is a measure of consciousness. (p. 60)

In addition to these four basic concepts, *pattern recognition, pattern,* and *expanding consciousness* are three concepts that are vital to the understanding of Newman's theory of health. These concepts are defined in the following paragraphs and are discussed in relation to the four paradigm concepts of nursing: *person, environment, health,* and *nursing* (Fawcett, 1989; Newman, 1983c).

Consciousness

Consciousness is defined by Newman (1986) as the

informational capacity of the system: the capacity of the system to interact with its environment. In the human system, the informational capacity includes all of our present and developing knowledge about the nervous system, the endocrine system, the immune system, the genetic code, and so on. (p. 33)

Consciousness can be observed in the quality and diversity of inter-actions: The more complex the informational capacity and the more varied and more numerous the responses to the environment, the more highly developed is the human system.

Time-Space

Newman (1979) asserts that the world must be viewed as "a com-plicated network of interrelated changing events, as dynamic pat-terns of activity, with space aspects and time aspects" (p. 60). She insists that time and space are inextricably linked, yet one can identify aspects of each. For example, there is subjective time, objective time, time perspective, use of time, private time, coordinated time, and shared time. There is also personal space, inner space, territorial space, shared space, geographical and physical space, maneuverable space, distance-regulating space, and life space (Newman, 1979, p. 61). Newman (1979) follows Bentov's (1978) lead in the study of subjective and objective time. Time perception, or the subjective sense of passing time, has been shown to vary with time of day and is thought to be synchronized with other circadian rhythms, particu-larly body temperature. An increase in body temperature is related to the subjective sense of a greater amount of time passing than is revealed by clock time (objective time) and thus the feeling that time is dragging (Newman, 1986, p. 51).

The complementarity of time and space is viewed on different levels of analysis. Newman (1979, p. 61) uses an example from astron-omy to illustrate the concept of the complementarity of time and space at the macrocosmic and microcosmic levels of systems analysis. That is, time flows in the opposite direction from human perspectives of time in the probability of antimatter galaxies, whereas, with the possible existence of black holes in space, time and space are viewed as being wrapped up by gravitation in unimaginable ways. Subatomic particles of matter, at the microscopic level, appear to be going backward in time.

Newman (1979, 1982) has also shown through study how the complementarity of space and time can be seen in everyday events. The highly mobile individual lives in a world of expanded space and compartmentalized time. When a person's life space is decreased, as by either physical or social immobility, the person's time is increased. When physical or social life space is decreased, there is an opportunity for the person to focus attention on inner space. As a person focuses on the space within and transcends the limitations of three-dimensional space, the experience of time and the level of consciousness for that person are changed. Concepts of life space, personal space, and inner space can also be examined in relation to time to show that the concepts of space and time are inextricably linked.

Movement

Newman (1979, p. 61) defines movement as the change occurring between two states of rest. It is an essential property of matter needed to bring about change. Without movement there is no manifest reality. Movement is the manifestation of consciousness and is the fundamental unit of analysis in Newman's theory of health. Movement represents "a pivotal choice point in the evolution of human consciousness" (Newman, 1986, p. 58). The task of the choice point is discovering new rules for living. Through movement, a person "discovers the world of time-space and establishes personal territory" (Newman, 1990a, p. 39). When persons no longer have the power of physical or social movement, they are forced to go beyond themselves. As persons "are able to recognize the boundlessness and timelessness of human existence," they are free to return "to the ground of consciousness" (Newman, 1990a, p. 40). Movement is seen as an awareness of self, as a means of communicating, and as a daily mode of expression in gesture and speech.

To illustrate the manifestation of consciousness from the perspective of a person's movement, time, space, and environment interactions, Newman (1986) cited several case examples of the interaction patterns of women who were interviewed by graduate students as part of a study of adult health. Two of these examples are described below:

Case 1: Mrs. V. made repeated attempts to *move* away from her husband and to *move* into an educational program to become more independent. She felt she had no *space* for herself and she tried to distance herself (*space*) from her husband. She felt she had no *time* for leisure (self), was overworked, and was constantly meeting other people's needs. She was submissive to the demands and criticisms of her husband.

Case 2: Mrs. K. decreased her activities (*movement* outside of home (such as work and church) and appeared to be separating herself from others (building up *space* around herself). Her husband was away from home most of the time (*spatial distance*). There were indications that she was taking some form of sedatives or alcohol and slept most of the time (altering *time*) (Newman, 1986, p. 56).

In applying her theory to these cases Newman (1986) explains,

> These examples reflect a diminished sense of self as reflected in contracted, almost nonexistent space-time dimension. They illustrate the relevance of the space time dimension in the sense of self. The point of intersection of the time, space, and movement dimensions represents the pattern of consciousness, the quality and quantity of interaction. In these examples the interaction . . . could be regarded as a low level of consciousness as defined by this model. (pp. 56-57)

It is at this juncture (pivotal point) that the nurse, in mutual collaboration with both of these women, could act to facilitate their expanding consciousness through pattern recognition and the discovery of new rules as the women move beyond the physical restrictions of space and time.

Pattern Recognition

Pattern recognition is key in the process of evolving to higher levels of consciousness. It occurs instantaneously and is the realization of a truth, recognition of an insight, a principle, or an intuition (Newman, 1990a, p. 40). Insight has been "equated with the inner voice that some people consider their intuition" (Newman, 1986, p. 42). When pattern recognition occurs, it illuminates the possibilities for action. Newman (1990) uses a metaphor of being in the light or dark to describe the process of pattern recognition:

> It is like the difference between being in the dark and turning on the light: when the light comes on, one can see the possibilities for movement. Nursing facilitates this process by rhythmic connecting of the nurse with the client in an authentic way for the purpose of illuminating the pattern and discovering the new rules of a higher level of organization. (p. 40)

Pattern

Pattern is defined as relatedness, and is characterized by movement, diversity, and rhythm (Newman, 1986, p. 14). Pattern is intimately involved in energy exchange and transformation. Pattern is dynamic, in constant movement or change. The parts of pattern are diverse and are changing in relation to each other, and rhythm identifies the pattern. Pattern is recognized on the basis of variation in contrast and may not be seen all at once. Pattern unfolds over time, with one configuration evolving into the next configuration and so forth. Pattern is manifest in the way one moves, the way one speaks and talks, and the way one relates with others. The pattern of the person can be identified across space and time. Pattern identifies the wholeness of the person (Newman, 1986, p. 14; 1990a, p. 40; 1990b, p. 132).

Expanding Consciousness

Expanding consciousness is the evolving pattern of the whole. Expanding consciousness is health. It is the increasing complexity of the living system. Expanding consciousness is characterized by choice points, illuminations, and pattern recognition, resulting in a transformation and discovery of new rules of a higher organization (Newman, 1990a, p. 40).

34

Newman's Theory and Nursing's Paradigm Concepts

As Kuhn (1970) has noted, each discipline singles out certain phenomena with which it will deal in a unique manner. The concepts and propositions that identify and interrelate these phenomena comprise the paradigm of the discipline. Newman (1990b) uses the word *paradigm* to mean a worldview. The paradigm is the global perspective of a discipline and serves as a perspective from which the structure of the discipline develops.

Person, environment, health, and nursing are the four concepts that represent the basic components of nursing theory and are critical to the development of a paradigm for nursing (Fawcett, 1989; Newman, 1983b). According to Newman (1983c), "the domain of nursing has always included the nurse, the patient, the situation in which they find themselves, and the purpose of their being together, or the health of the patient" (p. 388).

The nursing theorists have placed different emphasis on each of the four basic concepts. *Person* has replaced *patient* as the concept used to represent humans. Humans are the "reason to be" for the discipline of nursing. This change in term from patient to person is reflective of the variety of settings within which nursing finds its practice domain. Newman (1979, 1986) has chosen to focus on health as the basic concept of nursing theory. In describing her theory, Newman explains person, environment, health, and nursing accordingly.

278

Person

Persons are dynamic patterns of energy and open systems in interaction with the environment. Persons are identified by their patterns
of consciousness. The person does not possess consciousness. The
person *is* consciousness (Newman, 1986, p. 33; 1990a, p. 40).

Environment

Environment is viewed as the event, situation, or phenomena with
which an individual interacts. Environment is represented as a universe of open systems. The pattern of person-environment interaction
constitutes health. These patterns of person-environment interaction
are manifest in such observable phenomena as body temperature,
pulse, and blood pressure; regimens of diet, rest, and exercise; neoplasms and biochemical variations; social relations and communications; cognition and emotions (Newman, 1986, p. 13).

A comprehensive portrayal of person-environment interactions
can be gleaned from the nine dimensions of the North American
Nursing Diagnostic Association (NANDA) assessment framework:
exchanging, communicating, perceiving, relating, choosing, moving,
valuing, feeling, and knowing (Kim & Moritz, 1982). These nine
dimensions are defined and illustrated later in this section.

Health

Health is the expanding of consciousness. Health is constituted by
the pattern of person-environment interaction. Health is *the evolving
pattern of the whole of life.* (This is the crux of Newman's theory.) Health
is the synthesis of disease/nondisease. Health is the process of transformation to higher levels of consciousness (Newman, 1979, 1986).

Nursing

Newman (1986) identified the critical task for gaining an understanding of her theory of health as the ability to view the concepts of

movement-space-time in relation to each other, simultaneously, as patterns of expanding consciousness. She sees the goal of nursing as one of assisting "people to utilize the power that is within them as they evolve toward higher levels of consciousness" (Newman, 1979, p. 67). Nursing practice, according to Newman, "is directed toward recognizing the pattern of the person in interaction with the environment and accepting it as a process of evolving consciousness" (Newman, 1986, p. 88). Nursing facilitates the process of pattern recognition by a "rhythmic connecting of the nurse with the client in an authentic way for the purpose of illuminating the pattern and discovering the new rules of a higher level of organization" (Newman, 1990a, p. 40).

Newman (1986) calls for nursing to employ a partnership model of nonintervention. She describes this relationship:

> The professional enters into a partnership with the client with the mutual goal of participating in an authentic relationship, trusting that in the process of its evolving, both will grow and become healthier in the sense of higher levels of consciousness. (p. 68)

According to Newman (1990b), "people need a partner" in the process of expanding consciousness," particularly when they are suffering and do not find any meaning in what is going on" (p. 136). Mutuality is key to the nurse-client partner relationship. Mutuality between nurse and client occurs in the process of the nurse's assisting the client in making and implementing the choices that emerge through pattern recognition (Newman, 1990b). The nurse connects with a client when the client is faced with a situation that she or he does not know how to handle, or when he or she is searching for new rules when old rules for living no longer work. The nurse releases the desire to control the situation, interacts with the client, shares his or her consciousness, and helps to identify the pattern that is manifest. The task of the nurse is to be free of a predetermined agenda, to be present with the client as the possibilities for transformation emerge, and to support the client as she or he makes decisions and choices (Newman, 1990b, pp. 136-137).

35

Propositions

Propositions are ideas brought forward for consideration, acceptance, or adoption. They are declarations of the design or intention of a theory. They are statements of truth to be demonstrated or operations to be performed.

The fundamental proposition in Newman's model is the view that health and illness are synthesized as health. In this proposition, Newman (1979, 1986) applies Hegelian dialectical logic; that is, "that thought proceeds by contradiction and the recognition of contradiction, the overall pattern being one of thesis, antithesis and synthesis" (Flew, 1984, p. 94). Newman proposes that one state of being (disease) unites with its opposite (nondisease) resulting in a synthesis of the two. The fusion of these two antithetical concepts brings forth a synthesis that can be regarded as health (Newman, 1979, p. 56).

The proposition that health is to be viewed as an evolving pattern of the whole is basic to the understanding of Newman's theory of health. Newman (1986) explains,

> The emerging paradigm of health is pattern recognition. It involves moving from looking at parts to looking at patterns. The pattern is information that depicts the whole, understanding of the meaning of all the relationships at once. It is a fundamental attribute of all there is and gives unity in diversity. (p. 13)

This conceptualization of health as pattern also finds root in Rogers's (1970) theory of unitary man. Rogers's insistence that health and illness are simply manifestations of the rhythmic fluctuations of the life process led Newman to the view that health and illness are a unitary process moving through variations in order-disorder. From this perspective it is no longer possible to view health as a continuum extending from illness to wellness. The illness-wellness continuum is part of the worldview of health as the absence of disease, because as one moves toward the wellness end of the continuum, one moves away from disease by either preventing the disease or promoting behaviors that are thought to promote health (Newman, 1990b). According to Newman's view, health encompasses disease as a meaningful aspect of health. In this view then, health and the evolving pattern of consciousness are one and the same (Newman, 1990a).

36

Overview of Newman's Theory

Newman (1979, 1986) posits that health is process. She claims that pattern is the essence of a holistic view of health. In this view, health is the flow of life. It is a kaleidoscopic evolution of patterning, with contradictions, ambiguities, and paradoxes, continually synthesized into insights that lead to an ever expanding consciousness (transformation). Movement is fundamental to this dialectical process of transformation. Pattern recognition is a spontaneous insight in relation to a shift in organizational complexity, affording greater freedom and variety of responses to any given situation. Expanding consciousness occurs as a process of pattern recognition (insights) following a synthesis of contradictory events or disturbances in the flow of daily living. Disease and nondisease serve as reflections of a larger whole. The proposition that health is the synthesis of disease and nondisease is a revolutionary way of conceptualizing health.

Newman (1986, 1990a, p. 39) describes the parallels between her theory of health as expanding consciousness and Young's (1976b) theory of the evolution of consciousness. For instance, Young claims that humans enter this world with a state of potential freedom and move through several stages of loss of degrees of freedom as they descend into a deterministic physical world. Young calls his first stage the stage of binding. In the binding stage, a person is bound into the larger network of the whole in which everything is regulated, and the individual is sacrificed for the good of the whole. There is very little individual identity or choice in the binding stage. The binding stage is followed by the centering stage, whereby a person establishes an identity, self-consciousness, and self-determination. In this centering stage, the self breaks with the authority of the binding stage. The centering stage is a competitive, persuasive stage in which a person seeks to gain power over others and gain power for him- or herself. The turning point is the stage called choice. In this stage, the things that worked in the past no longer work. What was formerly considered progress is no longer seen as progress. It is in the choice stage that the individual must master the task of learning new rules. Reformation or transformation is preceded by a realization of self-limitation. It is this realization that makes it possible for persons to begin the evolution back to freedom by going beyond themselves and entering into the stages of decentering and unbinding.

Newman (1990a) illustrates the similarity between her theory of health as expanding consciousness and Young's (1976b) evolving consciousness theory, as shown in Figure 36.1.

According to Newman (1990a),

> A person comes into being from the ground of consciousness and loses freedom as one is bound in time and finds one's identity in space. Matters of time-space are very much involved in one's struggles for self-determination and status. Movement represents the choice point. It is central to understanding the nature of reality. Through movement one discovers the world of time-space and establishes personal territory. It is also when movement is restricted that one becomes aware of personal limitations and the fact that the old rules don't work anymore. When one no longer has the power of movement (either physical or social), it is necessary to go beyond oneself. As one is able to recognize the boundarylessness and timelessness of human existence, one gains the freedom of returning to the ground of consciousness. (pp. 39-40)

To illustrate this process, Newman (1986) describes the restrictions of her own mobility and her transformation in terms of space and time during her experience as primary caregiver for her mother, who was incapacitated with amyotrophic lateral sclerosis. Not only was Newman's mother not free to move about in space or to control her own time, these restrictions also applied to Newman. The freedom to come and go as and when she chose was no longer an option. Usually taken for granted, these mobility options are altered by situations and

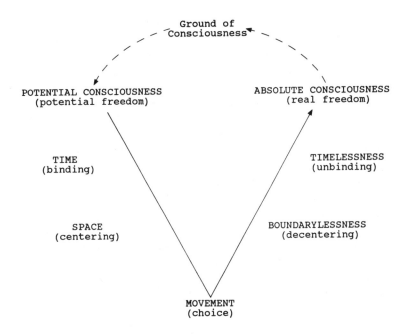

Figure 36.1. Parallel between Newman's theory of expanding consciousness and Young's stages of human evolution.
SOURCE: Adapted from "Newman's Theory of Health as Praxis," by M. A. Newman, 1990, *Nursing Science Quarterly, 3*(1), p. 39. Copyright 1990 by Chestnut House Publications. Reprinted with permission.

circumstances that render imprudent or impossible the freedom of movement. According to Newman (1986), restrictions of movement force a person into a realm beyond space and time. The old rules for relating no longer work. Persons find themselves faced with their selves and their own inner resources. They are confronted with the quality of their relationships and their ability to live in the present. Given these circumstances, the developmental task involves becoming open to the transformation, allowing it to occur as the person transcends space and time and moves to higher consciousness.

West (1984) observed this process in mothers of developmentally disabled children. Even though the mothers' care responsibilities of their disabled children restricted their independent movement outside the family, these mothers were able to compensate by constructing activities in which the family "moved" together. Time and space were undifferentiated by these mothers. Their days were usually filled with caring responsibilities. They discovered that time was not something they could control. They also noted that it was important to live one day at a time, that is, in the present dimension.

Caregivers of impaired or incapacitated family members have recently become the object of nursing's concern (Klein, 1989; Robinson, 1990). This concern has been expressed in the form of respite care. Respite care is temporary care of the impaired family member, provided by a professional, aimed at helping to relieve the burden of the caregiver by affording her or him the opportunity for freedom of movement. Family caregivers, especially the spouse or parent of an impaired family member, often experience restricted movement in the form of social isolation, career interruptions, financial drain, and lack of space-time for self, other family members, and friends. Newman's (1979, 1986) theory of health provides nursing with insights for an understanding of the movement restrictions of these family caregivers, and suggests directions for assisting them in finding new rules for living and transcending their movement restrictions.

37

Evolving the Pattern of the Whole

Newman (1987) claims that pattern recognition comes from within the observer, which means that with any set of data or sequence of events, "an infinite number of patterns are possible" (p. 38). Patterns unfold in time and cannot be predicted with certainty, because the additional information has not happened yet. The evolving pattern of the person is best portrayed as sequential patterns over time. To illustrate a person's pattern of the whole, Newman (1987) described a case of a client experiencing a crisis event. The example was obtained from the caseload of a community health nursing colleague. The analysis of the unfolding pattern is portrayed in three time frames: prior to the crisis, immediately following the crisis event, and fifteen weeks after the crisis.

A Case Study: Client K

This is the description of client K's pattern: She was a young divorced woman who was solely responsible for the care of her two preschool-aged children. K's means of support was generated through her provision of day care for three other preschool children and an infant. The event that brought K to the attention of the nurse was the sudden death of the infant while K was caring for him in her home. Shortly after the infant's death, the nurse contacted the client and offered information about Sudden Infant Death Syndrome (SIDS). The client asked for help in relating to her own two children, aged 2 and 5, who had witnessed the event and who had since manifested behavior changes. When the nurse visited the home, she found it in complete disarray. The children were fighting with each other and their mother. K complained of insomnia, fatigue, and loss of interest in her children. She was tearful and expressed a desire to be alone. The nurse provided suggestions for immediate action in relation to the children and was instrumental in steering K toward a SIDS support group. K later reported that she had received considerable comfort as a result of her attendance at the support group meetings.

The nurse maintained periodic contact with K. On visiting the home 15 weeks after the SIDS event, the nurse found that although K was still sad about the infant's death she had begun to reach out (move) to others in her family and in the community. She had obtained an instructor's license in cardiopulmonary resuscitation (CPR) and was already teaching a CPR class. K volunteered to serve on a local health service board. She helped present a program about SIDS for day-care providers, made contact with baby-sitters who had had similar experiences with SIDS, and arranged for the distribution of printed information about SIDS to licensed day-care providers.

Prior to the SIDS event, K was feeling bored with her life. She was relatively isolated from adult interactions. Contacts with her ex-husband were limited, and she was not close to her family of origin, even though her mother and brother lived nearby. At the time the nurse entered the situation, K's pattern of interaction could be described as one of disorganization. She expressed feelings of sadness and guilt related to the infant death and was frustrated with her child-care responsibilities. As she moved to a new level of consciousness through a synthesis of the SIDS experience and her interactions with the nurse and the SIDS support group, she was able to develop a new set of rules for living. For the first time, she was able to reach out for assistance to her mother-in-law, who began to participate with her in the care of the children. She reported that she had maintained a friendship with the parents of the infant who died suddenly. She encouraged her children to openly discuss the experience of the infant's death and to ask questions freely. K also expressed the feeling that she had become more outgoing and caring in her relationships with other people.

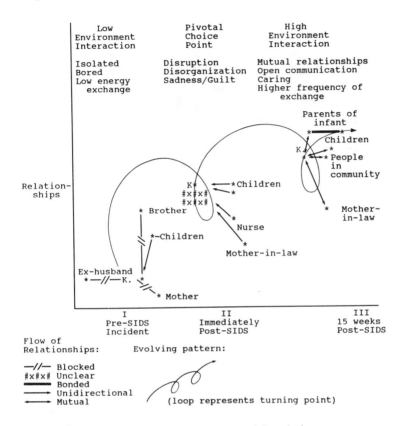

Figure 37.1. Case study of client K: Pattern of the whole.
SOURCE: Adapted from "Patterning," by M. Newman, 1987, p. 42 in M. Duffy and N. Pender (Eds.), *Conceptual Issues in Health Promotion: Report of Proceedings of a Wingspread Conference*, Indianapolis: Sigma Theta Tau. Reprinted by permission.

A diagram of three sequential patterns from client K's life can be seen in Figure 37.1.

The first pattern is seen as a relatively closed space-time, low-energy system in which K existed, almost entirely alone, with the young children in her life. Immediately following the death of the infant, her pattern is marked by disruption and disorganization. K begins to move through the events and confronts her feelings and the children's behavior changes. This period can be viewed as a beginning of the turning point for K. As she interacts with the nurse and the support group, she completes the turning point to discover new rules for relating with her environment. This discovery is depicted in the third pattern, which, for K, is one of reaching out to others to receive and give help. K has moved from a pattern of low energy to a higher-energy exchange between herself and her environment and, in so doing, has increased the quality of her relationships. In viewing this case study through the lens of Newman's theory, one can describe K's pattern of the whole as an increase in the quality of her family and community relationships and a transforming sense of self—an expanding consciousness.

38

Framework for Assessing the Pattern of the Whole

Newman (1986, 1987) has suggested that the assessment framework developed by nurse theorists for the North American Nursing Diagnostic Association (NANDA) can be used in initial efforts to identify pattern of the whole. Manifestations of the unitary pattern are expressed in the dimensions of the NANDA framework: exchanging, communicating, valuing, relating, choosing, moving, perceiving, feeling, and knowing.

Newman (1986, p. 74) has defined these nine assessment dimensions relative to her theory of health, as modified from those accepted by the nurse theorist group at the third and fourth conferences of NANDA (Kim & Moritz, 1982). Exchanging involves the interchange of energy and matter between person and environment. It also involves the transformation of energy from one form to another. Communicating involves the interchange of information from one system to another. Relating is the process of connecting with other persons and with the environment. Valuing is the process of assigning worth. Choosing involves the selection of one or more alternatives. Moving is the process of rhythmic alternating between activity and rest. Perceiving is the process of receiving and interpreting information. Feeling involves a sensing of physical and intuitive awareness. Knowing is the process of personal recognition of self and world.

The process of assessing the pattern of the whole proceeds in the following fashion: The nurse surveys the client-environment inter-action data in terms of the nine assessment dimensions, describes a nonjudgmental pattern of interaction, and searches for the underlying pattern of the whole. A case study illustrating this assessment process can be found in Newman's 1984 *American Journal of Nursing* article. A description of the case study assessment data, gathered from the client, using the NANDA framework, and interpreted from the perspective of Newman's theory, is included here.

A Case Study: Client X

Ms. X is 40 years old and is the youngest of five sisters. She is currently on a leave of absence from a recently acquired secretarial job due to right arm and right breast edema that interfered with her ability to work. She is 20 pounds overweight and does not engage in any routine exercise or recreation, even though she had formerly been a dancing instructor. She reverses the few decisions her husband makes and speaks angrily about him, describing him as a passive, incompetent person who is incapable of decision making. It is unclear to what extent she communicates this perception and anger to her husband. She says he is the only kind of man that she could live with because he provides her with the freedom to act alone and to do what she wants.

She speaks little of her two sons, who are 12 and 14 years of age. When she does mention them, her comments are also filled with criticism. Ms. X also describes her father, who is now dead, as a passive and invisible person.

Ms. X lost her mother to multiple myeloma. Ms. X was her mother's sole care provider during the last 3 months of her illness. She speaks frequently of her mother.

She views her nuclear family as totally dependent on her and presents herself as a martyr. For instance, she must take care of the house, clothing, and cooking with little assistance from her sons and husband.

She claims she is fatigued and has difficulty sleeping, suppressing her problems during the day and awakening during the night to ponder them. She has designated Saturday mornings as her private space-time and prohibits any intrusions. She indicates that she does not have friends. She makes phone visits with her sisters, but they are geographically distant. Her nieces have come to assist her during previous illnesses.

Her boss describes her as a creative, self-directive, and capable woman, who appears engrossed and stoic, yet tense beneath the surface. Outside the work setting, she does not associate with co-workers, although at work she is sensitive to their needs.

She has had two previous hospital admissions. Once, at age 20, she was admitted for dysmenorrhea, diagnosed with endometriosis, and told that she would be unable to conceive children. She had no trouble conceiving her two sons. She was hospitalized for a possible hysterectomy at age 36 but was found to have a right ovarian cyst. A right oophorectomy was performed instead. Following this surgery, she continued to experience painful dysmenorrhea and irregular periods. She disagreed with the surgeon's claim that it was not necessary to do the hysterectomy and was very distressed that it was not done.

According to Newman (1984), the data obtained from clients tend to cluster within two or three dimensions of the NANDA schema. The experienced nurse may identify the emerging pattern without collecting data in every dimension of the assessment framework. Even though many aspects of the life pattern of Ms. X are unknown, the experienced nurse may begin to visualize the emerging pattern (nursing diagnosis) even with only the sparsest of data. Newman (1984) identified the emerging pattern for Ms. X: retention of energy, characterized by trapped fluid in the right arm and breast, excess fat, and anger and self-pity; repulsion and control of others, characterized by criticism, distancing, and self sacrifice; and internal conflict with minimal channels for expression.

A more detailed account of this case can be seen in Table 38.1 (developed by Newman, 1982), depicting specific observations and organized according to the nine assessment dimensions described above. The assessment framework, based on a unitary pattern of person-environment interactions, provides a holistic approach toward nursing diagnosis. Ms. X's hospitalization may be viewed as a choice point. The task that Ms. X is now facing is how to discover new rules for engaging in meaningful, reciprocal relationships. She may not know how. This is where the nurse, through a mutual negotiation with the client, may help her to get in touch with her pattern of blocked energy. Through a process of mutual authentic relating, the nurse can facilitate the insight, the discovery of new rules for

TABLE 38.1 The Emerging Pattern of Ms. X

Dimension	Observation	Emerging Pattern
Exchanging	History of endometriosis. Right oophorectomy, cyst removal. Overweight 20 pounds. Trapped fluid in right arm and breast.	Retention.
Communicating	Directive, corrective, and critical communication with husband and sons. Maintains distance with co-workers with only business level interactions.	Repels outflow, distancing via space and time, building tension with no outlet.
Relating	Subordinate relationship to boss, dominant relationship to husband and sons, unclear relationship with sisters. No friends. Previous commitment to mother. Disregard of husband and father. Distances self from family.	Vertical relationships with distancing; bonding more easily with women than with men.
Valuing	Being alone. Doing what she wants to do. Being in control. Doing a good job.	Centered on self.
Choosing	To assume full responsibility for care of mother. To stay married to a man whom she does not respect. To work in subordinate role. To make family decisions on her own.	Unilateral. Apparently without any consideration of the alternatives.
Moving	Performs household tasks. Moved to sedentary job from job of dance teacher. Fatigued—insomnia. Arm restricted, can't do job.	Restricted. Diminished.
Perceiving	Sees husband as incompetent, physician as wrong, sisters as uncaring, self as responsible, and self-sacrificing.	Selective, self-centered.

TABLE 38.1 (Continud)

Dimension	Observation	Emerging Pattern
Feeling	Fatigue. Edema discomfort. Appears tense underneath calm. Dissatisfied, angry with regard to family relationships. Absence of self-regard. Previous dysmenorrhea.	Internal unrest.
Knowing	Recollects mother's illness and death. Suppresses concerns during day, tries to think them through at night. Knows something is wrong physically. Knows how to meet other people's needs but little about herself.	Internal turmoil. Lack of clarity regarding self.

SOURCE: Adapted from "Nursing Diagnosis: Looking at the Whole," by M. Newman, 1984, *American Journal of Nursing, 84*(12), 1496-1499. Copyright 1984 by American Journal of Nursing. Reprinted by permission.
NOTE: Newman no longer uses a table format to represent patterning of the whole.

living, and the empowerment that Ms. X needs to transform her emerging pattern into an evolving of health as expanding consciousness (Newman, 1984).

Practitioners in clinical settings may find the case of Ms. X useful in applying and interpreting the NANDA framework as Newman has defined it. However, it is necessary to note that the table in the 1982 *American Journal of Nursing* article was one of Newman's earliest attempts to illustrate a clinical example of the NANDA assessment framework relative to the identification of pattern. She has now revised her thinking on the use of this table illustration and claims that a better way to represent the emerging pattern of the whole is to record the development of sequential patterns over time (as seen in Figure 37.1). Table 38.1, depicting data from client X, fails to show the pattern in sequence. In critique of Table 38.1, Newman notes that the table combines information nonsequentially from different phases of Ms. X's life and, as such, does not reveal the emerging pattern. She claims that the organization of data in this way implies a more mechanical method of determining pattern than is actually the case. Her current thinking on pattern depiction is to organize data in a narrative form and let the pattern "fall out" from the data (Newman, personal communication, June 11 and July 4, 1991).

It may be of interest to students of nursing theory to see that the task of pattern identification/recognition is still being worked out by Newman. The 1982 journal article, chronicling the case study of Ms. X, as illustrated in Table 38.1, serves as a beginning point in the evolution of Newman's thinking on this task. She continues to work out better ways to discover this process of pattern recognition and to illustrate the emerging pattern of the whole.

Kalb (1990) applied Newman's theory of health and the pattern recognition model in a program of care developed with high-risk pregnant women who were hospitalized with adverse physiological manifestations of maternal-fetal health. For these women, their high-risk pregnancy represented a critical event that yielded alterations in their physical and social world. The alterations in each woman's pattern of health required energy from the environment to produce a higher level of organization and a new level of consciousness. Through the intervention of pattern recognition, Kalb (1990) claimed, the nurses caring for these women with high-risk pregnancy provided a source of the environmental energy.

Kalb (1990) portrayed the manifestations of pattern in pregnancy using, as her framework, the four concepts of Newman's theory of health: movement, time, space, and consciousness. The alterations created by pregnancy include changes in a woman's pattern of movement. Pregnant women move more slowly. The pregnant woman's perceptions are altered by hormonal changes that lead to feelings of fatigue. These feelings of fatigue may have significant effects on the woman's ability to continue her previous pattern of interaction with the environment and the control she has previously been able to maintain in the quality of her interactions. A woman's perceptions of her own rhythmicity and movement may be altered by the awareness of her unborn child's pattern of activity and movement, as well as the circadian pattern of the woman's uterine activity and contractions.

The pregnant woman's perception of time is frequently altered as she anticipates the birth of her child. Time seems to drag, especially in the third trimester when movement is slowed and fatigue is increased. Personal tempo and time experience of the pregnant woman may follow the basic rhythm or pattern used throughout the woman's life experiences and are linked to space and movement.

As the pregnancy continues and the unborn child develops, the woman's size and shape are altered and become larger. This increased body space frequently results in an altered self-image. It is also interesting to consider the space-time-movement-laden language used in describing a woman's pregnancy. Movement-space-time connotations are exemplified: for example, in the phrase "expected date of confinement." The notion of restricted movement and the perceptions of altered space-time during the experience of pregnancy are images explicitly created by our language (Kalb, 1990).

The awareness of new sensations within the pregnant woman's body, the feelings of fetal movement, the hormonal fluctuations, the alterations of her own bodily rhythms, and the synchronicity of self with the unborn child are all manifestations of an altered pattern of consciousness. Alterations in patterns of interaction with her partner, significant others, and in her internal and external environment are also critical attributes of consciousness in the woman's evolving pattern of pregnancy.

Pregnant women who are hospitalized for high-risk complications also experience changing patterns of movement, space, and time. Movement is restricted to bed or within the room, nursing unit, or hospital and may be further limited by the length of an intravenous tubing. Time becomes routinized according to the hospital schedule, as in prescribed times for visitors, vital signs, meals, grooming, nursing shift changes, and so on. The woman's typical routine, such as having baby showers, attending childbirth classes, and preparing a room for the baby, are frequently suspended during her hospital confinement. In the hospital, the pregnant woman must share space with nonsignificant others; is confined in an unfamiliar environment; separated from her partner, family, and friends; and is often forced to spend time alone or interacting with strangers. Her perceptions of space are often altered by the viewpoint of always being in a reclining or sitting position. Her awareness is shifted abruptly to self and to the unborn child's well-being. As the woman's perceptions of movement, time, and space are altered in the management of her high-risk pregnancy, her capacity to interact with her environment changes, thus indicating changes in her level of consciousness.

Kalb (1990) described a Minnesota hospital program, based on the concept of pattern recognition, designed for high-risk women to actively participate in the monitoring and management of their pre-term labor. The women, in partnership with a nurse, learn to recognize and identify the physical manifestations of pregnancy that they are experiencing and to integrate the characteristics of their experiences into their pattern of the whole. They are taught to keep a diary of self-palpations of uterine activity and contractions and pulse rates. Based on this record, the women are taught to self-administer subcutaneous drug therapy (terbutaline, a tocolytic medication) for labor control. The client, as "partner with the nurse and active participant in the experience of managing her high-risk pregnancy, is able to recognize and describe her pattern of the whole" (Kalb, 1990, p. 179). Therefore, the client with a high-risk pregnancy responds more fully in synchrony with her own pattern.

Recently, Newman, Lamb, and Michaels (1991) selected Carondelet Health Center in Tuscon, Arizona, as their demonstration site to show how Newman's theory of health applies to nursing care delivery in the new nursing role of the case manager. These authors recommend the blending of theory and practice as an initial step toward defining and documenting the nursing practice needed to satisfy third-party payers. The bibliography contains other examples of applications of Newman's theory in clinical settings.

39

Newman's Theory and Family Health

Newman (1983b) extended her theory of health as expanding consciousness to explain the health of the family. According to Newman, family health is the expansion of consciousness of the family. Consciousness for the family system is the increase in the quantity and quality of responses of the family members manifested in greater spontaneity within the family. The spontaneous interactive pattern of the family, expressed through movement, is seen as a manifestation of expanding consciousness.

Family space, time, and movement dimensions have been reconceptualized in terms of the family. Family applications of Newman's theory of health can be found in a chapter by Marchione (1986b) in Winstead Fry's edited text titled *Case Studies in Nursing Theory*. A community application is also described by Marchione (1986a) in her supplemental chapter to the Newman (1986) text.

40

Research and Newman's Theory

Newman's (1966) earliest research effort was qualitative in nature, based on individualized, reciprocal interaction with hospitalized patients, and it incorporated her thoughts and feelings as factors that made a difference in the findings. Newman intended to identify needs of patients (content), but in the course of doing so, the more significant finding was the process used in identifying the needs. That particular study "contributed directly to the knowledge of nursing practice," and Newman (1990a) claims, "it was also personally meaningful [to her] as the investigator" as well as "to the patients who participated as subjects" (p. 37).

Later, Newman (1972, 1976) converted holistic parameters of a person's living experience into manipulable artifacts in the laboratory in an attempt to test several very basic relationships of movement, time, and consciousness. The outcomes of these studies were tangential to the meaningful experiences that were their source. The aspect of her research that stimulated insight regarding the relevance to nursing practice was the debriefing interviews in which Newman sought a greater understanding of the person's experiences in movement-time-space. She continued to pursue this line of investigation in an attempt to demonstrate the expansion of consciousness with age (Newman, 1982; Newman & Gaudiano, 1984). She claims her inability in these studies to adequately capture the major variables or to rule out intervening variables raised questions regarding the validity of the methods to test the theory and pointed her toward other modes of inquiry. Gradually, she moved to a method of inquiry that was consistent with her theoretical assumptions, that is, the open, interactive nature of the evolving pattern. She concluded that the important part of her research was the process involved in interacting with patients. Newman (1990a) asserts that "the *process* in nursing, and in nursing research, is the *content*" (p. 38).

Newman (1983a) proposes that pattern recognition is the appropriate method for nursing research. In an editorial to the readers of *Advances in Nursing Science*, she calls for nurse researchers to use the method of pattern in the development of nursing knowledge.

Schorr, Farnham, and Ervin (1991) used Newman's theory of health as expanding consciousness in their study of the phenomenon of powerlessness among aging women. Using a survey design and quantitative analysis, they sought to identify a pattern of relationships among the impact of chronic illness, frame of temporal reference, death anxiety, hopelessness, and powerlessness. Among their sample of 60 women, ranging in age from 65 to 93 years, they found that a majority of the women manifested high levels of perceived situational control or powerfulness. The majority of their subjects, using their chronic illnesses, diminished functional ability, and decreased control over daily activities as choice points, synthesized this situation into a pattern of powerfulness and hopefulness for the future. It was not stated whether the clients in this study synthesized their choice points as a result of their partnerships with a nurse or whether the synthesis occurred independently. The authors interpreted their findings of powerfulness and hopefulness patterns in aging women as reflections of expanding consciousness and awareness of health as the pattern of the whole (Schorr et al., 1991, p. 62).

Recently, Newman (1990a) described the elements of a qualitative praxis research method that are necessary to elaborate the pattern of a person's expanding consciousness. These elements are (a) establishing the mutuality of the process of inquiry, (b) focusing on the most meaningful persons and events in the interviewee's life, (c) organizing the data in narrative form and displaying it as sequential patterns over time, and (d) a sharing of the interviewer's perception of the pattern with the interviewee and seeking revision or confirmation.

According to Newman (1990a), in praxis research the interviewees gain insight into their own pattern and concomitant illumination of their action possibilities. These insights and illuminations are inherent in the research process. Praxis research requires negotiation, reciprocity, and empowerment. Praxis research requires a mutual relationship between interviewee and researcher. These are the characteristics of praxis whereby research, practice, and theory are inseparable.

Moch's (1990) study is one example of the use of praxis research. Her research was designed for the purpose of describing and explaining the manifestation of health in illness. She collaborated with 20 women, ranging in age from 38 to 60 years, who had experienced breast cancer. The women were asked to describe their experiences with breast cancer through two open-ended interviews. Patterns of their person-environment interaction were identified by extracting themes from the interview data. Changes in their relatedness to others and to the environment were apparent as a predominant theme. The women experienced increasing richness in their relatedness to others. They were increasingly receptive to and felt closer to others, particularly members of their family; they were more open to experiencing others' expressions of caring. As they became aware of their own mortality, they found new meaning and value in their lives. They were more open to their surroundings and experienced greater enjoyment in life. These manifestations of the increasing quality and diversity of their lives are examples of their expanding consciousness in the experience of breast cancer.

Regardless of the level of disease or disability of given persons, the action potential of their patterns of interaction focus on their relationships with other people. The task they are facing is how to engage in meaningful, reciprocal relationships through the discovery of new rules. They want to talk about things that are important to them, to express a full range of emotions, and to be truly themselves. But often they do not know how. According to Newman (1990a), it is at this point that nursing, using praxis research, comes into the picture. Praxis research involves a mutuality between researcher and interviewee. This research method is an embodiment of negotiation, reciprocity, and empowerment. Through praxis research nurses can assist people in discovering the new rules and in recognizing the action potential of the pattern, thus opening the way for transformation and for the unfolding of a higher level of consciousness. Praxis research intertwines theory, practice, and research. As Lather (1986) has explained, in praxis research there must be an intersection between people's self-understanding and the researcher's theoretical stance, which seeks to provide a change-enhancing context. The praxis researcher seeks theory that grows out of context-embedded data. Nurse researchers are urged to use praxis research to help participants understand and change their situations. Newman's theory of health as expanding consciousness is conducive to the method of praxis research (Newman, 1990a).

Newman and Moch (in press) applied praxis research, explicating Newman's theory of health, in a recent study of person-environment patterns of 11 people with coronary heart disease (CHD). The study emphasized the meaning of the disruption that CHD represented for each person. Narratives of evolving patterns of meaning based on the clients' descriptions were later confirmed or revised by the clients. Similarities in meaningful patterns described by the clients who participated in the study were (a) a sense of who they were, (b) a need to develop better relationships with members of their family, and (c) the desire to discover new ways of living.

The mutual process of pattern recognition in this study was seen as a rhythmic coming together and moving apart of client and nurse in a shared consciousness until the client was able to see clearly and take action to express her or his meaning. This method of cooperative inquiry was recommended as a model for nursing research and practice.

41

Conclusion

In this section, the Newman theory of health as expanding consciousness has been explained. Major propositions, assumptions, and concepts of the theory have been identified, described, and defined. Case studies have been included to illustrate the application of the theory in practice. Research applications by Newman and others have been noted. Newman's praxis research method has been explicated.

Newman's theory of health can be useful as a guide for nursing practice and research. The praxis research method identified by Newman has begun to take hold in academic and practice settings. According to Newman (1990a), current research focuses on the unfolding pattern of person-environment over time and incorporates the authentic involvement of the nurse researcher as a participant with the client in the process of expanding consciousness.

Newman's (1986) book on the theory of health as expanding consciousness has been critiqued by Watson (1987), Cowling (1988), Pearson (1988), Silva (1988), and Smith (1990). Newman's theory of health as praxis research has been critiqued by Boyd (1990), Ray (1990), and Batey (1991). Readers are encouraged to study the original writings of Newman and the critiques of her works for a complete understanding of this revolutionary theory of health.

Glossary

Consciousness

Consciousness is the informational capacity of the system (individual, family, or community). It is the ability of the system to interact with the environment. Consciousness includes cognitive and affective awareness, and the interconnectedness of the entire living system, which includes growth processes and physiochemical maintenance as well as the immune system, the genetic code, the nervous system, and so on. Consciousness is an indivisible pattern of information that is part of a larger undivided pattern of an expanding universe (Newman, 1986, p. 33; 1990a, p. 38).

Environment

Environment is represented as a universe of open systems. Environment is an energy field, and is viewed as the event, situation, or phenomena with which an individual interacts. The pattern of environment-person interaction constitutes health. Manifestations of the environment-person interaction are seen in such observable phenomena as body temperature, pulse, and blood pressure; neoplasms and biochemical variations; regimens of diet, rest, and exercise; social relations, communications, cognition, and emotions (Newman, 1986, p. 13). A comprehensive portrayal of patterns of person-environment interaction can be viewed through the nine assessment dimensions of the North American Nursing Diagnosis

Association framework, that is, exchanging, communicating, valuing, relating, choosing, moving, perceiving, feeling, and knowing
(Kim & Moritz, 1982). In this glossary these terms are defined separately under the concept "NANDA Assessment Framework."

Expanding Consciousness

Expanding consciousness is the evolving pattern of the whole. Expanding consciousness is the increasing complexity of the living
system. Expanding consciousness is characterized by a choice point,
an illumination, and pattern recognition, resulting in a transformation and discovery of new rules of a higher level of organization.
Expanding consciousness is health (Newman, 1990a, p. 40).

Health

Health is the expanding of consciousness. Health is the evolving
pattern of the whole of life. (This is the crux of Newman's theory.)
Health is a synthesis of disease-non-disease. Health is the process of
transformation to higher levels of consciousness (Newman, 1979,
p. 58; 1990a, p.40).

Hegelian Dialectical Logic

Dialectic is a term derived from the Greek word that means to con-
verse or to discourse. The dialectic that is ascribed to the Greek
philosopher Socrates is close to this sense. It refers to his conversa-
tional method of argument, involving thought as question and answer. Hegel, a late 18th- and early 19th-century philosoper, described
a pattern of dialectical logic that thought must follow. Hegel argued
that thought proceeds by contradiction and the reconciliation of
contradiction. This dialectical logic and overall pattern of thought is
one of thesis, antithesis, and synthesis. For Hegel, thought is reality,
and the laws that thought must follow are also the laws that govern
reality (Flew, 1984, p. 94).

Movement

Movement is the change occurring between two states of rest. It is an
essential property of matter needed to bring about change. Movement
represents the choice point in transcending physical determinism.
Movement is central to understanding the nature of reality. Movement is a manifestation of consciousness. Movement is an awareness
of self and a means of communicating (Newman, 1979, pp. 61-63;
1990a, p. 39).

NANDA Assessment Framework

Nurse theorists developed a framework for the North American Nursing Diagnostic Association (NANDA) by delineating nine assessment dimensions for use in nursing diagnosis (Kim & Moritz, 1982). Manifestations of unitary pattern are expressed in the nine dimensions of the NANDA framework. Newman (1986) has recommended that the NANDA assessment framework be used in initial efforts to identify pattern of the whole, and has specifically defined these nine assessment dimensions relative to her theory of health:

Choosing. Choosing involves the selection of one or more alternatives.

Communicating. Communicating involves the interchange of information from one system to another.

Exchanging. Exchanging involves the interchange of energy and matter between person and environment. Exchanging also involves the transformation of energy from one form to another.

Feeling. Feeling involves a sensing of physical and intuitive awareness.

Knowing. Knowing is the process of personal recognition of self and world.

Moving. Moving is the process of rhythmic alternating between activity and rest.

Perceiving. Perceiving is the process of receiving and interpreting information.

Relating. Relating is the process of connecting with other persons and with the environment.

Valuing. Valuing is the process of assigning worth. (Newman, 1986, p. 74).

Nursing

Nursing is the act of assisting people to use the power that is within them as they evolve toward higher levels of consciousness. Nursing is directed toward recognizing the pattern of the person in interaction with the environment and accepting the interaction as a process of evolving consciousness. Nursing facilitates the process of pattern recognition by a rhythmic connecting of the nurse with the client in an authentic way for the purpose of illuminating the pattern and discovering the new rules of a higher level of organization. Nursing is relating in mutual partnership with a client in the expansion of consciousness (Newman, 1979, p. 67; 1986, pp. 68, 88; 1990a, p. 40; 1990b, p. 136).

Pattern

Pattern is relatedness. Pattern is characterized by movement, diversity, and rhythm. Pattern is a scheme, a design, or framework, a series of acts and aspects regarded as characteristic of persons or environments. Pattern is seen in person-environment interaction. Pattern is recognized on the basis of variation and may not be seen all at once. Pattern unfolds over time with one configuration evolving into the next configuration and so forth. Pattern is key to understanding reality and is manifest in the way one moves, speaks, talks, and relates with others. Pattern identifies the wholeness of the person (Newman 1986a, p. 14; 1990a, p. 40; 1990b, p. 132).

Pattern Recognition

Pattern recognition is the insight or instantaneous recognition of a principle, a realization of a truth, or reconciliation of a duality. Pattern recognition illuminates the possibilities for action. Pattern recognition is key to the process of evolving to higher levels of consciousness (Newman, 1983a, pp. x-xi; 1990a, p. 40).

Person

A person is a dynamic pattern of energy and an open system in interaction with the environment. Persons are identified by their patterns of consciousness. The person does not *possess* consciousness. The person *is* consciousness (Newman, 1986a, p. 33; 1990a, p. 40).

Praxis Research

Praxis research is a process whereby theory, practice, and research are one. Praxis research requires a mutual relationship between interviewee and researcher within a process of inquiry requiring negotiation, reciprocity, and empowerment. In praxis research, the interviewees gain insight into their pattern and concomitant illumination of their action possibilities. An intersection occurs between the interviewee's self-understanding and the researcher's theoretical stance, which provides a change-enhancing context (Lather, 1986, p. 262; Newman, 1990a, p. 38).

Space
Space is inextricably linked with time. There is personal space, inner space, territorial space, shared space, physical and geographical space, maneuverable space, distance-regulating space and life space (Newman, 1979, p. 61).

Time
Time is inextricably linked with space. There is subjective time, objective time, time perspective, utilization of time, private time, coordinated time, and shared time (Newman, 1979, p. 61).

References

Batey, M. (1991). Response: Research as practice. *Nursing Science Quarterly, 4*(3), 101-103.

Bentov, I. (1978). *Stalking the wild pendulum.* New York: Dutton.

Bohm, D. (1980). *Wholeness and the implicate order.* London: Routledge.

Boyd, C. O. (1990). Critical appraisal of developing nursing research methods. *Nursing Science Quarterly, 3*(1), 42-43.

Cowling, W. R. (1988). Book reviews: Newman, M. A. (1986). Health as expanding consciousness. *Nursing Science Quarterly, 1*(3), 133-134.

Fawcett, J. (1989). *Conceptual models of nursing* (2nd ed.). Philadelphia: F. A. Davis.

Flew, A. (Ed.). (1984). *A dictionary of philosophy* (2nd ed.). New York: St. Martin's.

Kalb, K. A. (1990). The gift: Applying Newman's theory of health in nursing practice. In M. E. Parker (Ed.), *Nursing theories in practice* (pp. 163-186). New York: National League for Nursing.

Kim, M. J., & Moritz, D. A. (Eds.). (1982). *Classification of nursing diagnosis: Proceedings of the third and fourth national conferences.* New York: McGraw-Hill.

Klein, S. (1989). Caregiver burden and moral development. *Image, 21*(2), 94-97.

Kuhn, T. (1970). *The structure of scientific revolutions* (2nd ed.). Chicago: University of Chicago Press.

Lather, P. (1986). Research as praxis. *Harvard Educational Review, 56*(3), 257-277.

Marchione, J. M. (1986a). Application of the new paradigm of health to individuals, families and communities [Special supplement]. In M. Newman (Ed.), *Health as expanding consciousness* (pp. 107-134). St. Louis: C. V. Mosby.

Marchione, J. M. (1986b). Pattern as methodology for assessing family health: Newman's theory of health. In P. Winstead-Fry (Ed.), *Case studies in nursing theory* (pp. 215-240). New York: National League for Nursing.

Moch, S. D. (1990). Health within the experience of breast cancer. *Journal of Advanced Nursing, 15,* 1426-1435.

Moss, R. (1981). *The I that is we*. Millbrae, CA: Celestial Arts.

Newman, M. A. (1966). Identifying patient needs in short-span nurse-patient relationships. *Nursing Forum, 5*(1), 76-86.

Newman, M. A. (1972). Time estimation in relation to gait tempo. *Perceptual and Motor Skills, 34*, 359-366.

Newman, M. A. (1976). Movement tempo and the experience of time. *Nursing Research, 25*, 273-279.

Newman, M. A. (1979). *Theory development in nursing*. Philadelphia: F. A. Davis.

Newman, M. A. (1982). Time as an index of consciousness with age. *Nursing Research 31*, 290-293.

Newman, M. A. (1983a). Editorial. *Advances in Nursing Science, 5*(2), x-xi.

Newman, M. A. (1983b). Newman's health theory. In I. Clements & F. Roberts (Eds.), *Family health: A theoretical approach to nursing care* (pp. 161-175). New York: John Wiley.

Newman, M. A. (1983c). The continuing revolution: A history of nursing science. In N. L. Chaska (Ed.), *The nursing profession: A time to speak* (pp. 385-393). New York: McGraw-Hill.

Newman, M. A. (1984). Nursing diagnosis: Looking at the whole. *American Journal of Nursing, 84*, 1496-1499.

Newman, M. A. (1986). *Health as expanding consciousness*. St. Louis: C. V. Mosby.

Newman, M. A. (1987). Patterning. In M. Duffy & N. J. Pender (Eds.), *Conceptual issues in health promotion: Report of proceedings of a wingspread conference* (pp. 36-50). Indianapolis: Sigma Theta Tau.

Newman, M. A. (1990a). Newman's theory of health as praxis. *Nursing Science Quarterly, 3*(1), 37-41.

Newman, M. A. (1990b). Shifting to higher consciousness. In M. Parker (Ed.), *Nursing theories in practice* (pp. 129-139). New York: National League for Nursing.

Newman, M. A. (1991). Commentary: Research as practice. *Nursing Science Quarterly, 4*(3), 100.

Newman, M. A., & Gaudiano, J. K. (1984). Depression as an explanation for decreased subjective time in the elderly. *Nursing Research, 33*(3), 137-139.

Newman, M. A., Lamb, G. S., & Michaels, C. (1991). Nurse case management: The coming together of theory and practice. *Nursing and Health Care, 12*(8), 404-408.

Newman, M. A., & Moch, S. D. (in press—still ??). Life patterns of persons with coronary heart disease. *Nursing Science Quarterly, [vol. ??], [pp. ???]*.

Pearson, B. D. (1988). Book reviews: Newman, M. A. (1986). Health as expanding consciousness. *Nursing Science Quarterly, 1*(3), 134-136.

Ray, M. A. (1990). Critical reflective analysis of Parse's and Newman's research methodologies. *Nursing Science Quarterly, 3*(1), 44-46.

Robinson, K. M. (1990). Predictors of burden among wife caregivers. *Scholarly Inquiry for Nursing Practice: An International Journal, 4*(3), 189-203.

Rogers, M. E. (1970). *An introduction to the theoretical basis of nursing*. Philadelphia: F. A. Davis.

Schorr, J. A., Farnham, R. C., & Ervin, S. M. (1991). Health patterns in aging women as expanding consciousness. *Advances in Nursing Science, 13*(4), 52-63.

Silva, M. C. (1988). [Book review of] Newman, M. A. (1986). *Health as Expanding Consciousness. Nursing Science Quarterly, 1*(3), 136-138.

Smith, M. C. (1990). Pattern in nursing practice. *Nursing Science Quarterly, 3*(2), 57-59.

Teilhard de Chardin, P. (1959). *The phenomenon of man.* New York: Harper & Brothers.

Watson, J. (1987). Book reviews: Health as expanding consciousness. *Journal of Professional Nursing, 3*(5), 387.

West, M. C. (1984). *Patterns of health in mothers of developmentally disabled children.* Unpublished master's thesis, Pennsylvania State University, University Park.

Young, A. M. (1976a). *The geometry of meaning.* San Francisco: Robert Briggs.

Young, A. M. (1976b). *The reflexive universe: Evolution of consciousness.* San Francisco: Robert Briggs.

Bibliography

Theory Development—Classic and Contemporary Works

Newman, M. A. (1979). *Theory development in nursing.* Philadelphia: F. A. Davis.

Newman, M. A. (1983a). Editorial. *Advances in Nursing Science, 5*(2), x-xi.

Newman, M. A. (1983b). Newman's health theory. In I. Clements & F. Roberts (Eds.), *Family health: A theoretical approach to nursing care* (pp. 161-175). New York: John Wiley.

Newman, M. A. (1984). Nursing diagnosis: Looking at the whole. *American Journal of Nursing, 84,* 1496-1499.

Newman, M. A. (1986). *Health as expanding consciousness.* St. Louis: C. V. Mosby.

Newman, M. A. (1987a). Nursing's emerging paradigm: The diagnosis of pattern. In A. M. McLane (Ed.), *Classification of nursing diagnoses: Proceedings of the Seventh Conference* [of the North American Nursing Diagnosis Association] (pp. 53-60). St. Louis: C. V. Mosby.

Newman, M. A. (1987b). Patterning. In M. Duffy & N. J. Pender (Eds.), *Conceptual issues in health promotion: Report of proceedings of a wingspread conference* (pp. 36-50). Indianapolis: Sigma Theta Tau.

Newman, M. A. (1989). The spirit of nursing. *Holistic Nursing Practice, 3*(3), 1-6.

Newman, M. A. (1990a). Newman's theory of health as praxis. *Nursing Science Quarterly, 3*(1), 37-41.

Newman, M. A. (1990b). Shifting to higher consciousness. In M. E. Parker (Ed.), *Nursing theories in practice* (pp. 129-139). New York: National League for Nursing.

Newman, M. A. (1990c). Professionalism: Myth or reality. In N. L. Chaska (Ed.), *The nursing profession: Turning points* (pp. 49-52). St. Louis: C. V. Mosby.

Newman, M. A. (1991). Commentary: Research as practice. *Nursing Science Quarterly, 4*(3), 100.

Newman, M. A., Lamb, G. S., & Michaels, C. (1991). Nurse case management: The coming together of theory and practice. *Nursing and Health Care, 12*(8), 404-408.

Newman, M. A., & Moch, S. D. (in press ???). Life patterns of persons with coronary heart disease. *Nursing Science Quarterly.*

Influencing Sources

Bentov, I. (1978). *Stalking the wild pendulum.* New York: Dutton.

Bohm, D. (1980). *Wholeness and the implicate order.* London: Routledge.

Lather, P. (1986). Research as praxis. *Harvard Educational Review, 56*(3), 257-277.

Moss, R. (1981). *The I that is we.* Millbrae, CA.: Celestial Arts.

Rogers, M. E. (1970). *An introduction to the theoretical basis of nursing.* Philadelphia: F. A. Davis.

Teilhard de Chardin, P. (1959). *The phenomenon of man.* New York: Harper & Brothers.

Young, A. M. (1976a). *The geometry of meaning.* San Francisco: Robert Briggs.

Young, A. M. (1976b). *The reflexive universe: Evolution of consciousness.* San Francisco: Robert Briggs.

Research and Application References

Gustafson, W. (1990). Application of Newman's theory of health: Pattern recognition as nursing practice. In M. E. Parker (Ed.), *Nursing theories in practice* (pp. 141-161). New York: National League for Nursing.

Kalb, K. A. (1990). The gift: Applying Newman's theory of health in nursing practice. In M. E. Parker (Ed.), *Nursing theories in practice* (pp. 163-186). New York: National League for Nursing.

Jonsdottir, H. (1988). *Health patterns of clients with chronic obstructive pulmonary disease,* Unpublished master's thesis, University of Minnesota, Minneapolis.

Marchione, J. M. (1986a). Application of the new paradigm of health to individuals, families and communities [Special supplement]. In M. Newman, *Health as expanding consciousness* (pp. 107-134). St. Louis: C. V. Mosby.

Marchione, J. M. (1986b). Pattern as methodology for assessing family health: Newman's theory of health. In P. Winstead-Fry, (Ed.), *Case studies in nursing theory* (pp. 215-240). New York: National League for Nursing.

Moch, S. D. (1988). Health in illness: Experiences with breast cancer (Doctoral dissertation, University of Minnesota). *Dissertation Abstracts International, 50,* 47B.

Moch, S. D. (1990). Health within the experience of breast cancer. *Journal of Advanced Nursing, 15,* 1426-1435.

Newman, M. A. (1966). Identifying patient needs in short span nurse-patient relationships. *Nursing Forum, 5*(1), 76-86.

Newman, M. A. (1972). Time estimation in relation to gait tempo. *Perceptual and Motor Skills, 34,* 359-366.

Newman, M. A. (1976). Movement tempo and the experience of time. *Nursing Reserrch, 25,* 273-279.

Newman, M. A. (1982). Time as an index of consciousness with age. *Nursing Research, 31,* 290-293.

Newman, M. A. (1991). Commentary: Research as practice. *Nursing Science Quarterly, 4*(3), 100.

Newman, M. A., & Gaudiano, J. K. (1984). Depression as an explanation for decreased subjective time in the elderly. *Nursing Research, 33*(3), 137-139.

Newman, M. A., Lamb, G. L., & Michaels, C. (1991). Nurse case management: The coming together of theory and practice. *Nursing and Health Care, 12*(8), 404-408.

Newman, M. A., & Moch, S. D. (in press ???). Life patterns of persons with coronary heart disease. *Nursing Science Quarterly.*

Schorr, J. A., Farnham, R. C., & Ervin, S. M. (1991). Health patterns in aging women as expanding consciousness. *Advances in Nursing Science, 13*(4), 52-63.

West, M. C. (1984). *Patterns of health in mothers of developmentally disabled children.* Unpublished master's thesis, Pennsylvania State University, University Park.

Critique of Newman's Theory

Batey, M. (1991). Response: Research as practice. *Nursing Science Quarterly, 4*(3), 101-103.

Boyd, C. O. (1990). Critical appraisal of developing nursing research methods. *Nursing Science Quarterly, 3*(1), 42-43.

Cowling, W. R. (1988). [Book review of] Newman, M. A. (1986). *Health as expanding consciousness. Nursing Science Quarterly, 1*(3), 133-134.

Pearson, B. D. (1988). [Book review of] Newman, M. A. (1986). *Health as expanding consciousness. Nursing Science Quarterly, 1*(3), 134-136.

Ray, M. A. (1990). Critical reflective analysis of Parse's and Newman's research methodologies. *Nursing Science Quarterly, 3*(1), 44-46.

Silva, M. C. (1988). [Book review of] Newman, M. A. (1986). *Health as expanding consciousness. Nursing Science Quarterly, 1*(3), 136-138.

Smith, M. C. (1990). Pattern in nursing practice. *Nursing Science Quarterly, 3*(2), 57-59.

Watson, J. (1987). [Book review of] *Health as expanding consciousness. Journal of Professional Nursing, 3*(5), 387.

Videotapes

Helene Fuld Health Trust (Producer), & Fawcett, J. (Interviewer). (1990). *Portraits of excellence: Margaret Newman* [VHS videocassette]. Oakland, CA: Studio III.

Kerr, J. (Director). (1990). *Interview of Margaret Newman* (Part of a series on Nursing as a Practical Science). (Available from the University of Alberta, Faculty of Nursing, Edmonton, Alberta, Canada)

Stearns, S. (Producer), & Marchione, J. (Interviewer). (1983). *A conversation with Margaret Newman, explaining her theory of health* [JVC videocassette]. (Available from the University of Minnesota, School of Nursing; Pennsylvania State University, Division of Nursing; and the University of Akron, College of Nursing)

PART VII

Paterson and Zderad

Humanistic Nursing Theory

NANCY O'CONNOR

Biographical Sketches of the Nurse Theorists:
Josephine G. Paterson (DNS, RN)

Born: September 1, 1924, in Freeport, New York
Position: Retired from nursing, 1985; position prior to
    retirement as "nursologist" at the Northport Veterans
    Administration Hospital in Northport, New York
Diploma: Lenox Hill Hospital School of Nursing, New York,
    August 1945
BS Nursing Education, St. John's University, Brooklyn, New
    York, August 1954
MPH, Johns Hopkins School of Hygiene & Public Health,
    Baltimore, Maryland, June 1955
Specialty: mental health; fieldwork completed April 1956
DNS, Boston University, 1969; specialty: psychiatric mental
    health

Loretta Zderad (PhD, RN)

Born: June 7, 1925, Chicago, Illinois
Position: Retired from nursing, 1985; position prior to
    retirement as "nursologist" at Northport Veterans
    Administration Hospital, Northport, New York
Diploma: St. Bernard's Hospital School of Nursing, Chicago,
    Illinois, June 1947
BS Nursing Education, Loyola University, Chicago, Illinois,
    June 1947 (concurrent with receipt of diploma from St.
    Bernard's)
MS Nursing Education, Catholic University, psychiatric
    nursing major, June 1952
MA Philosophy, Georgetown University, 1960
PhD Philosophy, Georgetown University, 1968

Foreword

The purpose of this section is to systematically relate humanistic nursing theory to the identified metaparadigm elements in nursing. Consequently, the humanistic nursing conceptualization with regard to person, nurse, health, and environment is recounted. Starting with (a) the individual lived experiences and lives of Josephine Paterson and Loretta Zderad, (b) the historical development of the theory, (c) the implicit assumptions, and (d) a glossary of terms, the *content* and *process* of the theory are examined.

The major phenomena of interest to creators of humanistic nursing theory are person and nurse. The theory also provides for the placement of health and environment but to a less well developed degree. Nursing is viewed as an authentic dialogue involving meeting, relating, and presencing in a world of people, things, time, and space. All of these concepts are explained in detail. The existential foundations of humanistic nursing include the uniqueness and sameness of each individual person along with human relating for development of potentials. The potentials, when developed by choice and authentic awareness, lead to more being and growth (health). The outcome of authentic encountering, according to Paterson and Zderad, is comfort.

Nursing occurs all at once with multifarious multiplicities, and the value of diversity with regard to setting for nursing practice is related by *inclusion* of role function and clinical focus. The weaving of the objective-subjective-intersubjective relating of the situation is suggested for phenomenological description of the lived human event of nursing. Thus the expression attributed to R. D. Laing that theory is "the articulated vision of experience" is given credence by the theorists. *Nursology* is the name given to the theorizing process. The process of nursology answers the question "How can the nurse, a subjective-objective human being, know the other and compare and complementarily synthesize the exchanges between these known others?" The section explains the five phases of this process and the results that are transforming and inclusive for a unified insight. New creation happens as one reality from the lived situation illuminates another for additive development of general knowledge principles.

Within the section, the concepts of presence and dialogue are presented as examples of nursing involving doing and being in relationship. The confirming of the persons (nurse and patient) happens during "presencing." The presencing enfolds the skill or technical "doing" part of the nursing care for goal attainment. The attributes of presence are fully described within the context of the nursing situation. Dialogue as nursing is a transactive process implied as a special kind of meeting of humans for a purposeful "call and response" situation. A deep encountering happens as a result of the interchange. For future connection and direction, an example using humanistic nursing practice components is provided. The current resources and projects that involve concepts or aspects of humanistic nursing theory are listed.

Acknowledgment is given to Josephine Paterson and Loretta Zderad for the development of a theory and an explication of a phenomenological process that expresses value, commitment to, and investment in the lived experience of the patient and the nurse.

Doris R. Hines, PhD, RN

Preface

I first became acquainted with the thinking and writing of Paterson and Zderad in 1976 upon publication of their text *Humanistic Nursing*. At that time I had the good fortune of being a registered nurse enrolled in a BSN completion program at a private college in which the educational philosophy included both a strong liberal arts thread within all majors and a pragmatic focus on preparation of baccalaureate graduates for the world of work. This institution had achieved an understanding of the appropriate blend of thinking and doing that characterizes meaningful work and sustains persons engaged in such work. Conditions were thus favorable for my first reading of *Humanistic Nursing*. I came to it as a seasoned nurse with an understanding of the practice world of nursing and as a learner receptive to new ways of thinking about my work. My readiness to learn was supported by an environment that honored both practical and conceptual ways of knowing. Thus the essential themes in *Humanistic Nursing* made sense to me at that time in my nursing world. Reading and discussing this text with classmates and faculty was extremely influential both in making explicit our shared nursing experiences and in ushering in a glimpse of the possibility of a lifetime pursuit of nursing scholarship.

As with all enduring works, *Humanistic Nursing* both anticipates and continues to speak to important issues in contemporary nursing. For example, the value of explicating that knowledge which is unique to nursing, the creation of research methodologies that are consonant with the nursing world, the understanding of the multiple ways of knowing necessary in nursing contexts, the grounding of nursing knowledge in the nursing situation, the importance of the knower in knowledge development, and the integration of thinking, doing, and being within the nursing world are but a few topics about which readers of the original work will gain insight. I believe that *Humanistic Nursing* will continue to be studied as a foundational work in nursing epistemology. It is my pleasure to present to the reader an abbreviated and interpreted version of this work that has been so influential in my nursing world and that continues to illuminate our collective nursing worlds. I would like to thank editors Chris McQuiston and Adele Webb for this reader-friendly text on nursing theory. We in nursing continue to be ambivalent about the role of ease and pleasure in matters of nursing knowledge construction.

NANCY O'CONNOR

42

Historical Development of the Model

Paterson and Zderad began theorizing about the nature of nursing amidst the clamor within the profession to develop a scientific basis of nursing practice. During the 1950s and 1960s, many nurses began to ask fundamental questions regarding the nature of nursing. Many psychiatric nurses explored in particular the nature of the nurse-patient relationship and viewed nurse-patient relations as the central phenomenon to be addressed in nursing theory development. Newman (1983) suggests that the 1950s and 1960s were dominated by this focus in nursing theory development. This is certainly true of Paterson and Zderad's (1988) model.

It was during this time that Paterson and Zderad began their "dialogue with reality" (Zderad, 1978, p. 39), which they later called theorizing. They did not set out deliberately and consciously with the intention to develop nursing theory. Nonetheless, they both describe a certain unrest in their teaching that stemmed from including bits and pieces from many nonnursing disciplines as opposed to teaching from nursing's theoretical base. This spurred their efforts to develop the theoretical basis of nursing. They describe their process of theorizing as a slow evolution toward nursing theory. Paterson (1978) has described the process of theory development in nursing as "tortuous" (p. 49), by which she conveys the nonlinear and somewhat mazelike nature of humanistic nursing practice theory development. Theorizing is thus filled with meanderings, scenic paths, and seeming detours. Yet it remains intent on seeking a clearing in the maze, an articulated vision of the reality of the lived nursing act.

Early in theory development, Paterson and Zderad became disillusioned with what they felt was an overemphasis on scientific processes of theory building. They did not feel that this scientific theory-building process was able to express fully the complexity or the aesthetic qualities of the nursing situation. Paterson and Zderad therefore developed a process of theorizing that was more akin to the nature of nursing itself.

> By analogy the model or form or phases of this method can be correlated with the model or form or phases of a clinical nursing process. This is an attempt to apply a method of study to nursing which corresponds to the nature of nursing as perceived by this author . . . this is a subjective-objective method of study that conforms to the nature of professional nursing. It attempts to describe the nature of the complex mobile spirit of nursing by a process which preserves this spirit intact. (Paterson, 1971, pp. 143, 146)

Therefore they experienced what all theorists, writers, and artists experience to some degree: namely, the limitations of words or images to convey the fullness of human experience. A quote by Bergson conveys their concern with this: "Fixed concepts can be extracted from our thought from the mobile reality; but there is no means whatever of reconstituting with the fixity of concepts the mobility of the real" (Bergson, 1962, cited in Paterson, 1971, p. 144). This concern led them to examine the discipline of philosophy wherein they learned different ways to explore the nature of things. They soon recognized their concerns as being more consistent with a phenomenological method of inquiry as compared with the scientific method. Later, they formulated a position that viewed phenomenological inquiry and scientific inquiry as complementary (Paterson & Zderad, 1978). Both theorists began the process of theorizing about nursing while actively engaged in the practices of clinical nursing and nursing education. The need to "root" (Zderad, 1978, p. 35) nursing theory in the clinical setting was another major goal of the theorists. Paterson (1978) describes theory and practice as "two sides of one indivisible coin" (p. 51). The threefold process of (a) experiencing, (b) reflecting upon, and (c) describing their nursing experiences emerged from their conscious attentiveness to the nature and meaning of these practices and ultimately became the cornerstone of the process of clinical theorizing that they termed *nursology* (Paterson, 1971). Recognition of and cultivation of the interrelationships of nursing practice, nursing education, and nursing research became both a hallmark of and the goal of humanistic nursing practice theory development. Indeed, the culmination of their careers as "nursologists" at the Northport Veterans Administration Hospital enabled them to engage simultaneously (all at once) in the three-pronged practices of clinical nursing (practice, education, and research) as they lived and articulated their vision of humanistic nursing practice theory.

Thus the theorizing efforts of Paterson and Zderad began with the recognition at some level that they themselves are, and indeed each practicing nurse is, a "noetic locus" (Desan, 1972, cited in Paterson & Zderad, 1988, p. 39), or a knowing place. It is the professional responsibility of each nurse to contribute to the evolution of nursing theory by attending knowingly to his or her practice and by asking questions of that practice—such as what, why, how, how better, ought, and ought not—by reflecting on possibilities and by articulating this vision in an enduring form to be shared both with other nurses and with humanity in general (Paterson & Zderad, 1978). Through such thoughtful attending and sharing by each nurse, a wide variety of nursing experiences can be brought under the umbrella of fewer enduring phenomena that will reflect the essential core of nursing as it is lived across diverse nursing contexts.

Staying with a chosen phenomenon over time by weaving back and forth between the experiencing, reflecting, and describing realms will generate rich phenomenological descriptions of essential nursing concepts and will reveal the relatedness among these concepts. The development of humanistic nursing practice theory proceeded along just these lines as Paterson and Zderad engaged themselves with in-depth study of their initially chosen and ever evolving phenomena of interest. For example, Paterson began studying the phenomenon of ambivalence, moved through such concepts as growth, health, freedom, and openness promotion, and finally focused on the concept of comfort (Paterson & Zderad, 1978). Zderad began with wondering how it is possible to know another person and traveled through such phenomena as empathy and presence to the notion of "withness" (Zderad, 1978, p. 44). The fruits of their individual and collective efforts are expressed as their major text, *Humanistic Nursing*, first published in 1976 and reprinted in 1988. The text is presented by the theorists as the culmination of their experience of teaching a continuing education course entitled "Humanistic Nursing" at the Northport Veterans Administration Hospital over a period of years.

The development of humanistic nursing practice theory by Paterson and Zderad was thus a response to a call from within themselves to search for and to articulate the meaning and value of their own nursing practices. Nursing "undescribed and unappreciated" (Paterson, 1978, p. 51) is nursing inadequately conceptualized and uncommunicated to others. Thus their personal call resonated with the call within the profession of nursing to explicate the nature and significance of nursing as a professional discipline. Paterson and Zderad were thus among the pioneers in nursing who readily understood the value and nature of theory in a practice discipline and responded by developing a method of theorizing that is congruent with the practice of nursing.

The capstone summary statement of their view of theory is that of R. D. Laing, who stated that "theory is the articulated vision of experience" (quoted in Zderad, 1978, p. 45). Zderad stresses the meaning of each key word in Laing's definition. She states that *articulated* means that the theory is expressed in an enduring form so that it can be shared with others and also means that the connectedness among the concepts in the theory is evident. *Vision* refers to the heuristic nature of the theory; it calls us forth to enact the possibilities as envisioned by the theory and goes beyond merely summarizing past concrete experiences. *Experience* refers to the nurse's lived acts as a nurse in the health-illness community from multiple vantage points. Finally, they maintain that nursing theory is a valued resource for nurses as educators, practitioners, and researchers and for humanity in general.

In their seminal work, *Humanistic Nursing,* Paterson and Zderad convey their vision of nursing expressed as humanistic nursing practice theory and as a general theory of nursing. In addition, they provide a rich metatheoretical landscape from which other theories can be sculpted. Paterson (1978) defined *metatheory* as a "systematized body of knowledge formulated for the purpose of making something else possible" (p. 50). The most general forms of nursing's phenomena of concern have been asserted by some nursing scholars (Fawcett, 1980, 1984; Flaskerud & Halloran, 1980; Newman, 1983) to form the metaparadigm of nursing. Flaskerud and Halloran (1980) have termed the four elements of nurse, person, health, and environment areas of agreement in nursing theory; that is, across time, these elements have formed the substance of nursing theory. It is common in nursing theory discourse to refer to metatheory as a conceptual framework. According to Fawcett (1980, 1984), a conceptual framework of nursing provides a distinct perspective on the elements of nursing's metaparadigm: namely, person, nursing, health, and environment. The perspective of Paterson and Zderad on the elements of the metaparadigm is first presented. This presentation is followed by a discussion of their general theory of nursing. This division is consistent with the theorists' assertion that there are two levels of nursing theorizing. The first is the phase of conceptualizing significant nursing phenomena phenomenologically. The second is the phase of interrelating the concepts into a coherent whole (Zderad, 1978, p. 45). The metatheory is more highly developed by the theorists than is the general theory of nursing. Nonetheless, the major concepts that are identified and explored within the metatheory are readily identified within the general theory of nursing.

Overview of Metatheory

Humanistic nursing as a metatheory of nursing provides highly developed viewpoints on the two metaparadigm elements of nursing and person and less well developed views of health and environment. The development of the view of nursing as a particular kind of human relating is perhaps its major contribution. The essence of the metatheory provides "a perspective of nursing as a happening between persons, an approach to nursing as existential presence and awareness, and a method of describing nursing as phenomenology" (Paterson, 1978, p. 49). This statement provides insight on the assumptions that are implicit within the metatheory. *Assumptions* are assertions of basic beliefs that "are taken as givens" (Fawcett, 1984, p. 2) prior to the presentation of the major ideas within the metatheory. Assumptions reflect philosophical positions about human ways of being, knowing, and doing. Within the metatheory, several implicit assumptions can be discerned; none has been deliberately put forward by the theorists as assumptions. They do, however, make the following comments regarding an apt starting point for humanistic nursing practice theory:

Nursing situations make available human existence events significantly worthy of description. Only human nurses can describe them. Humans' ability to describe reality adequately has its limits. We should describe since pridefully we humans are the only existing beings capable of giving meaning to, looking at, and expressing our consciousness. In the long run this effort could yield a nursing science. (Paterson & Zderad, 1988, p. 70)

43

Implicit Assumptions

Nature of Reality

For Paterson and Zderad (1978), the nature of nursing reality is held
to be objective, subjective, and intersubjective all at once. Objective
reality can be thought of as occurring "out there" (Paterson & Zderad,
1978). It can be observed, pointed at, held at a distance, and examined.
An object can be "apprehended intellectually" (Paterson & Zderad,
1988, p. 27). Subjective reality is known from the inside out; it is the
reality that can be thought of as awareness of one's own experience.
Intersubjective reality is experienced in what Paterson and Zderad
term the *between* (Paterson & Zderad, 1988, p. 4). Intersubjective
reality can be thought of as subject-to-subject relating. One's inherent
capacity to respond to other beings-as-beings is what gives rise to the
realm of the between as a facet of reality.

Humanistic nursing dwells primarily in the intersubjective realm
of nursing even while recognizing the trifold (objective, subjective,
intersubjective) nature of the nursing world. Similarly, the metatheory seems to accentuate the "being" qualities of nursing even
while recognizing the integrality of its "being and doing" (Paterson
& Zderad, 1988, p. 13). At the time that they were developing their
theory, Paterson and Zderad felt that the "doing" aspects of nursing
had been more commonly examined.

It is not difficult to follow the evolution of Zderad's journey from empathy through presence toward "withness" as a central phenomenon of inquiry; the preposition *with* thus becomes central within the metatheory. *With* also becomes a central concept within the intersubjective realm. Nonetheless, it is important to underscore that these aspects of nursing that come under closer scrutiny within the metatheory are not held to exhaust the reality of the nursing world as it is lived. Objective reality and doing with patients continue to be viewed as appropriate ways of knowing and being in the nursing world.

One Becomes Ever More

Another basic belief that underpins the metatheory is that the nature of person is both to be and to become ever more. The "beingness" of persons is discussed within the metatheory under "adequacy." Adequacy is one aspect of their view of the person. This basic belief also gives rise to two other related concepts within the metatheory known as "well-being" and "more-being," which speak to persons being and becoming ever more, respectively. These are discussed as health-related terms within the metatheory.

These and other basic beliefs within the metatheory can best be understood by examining the philosophical tenets of existentialism and phenomenology. Thinkers holding these philosophical views clearly influenced the development of Paterson and Zderad's thinking as did the two psychiatric mental health nurses Theresa G. Muller and Ruth Gilbert (Paterson & Zderad, 1988, p. 96). Nonetheless, the theorists' basic position on knowing underscores the new synthesis of thought that occurs within the knower through repeated cycles of experiencing, reflecting, and describing. The knower as a "noetic locus" synthesizes the thoughts of others with his or her own experience and reflection, giving rise to a new creation. Thus humanistic nursing practice theory should not be construed as an application of existential thought and phenomenological method within nursing as much as the "complementary synthesis" (1988, p. 73).

Humanistic nursing practice theory can be thought of as a blossoming of existential-phenomenological thought rather than as the plant that is firmly rooted in such thought. Nonetheless, as Paterson and Zderad (1978) maintain, while one can move from a philosophy to a theory realm, one cannot take the philosophy out of humanistic nursing practice theory. Persons are their history (past) as well as their choices (future); thus the theory is both distinct from and also related to the line of thought from which it arose.

The name given to this process of theorizing and to the resultant body of abstract knowledge in which it will ultimately result is *nursology*. The title given to nurses who undertake its development is *nursologist*.

Summary of Existential Thought

One thinker who is commonly associated with existentialism and who consents to be grouped with existentialists is Jean-Paul Sartre (1948, cited in White, 1983). According to Sartre (1948, cited in White, 1983), the central theme of existentialism is that "*existence* comes before *essence*" (p. 122). Existentialists believe that human beings do not have any predetermined nature or ultimate essence that thinkers through the years have called "human nature." Individuals are thus neither ultimately good nor ultimately evil. Instead, they come into the world and become all they will be based on choices that they continually make. They are not fulfilling any grand plan but are constantly free to make whatever choices they will. Paterson and Zderad (1988) depict the human as "lacking a fixed nature with his [or her] own mode of being as his [or her] fundamental project" (p. 78). This idea is commonly referred to as being "thrown" into the world and it underscores the freedom within the human condition. Sartre speaks of this "terrible freedom" (Sartre, cited in Guigan, 1986) that results from realization that individuals are free to become who they will. Coupled with this individual freedom is the responsibility for personal choices and this gives rise to the other central themes in existential thought: anxiety, dread, and abandonment. Capability unrealized is not treasured in this viewpoint. Sartre (1948, cited in White, 1983) states that, in the final analysis, "man [*sic*] is no other than a series of undertakings, that he [or she] is the sum, the organization, the set of relations that constitute these undertakings" (p. 135).

Many existential thinkers highlight the redemptive value of human relatedness. If it is one's plight to endure the "terrible freedom," it is also one's promise to do so in the company of others. Thus an important theme in existential writings is one's relation to others and one's responsibility to cultivate communities of dialogue. Dialogue becomes the primary way to experience community. The existential experience thus becomes one of both solitude and solidarity, which is perhaps the central paradox within existential thought.

Threads of existential thought can be seen in the centrality of choice within the metatheory of Paterson and Zderad (1988). They also espouse the primacy of action perspective that is essential to such thought. For example, they treasure the practices of humanistic nursing and highlight their interrelatedness to the knowing aspects of nursing. Finally, their general theory of nursing rests on a central premise of existential thought, that of the possibility of individual growth through authentic relating.

The use of the term *humanistic nursing* to describe their continuing education class was deliberately chosen by the theorists after first experimenting with longer titles that included the term *phenomenology*. The theorists (1988) state that they used the term *humanistic* to refer to an approach that encompasses an existential concept of person and a phenomenological approach to inquiry. Furthermore, they intended for this term to convey all ways of being and becoming. The place of technology is not negated in the use of the term *humanistic nursing*. Instead, technology is seen as a human capability.

Summary of Phenomenological Tradition

The central slogan of the phenomenological tradition might be held to be "to the things themselves." This saying is attributed to Husserl, the father of phenomenology (Paterson & Zderad, 1988). Phenomenological methods are primarily concerned with describing human experience in such a way that the fullness of experience is preserved. These methods cultivate knowing from within an experience rather than from looking at the experience from the outside.

For Paterson and Zderad (1988), the lived nursing act thus becomes the "thing itself" to which nursing theory must return. These lived acts of nursing become the fountainhead of humanistic nursing practice theory. The acts, when subjected to phenomenological description and inquiry by the community of nurses over time, will reveal the phenomena of central concern to nursing as a practice discipline. Paterson and Zderad's phenomenological method of nursology will be further described within their view of nursing as knowing.

44

Perspectives on Metaparadigm Elements

Person

Paterson and Zderad's view of persons is meant to apply to both the nurse and the patient and can be thought of as fleshing out their implicit assumptions. Within the metatheory, the patient is commonly referred to as *the nursed*. The use of this term underscores aspects of persons with which nurses are distinctly concerned, namely, persons-as-nursed. The use of the term also underscores the relational quality of the nurse-nursed relationship. One of the most important features of their view of persons is that they distinguish between ways of being-as-nurse and being-as-patient. This has implications for their conceptualization of nursing as a distinct form of human relating that is both similar to and yet distinct from other forms of human relating.

Freedom

According to Paterson and Zderad (1988), a major aspect of human nature is its nondeterminedness. Closely related to this premise is the notion that humans are "responsible for their condition of being" (Paterson & Zderad, 1988, p. 3). As a person, "I am my choices"

(Paterson & Zderad, 1988, p. 15). Paterson and Zderad interpret this existential dictum to mean that persons have an inherent capacity to choose to respond and to choose how to respond to situations presented by life. Therefore a person is not seen as choosing the situation but is held accountable for personal response to it. While this response influences the emerging situation as it changes over time, the response alone is an insufficient determinant of the health or illness situation. This distinction is important when considering the health and illness quality of life, because health and illness are influenced by multiple other factors not within the realm of individual accountability such as heredity, exposure to environmental agents, or natural disasters. The description of choice within Paterson and Zderad's (1988) conceptual model occurs in three phases. Phase 1 of the choice process is an awareness phase in which one recognizes that possibilities exist. In other words, the possibilities must become relevant. This openness to possibility is characterized by a freedom from "the bonds of habit and stereotyped response" (Paterson & Zderad, 1988, p. 16) and conveys a sense of openness to spontaneity and availability. In addition, this first phase of choice involves "getting in touch with one's experience, one's subjective-objective world" (Paterson & Zderad, 1988, p. 16) and one's situation. In Phase 2, one engages in reflection. In this phase of choice, one considers one's "unique situation . . . possible alternatives, . . . the values inherent within them" (Paterson & Zderad, 1988, p. 16). This reflection bears elements of the past (values), the current time (unique situation), and the future (possible alternatives). Finally, the person responds with a choice that is "expressed . . . as a willingness to accept responsibility for its foreseeable consequences" (Paterson & Zderad, 1988, p. 16).

Uniqueness

Paterson and Zderad underscore the distinctiveness of the person. Every person holds his or her own "angular view" (Paterson & Zderad, 1988, p. 37). This refers to the fact that every person sees, hears, feels, tastes, and experiences the world differently. These different experiences, which include the influence of family and history, give rise to a particular viewpoint or way of seeing the world.

Another belief of Paterson and Zderad (1988) regarding human nature is that, while every person is unique, it is this shared fact of uniqueness that persons have in common with each other. This uniqueness results in choices that appear somewhat lonely in that "only each person can describe or choose the evolvement of the project which is himself-in-his-situation" (Paterson & Zderad, 1988, p. 4).

Adequacy

Although human choice might be lonely, it is linked to the critical human capacity of hope, which inspires one to envision alternatives beyond those immediately apparent. While envisioning possibilities, one is confronted by conflicting and seemingly competing alternatives and by human limitation. Paterson and Zderad (1988) refer to the resolution of the polarity of human potential and limitation as "humanness," or the notion that it is "just how man [*sic*] is" (Paterson & Zderad, 1988, p. 5). *Humanness* also refers to the presence within humans of "the spiritual and the animal" (Paterson & Zderad, 1988, p. 55). Elsewhere, Paterson (1978) refers to this aspect of persons as a sense of human "adequacy" (p. 54).

Relatedness

Finally, one's capacity for relationship with others is a key attribute of individuals within this metatheory. This capacity for person-to-person relating Paterson and Zderad (1988) discuss as a capacity for presence, or being with another human being. Through relating with other persons as presences (intersubjectivity), individuals become more and realize their uniqueness. The choice to relate in such a way is made deliberately. Thus two interrelated processes are seen by Paterson and Zderad to contribute to human moreness, namely, choice and intersubjectivity.

Historicity

Nurses are their history and of necessity this affects their inner responses to their nursing world. Awareness of the meaning of their personal history enables them to be "in charge of it" (Paterson, 1978, p. 63) rather than for it to be in charge of them. Being in charge also applies to patients. Historicity contributes to the situatedness of choice. Thus one can choose within the limits of what one sees as possibilities. Part of the nursing process is engaging the patient's capacity to envision for him- or herself unseen possibilities.

Person-as-Nurse

Person-as-nurse is one who responds to the call of human beings with needs within the health-illness quality of life. According to Paterson (1978), nursing is a unique way of responding that will continue as a human response even if the nursing profession were to stop using the word *nursing* to describe its activity. Paterson (1978) also maintains that nursing as a profession survives because all humans have the potential to become patients.

Person-as-nurse is a presence with others whose health and survival are at issue. According to Paterson (1978), the nurse's existence is confirmed because of the difference made in the situation. Therefore person-as-nurse needs to nurse just as person-as-patient (nursed) needs to be nursed. Furthermore, a person-as-nurse identifies with the profession and is responsible to it. Person-as-nurse is therefore committed to strive to express the fullest meaning of humanistic nursing, which is seen as "existential engagement directed toward nurturing human potential" (Paterson & Zderad, 1988, p. 14). The key idea is that the nurse's commitment is to strive continually toward humanistic nursing as a goal despite the fact that in practice it may occur in various degrees.

Person-as-Patient

Within the metatheory, the person-as-patient is referred to as "the nursed" (Paterson & Zderad, 1978). The theorists assert that because of the limitations inherent in the human condition we all have the capacity to become patients. Paterson states,

> To be a patient is to worry, hurt, and suffer to a degree beyond one's own ability to heal or bear alone. . . . I am a being in a body; through my body my being is touched and affected. Because of this body it is necessary to lean, to depend. I am very aware of and alert to those other beings who touch and affect me, who support me. . . . I may experience them as being more or less powerful or benevolent than they really are. (1978, pp. 54-55)

Nursing

The metaparadigm element of nursing is the most highly developed one within the metatheory. Thus several different views of nursing are found within the metatheory. Integral to the theorists' thinking is that nursing is a way of knowing, being, and doing. The most general view about nursing is that the three practice realms in nursing (education, practice, and research) are intimately connected and together constitute clinical nursing. Paterson and Zderad (1988) maintain that humanistic nursing is concerned "with the phenomenon of nursing wherever it occurs regardless of its specialized clinical, functional or sociocultural form" (p. 18). Knowing and doing are thus interconnected processes that cut across all aspects of clinical nursing. Nursology is the successful weaving together of the three strands of clinical nursing.

Nursing as Knowing

Nursing as art-science. The notion of nursing as art-science is meant to convey the interrelated processes of art and science as they occur all at once in the nursing situation. Even the hyphen does not convey the synthesis of art and science that Paterson and Zderad hold as integral to nursing. They define the art-science quality of nursing as "a symbolic behavioral expression of intuitive logical knowledge derived from subjective, objective, and intersubjective experiences with reality" (1978). The notion of art-science highlights the multifaceted nature of knowing in nursing.

Nursing as a unique knowledge form. Highlighting the dynamic of distinctiveness within relatedness, Paterson and Zderad take the position that *nursing* used as a noun is a unique form of knowledge yet is related to general knowledge. The unique contribution of nursing to human science is expressed first in a question: "What knowledge gained through the study of nursing, a particular form of the human situation, could be contributed to the general body of human sciences?" (Paterson & Zderad, 1976, p. 20). Later in the metatheory, the unique knowledge of nursing and its potential contribution to general knowledge are expressed in the uniqueness of the dialogical process of nursing as it occurs through nursing acts. The potential contribution of nursing to general knowledge of dialogical human processes is "staggering" (Paterson & Zderad, 1976, p. 34). It is a combination of being with and doing with the patient in the nursing situation.

The value of conceptualizing this knowledge, embodied within concrete practice situations, and of articulating it in enduring form is echoed repeatedly by the theorists. For example, Zderad (1978) states: "Nursing, as every discipline, has its own distinctive encounter with reality; and in its encounter, each seeks meaning" (p. 48). This meaning in nursing science reflects both a body of substantive knowledge and a method for discovering and verifying new knowledge. "Each science, then, bears these twin hallmarks: its particular area of concern with reality and its particular approach to theorizing about it" (Zderad, 1978, p. 48). These concrete practice descriptions are seen as building blocks for nursing science. Articulation of the unique knowledge of nursing, however, is seen by Paterson and Zderad (1976) to have yet broader ramifications for human knowledge development: "If we truly experience nursing as a kind of art-science, as a particular dyad of flowing, synthesizing, subjective-objective intersubjective dialogue, then nursing offers a unique path to human knowledge and it is our responsibility to try to describe and share it" (p. 102).

Nursology. Nursology is the name given to a process of scientific inquiry in nursing that was first introduced by Paterson in 1971. She defined it as "the study of nursing aimed towards the development of nursing theory" (Paterson, 1971, p. 143). Viewed by Paterson as a form of phenomenology, it was also seen as a new creation that resulted from a "complementary synthesis" (p. 73) of phenomenological thought and nursing experience.

The method of nursology surfaced in true phenomenological fashion after Paterson reflected upon her experiences of trying to conceptualize the term *clinical*. Intent upon the outcome of her conceptualization of this term, the process by which this occurred went largely unnoticed. Of interest, it was the elucidation of the process of conceptualizing known as nursology that made its more enduring impact on nursing than the original conceptualization of the term clinical. The process of inquiry known as nursology is among the forerunners of methodologies distinct to nursing science. Paterson and Zderad were pioneers among nurse scholars in recognizing the need for congruence in philosophy, science, and method. The tradition has continued in nursing science with Parse's (1987) Man-Living-Health research methodology, a variant of phenomenology, and Leininger's (1985) ethnonursing method, which is derived from ethnographic methods.

A noteworthy characteristic of nursology is its similarity to the practice of clinical nursing. This view is consistent with Paterson and Zderad's beliefs in the integrality of nursing education, research, and clinical practice. Thus research was not held as something to be conducted only by academics but as part of the lived experience of all professional nurses, who weave the three threads of knowing, being, and doing into the art-science of practice.

The method of nursology seeks to answer the following question: "How can the nurse, a subjective-objective human being, know the other, be it person, thing, or spirit, and compare and complementarily synthesize these known others?" (Paterson, 1971, p. 144). The five overlapping and nonsequential phases of the method are (a) preparation of the knower for knowing, (b) knowing the other intuitively, (c) knowing the other scientifically, (d) complementarily synthesizing known others, and (e) succeeding from the "many" to the "paradoxical one" (Paterson, 1971, pp. 144-145; Paterson & Zderad, 1988, pp. 70-74).

Phase 1 (preparation of the knower) is a phase of receptivity and openness on the part of the knower. It is not a passive waiting but an active response to the invitation to know. The knower embraces an attitude of inquisitiveness and hopefulness and resists habitual response within situations. Paterson (1971) describes this as a risk-taking phase in which one dares to see the world as it presents itself rather than through an already established theoretical scheme. The "bracketing" (holding in abeyance) of one's prior assumptions, categories, and conceptions is attempted in this phase, although the impossibility of attaining a state of being without perspective is readily acknowledged. Instead, one attempts to gain maximal awareness of one's "angular view" such that one's shaded view of reality is recognized and considered. The outcome of this phase is the recognition and presentation of one's angular view of something.

Phase 2 (knowing the other intuitively) refers to the intuitive aspects of knowing in which the knower grasps the whole of the other through an imaginative process of getting in touch with the other's "rhythm and mobility" (Paterson, 1971, p. 144). The knower does not analyze the other. Intuition comes in the form of insight and understanding while analysis comes through a deliberate process of explaining or examining the other. This phase of knowing is comparable to the "I-Thou" moment in the transactive nursing process. Citing Buber, Paterson (1971, p. 144) states that intuitive-type knowing requires an "I" capable of both distance and relation with the other. The combination of distance and relation highlights the tension between merging with the other and maintaining a sense of one's own distinctiveness from the other. In this phase of knowing, the knower "does not superimpose, maintains a capacity for surprise and question, and is with the other as opposed to 'seeming to be' " (Paterson, 1971, p. 144). This intuitive phase necessarily precedes any meaningful analytic phase.

Phase 3 (knowing the other scientifically) highlights the kind of knowing that is a "looking at." It compares with the "I-It" moments in the transactive nursing process wherein the other is held at a distance and examined in its objectness. It is a phase of analysis and of interpretation. In this phase, a "name" is given to the lived experience and it is seen no longer primarily in its uniqueness but in its similarities to and differences from other experiences. It may become part of a categorization scheme. Its outcome is a relatively fixed symbolic representation of what had been the "mobile reality" (Bergson, cited in Paterson, 1971, p. 144) of the nursing situation.

Phase 4 (complementary synthesis) is the phase in which the knower as "noetic locus" (Paterson, 1971, p. 145) conducts an internal dialogue between the singular reality as conceptualized in Phase 3 and multiple other known realities. Within the knower, similarities and differences are noted among the multiple realities and a new creation emerges from this internal dialogue. This dialogue may lead to a statement of a general principle that includes, but is not exhausted by, the original experience. Complementary synthesis is thus described as "being more than additive because it allows mutual representation and illumination of one reality by another" (Paterson & Zderad, 1988, p. 74). In nursing process, this phase is likened to the noting of similarities and differences by the nurse across individual patients or within individual patients over time.

The fifth and final phase of nursology—succession from the "We" (Paterson, 1971, p. 145) or the "many" (Paterson & Zderad, 1988, p. 74) to the "paradoxical one"—refers to the phase in which the knower's original angular view of the other is changed as a result of participation in the first four phases of knowing. It is an acknowledgment of the transformative power of knowing. Its form is to be "ever more inclusive" (Paterson & Zderad, 1988, p. 74). This statement means that the transformed view of the other includes, but is not exhausted by, the newly formed insight. It is a view from the other side of the paradox that is obtained by struggling through the multiplicities toward a unified insight that moves knowledge forward. This temporary resting place can be likened to a moment of well-being in knowing; a moment in which the struggle to move beyond the achieved insight is suspended until one confronts in the clinical world something that cannot be included within the insight. Then begins the struggle toward more-being in knowing as the continuous refrain begins yet again.

Nursing as Doing and Being

Nursing as presence. Paterson and Zderad (1988) were among the first nursing theorists to explicate the concept of presence in nursing. Zderad (1978) suggests that the phenomenon as experienced in nursing situations is distinct from, yet related to, the phenomenon in general.

> Its occurrence or absence can be experienced. Both nurse and patient are aware of it. It is important to both. It makes one aware of oneself and of the other. It reveals a person to himself and to the other. Through it the nurse and the patient can show respect, closeness, caring—in short can confirm each other. In nurse-patient situations, the nurse's presence is expected by both. . . . [I]s "presence" a depreciable intangible in nursing that is more obvious in its absence? (Zderad, 1978, p. 42)

The theorists maintain that presence in nursing is a most exquisite rendition of "being with and doing with" (Paterson & Zderad, 1976, p. 13) patients. They suggest that "doing" aspects had previously been described in nursing. Their discussion of presence therefore focused on the quality of the nurse's being while recognizing that one of the distinct features of being present as a nurse is the inextricability of the threads of both being and doing. They further clarify the nature of this quality of being (which is expressed also in the doing) as involving one's whole being, as being given freely and chosen freely, and as being both personal and professional. The personal dimension attests to the unique quality of presence that each nurse brings to the nursing situation given her "angular" (Paterson & Zderad, 1976, p. 37) or unique perspective. Professional quality refers both to the goal-directedness of the situation and to the professional accountability of the nurse. Paterson and Zderad see nursing as being goal directed. The goal is "nurturing well-being and more-being" (Paterson & Zderad, 1976, p. 28) of patients within the "domain of health and illness" (p. 28). The accountability of the nurse to the patient, while experienced personally as human to human, is magnified and colored by the professional nature of the relationship. This professional accountability is influenced by the "limits of safe and sound practice" (Paterson & Zderad, 1976, p. 17) and is manifested by the nurse's "responsible choosing of overt responses based in knowledge and on nursing values" (Paterson & Zderad, 1976, p. 57).

A particularly important contribution of Paterson and Zderad's discussion of presence in the nursing situation is its ability to limit the concept within nursing's scope. The boundedness of the concept of presence is perhaps best seen in Paterson and Zderad's (1988) discussion of the attributes of presence such as spontaneity, availability, reciprocity, and mutuality. Although the foregoing are seen as critical attributes of presence, they are distinctly colored by the purpose of the nursing situation.

Paterson and Zderad's discussion of the attribute of spontaneity suggests their recognition of the tension between the goal-directedness of professional nursing presence and the inability to call forth presence on demand. Instead, presence can only be invoked or evoked and is a "gift of oneself" (Paterson & Zderad, 1988, p. 16) that is "revealed in a glance, touch or tone of voice" (Paterson & Zderad, 1988, p. 88). Therefore, immediately preceding presence, they recognize a "certain openness, a receptivity, readiness or availability" (Paterson & Zderad, 1988, p. 28). Said another way, being with in its fullest sense (presence) requires "turning one's attention toward the patient, being aware of and open to the here and now shared situation and communicating one's availability" (Paterson & Zderad, 1988, p. 14). It is the goal-directed nature of the nursing situation that modifies the quality of the availability, spontaneity, reciprocity, and mutuality that characterize nursing presence. *Availability* is modified as "availability-in-a-helping-way" (Paterson & Zderad, 1976, p. 28) and *openness* becomes an "openness to a person-with-needs" (Paterson & Zderad, 1976, p. 28).

Reciprocity, another critical attribute of nursing presence, is described as seeing both nurse (self) and patient (other) "as persons rather than as objects or functions" (Paterson & Zderad, 1988, p. 28). This reciprocity does not require that no differences be recognized between the presence of the nurse and the presence of the patient. Rather, the professional quality of nursing presence is "somehow colored by a sense of responsibility or regard for what is seen as the patient's vulnerability" (Paterson & Zderad, 1988, p. 28). The mutuality that characterizes nursing presence is not so much one of equality or of being "shared alike" as would be suggested by dictionary definitions of the term. Rather, reciprocity is seen as "flow between two persons with different modes of being in the shared situation" (Paterson & Zderad, 1988, p. 29).

Nursing as dialogue. The notion of nursing as dialogue conveys the back and forth ebb and flow of nursing as conveyed by Paterson and Zderad (1988). Nursing cannot take place without the nursed. Within this image of nursing, they discuss nursing lived as a "purposeful call and response" (p. 29), stating,

> Nursing implies a special kind of meeting of human persons. It occurs in response to a perceived need related to the health-illness quality of the human condition. Within that domain, . . . nursing is directed toward the goal of nurturing well-being and more-being (human potential). Nursing, therefore, does not involve a merely fortuitous encounter, but rather one in which there is purposeful call and response. In this vein, humanistic nursing may be considered a special kind of lived dialogue. (p. 24)

This discussion again calls attention to the fact that, for Paterson and Zderad, the mutuality that is involved in the nursing situation is experienced differently by the nurse and the nursed. This belief underscores the different modes of being in the situation that both bring.

They further describe dialogical nursing as a "transactive" process. By this description, they mean to convey the fact that the nursing process goes "both ways" (Paterson & Zderad, 1976, p. 132) between the participants (the nurse and the nursed). Even in the "intervention" phase of nursing, the nurse can call forth the possibilities seen within the patient, but "the patient must participate as an active subject to actualize the possibility (form) within himself [or herself]" (Paterson & Zderad, 1988, p. 92). Thus, within the transaction, there is always call and response. In another example, the theorists highlight the mutuality of the relation. They state, "Not only does the nurse see the possibilities in the patient but the patient also sees a form in the nurse (for example, possibility of help, of comfort, of support), and he [or she] responds in relation to bring it forth" (Paterson & Zderad, 1988, p. 92). In addition, they point out that the meaning of acts that occur in nursing situations are different for the nurse and the nursed. For instance, touch can be experienced as touching or being touched; the experience of feeding as feeding or being fed.

Health

Paterson and Zderad (1988) raise fundamental questions about whether health is the appropriate goal of nursing. They state that "the nursing act is always related to the health-illness quality of the human condition, or fundamentally to man's [sic] personal survival . . . that nursing is related to health and illness is self-evident. How it is related is not so apparent" (p. 12). Therefore they acknowledge the obviousness of nursing's involvement in health and illness but note that some of the most exquisite nursing acts occur in situations whereby health, taken in its narrow sense as the absence of disease, is not feasible as an aim. Some examples include dying patients, patients with incurable diseases, and those with chronic health conditions.

Comfort

Other nurses who have noted the poor fit between the definition of health as the absence of disease and nursing's focus have redefined health to include other meanings. Smith (1981) has pointed out some of these alternate meanings of health that have been commonly used in nursing discourse. Paterson and Zderad (1988), however, chose to define the aim of nursing as "comfort," which became "an umbrella term under which all other [health-related] terms could be sheltered" (p. 99). They reasoned that *comfort* was a term of historical importance in nursing and stated that it was also discussed in an ANA publication of their era as being of particular importance. Furthermore, it was a term that suggested itself to them as they sought to understand the major value that underlined their nursing practices (p. 98). Comfort was not chosen at whim; it emerged as an answer to the question as to "why" nurses are present in the health-illness situation.

The notion of comfort conveyed the sense that persons can be comfortable without being healthy and it is the promotion of this comfortable way of being that reflects nursing's most immediate concern. In other words, no matter what the state of health of a patient, a state of more or less comfort exists that is the proper aim of nursing. A patient can "be with" his or her health situation in a more or less comfortable way; this perhaps anticipated the American Nurses' Association's (1980) definition of nursing as being most concerned with the person's *response* to the health-illness situation.

The notion of comfort was also used to underscore the basic orientational belief that persons are capable of becoming ever more. Paterson and Zderad (1988) state, "Nursing's concern is not only with the well-being but with the more-being of patients" (p. 12). Thus comfort conveys the notion that a human being is "all he [or she] could be in accordance with his [or her] potential at any particular time in any particular situation" (p. 101).

Through their discussion of the similarities of the term *comfort* with the notion of contentment, Paterson and Zderad (1988) bring to light their particular understanding of the term *comfort:* It "does not imply passivity, resignation, retirement, or a simple avoiding of trouble" (p. 101). It is important that comfort not be equated with the absence of pain. Although the absence of pain can certainly be a comfortable state, it does not exhaust its possibilities. Because of the human capacity to become ever more, the natural state of human comfort is one of striving. Nonetheless, because of the notion of human adequacy and the tension between adequacy and possibility, it does not become what Benner and Wrubel (1989) have called "effortful striving." Boredom or lack of challenge can be as uncomfortable to humans as physical pain. Paterson and Zderad readily acknowledge that nurses at times encourage patients to experience stress or anxiety in the interest of growth. Zbilut (1980) has pointed out that this approach is common in holistic nursing practice. Achieving comfort is not akin to taking the easy way out of a situation or avoidance, although these possibilities remain open.

The ethics of this existentially grounded approach to comfort promotion have been questioned by Stevens (1990). She worries about the nurse imposing an existential view of comfort on patients. Does adopting this view of comfort mean that every patient should confront his or her situation and struggle to find its meaning? What about therapeutic denial? The key is to remember that, while the nurse might invite the patient to consider different possibilities, the nurse does not impose them on the patient. The mutuality of the nursing process as portrayed by these theorists would not allow such imposition of the nurses' intention on the patient. Nor would the patient's state of comfort-discomfort be solely determined by the nurse as a nursing diagnosis. Instead, the comfort-discomfort experience of the patient might be discerned by the nurse and then must be validated by the patient. It is highly likely that comfort goals will vary greatly both between patients and within a given patient over time. The important thing is to remain open to variation and choice within different contexts and understandings of comfort rather than stipulating what comfort will be. How much choice and variation is enough or too much within a professional relationship remains an ethical question of extreme importance within the discipline of nursing and one that is not limited to the problems posed by the existential viewpoint. Paterson and Zderad's view of the nurse-nursed relation identifies some limits within which such freedom is exercised, both on the part of the nurse and on the part of the patient. This view is consistent with their basic belief in situated versus radical freedom.

Well-Being and More-Being

Well-being and *more-being* are related terms within the metatheory and refer to human actuality and potential. Both are seen to contribute to the overall level of comfort of a given patient. In fact, they represent the essential tension between being and becoming, between what is and what might be, that characterizes the person within this metatheory. Well-being is closely related to the understanding of persons as "adequate" as described above. There is a sense in which humans are enough or just so. In addition, humans are free to choose to become more. Moreness is therefore a chosen way of being. It cannot be superimposed from the outside. The chief way in which persons become more is through relating to other persons in the various ways of "I-Thou," "I-It," and "We" (Paterson & Zderad, 1988, p. 44).

Environment

Views of the environment are not as fully explicated within this conceptual model as are the views of person and nursing. Nonetheless, references to relationships with the world in unique situations can easily be discerned. Paterson and Zderad (1988) state, "Nursing takes place in the real world of men [*sic*] and things in time and space" (p. 33). Further, they maintain that the meanings of these "things" vary between persons and that the time and space to which they refer are "as they are experienced" (p. 34). Human beings and the world are viewed as both distinct from each other and intimately related. Objective reality (something out there apart from one's experience of it) does exist even as subjective reality also exists. Paterson and Zderad thus avoid the idealist extreme of positing a *purely* subjective reality.

Despite the inclusion of objective reality, the main focus of Paterson and Zderad's (1988) view of the environment is that of time and space as experienced by both the patient and the nurse. Of particular concern is the subjective experience of both the patient and the nurse in a given situation such as crutch-walking or dealing with chronic illness and also with their intersubjective or shared experiences of the given situation (p. 19). In addition, while they acknowledge the environmental aspects of the nursing situation, Paterson and Zderad continue to hold the intersubjective nursing relationship as being of primary concern.

Here-and-Now

Paterson and Zderad's (1988) concept of the here-and-now always concerns a respect for the connectedness among one's past, current time, and future. It is always inclusive of both the nurses' and the patients' "origin, history, hopes, fears, and alternatives" (p. 68). Both participants in the nursing dialogue bring to the here-and-now their unique backgrounds and their hopes for the future. The notion of here-and-now builds upon the basic assumption of one's essential uniqueness and the responsibility this conveys. It can also refer to the fact that each here-and-now moment is significant and irreplaceable. Paterson and Zderad paraphrase Herman Hesse on this point: "Every nurse is more than just herself [or himself], she [or he] also represents the unique, the very special and always significant and remarkable point at which the nursing world's phenomena intersect, only once in this way and never again" (p. 69). Therefore it is the responsibility of each nurse to contribute to the development of general knowledge and nursing science by contributing his or her "nursing here-and-now to nursing's history through a lasting form of expression" (p. 69).

Nursing Situation

The nursing situation is a backdrop against which the intersubjective transaction that characterizes nursing dialogue occurs. It is a backdrop that at times becomes woven into the intersubjective transaction. Thus although Paterson and Zderad (1988) "place at the center of [their] universe . . . the nurse-patient intersubjective transaction" (p. 36), they readily acknowledge that this relationship does not take place in a vacuum. Indeed, they state that the "nursing dialogue is subjected to all the chaotic forces of life" (p. 31). Furthermore, they underscore that the health world is among the most complex, chaotic, and conflicted realms of existence. They present a summary statement of the nursing situation and hold it out as an inclusive yet open framework from which to explore more deeply the essential elements of humanistic nursing. They state that its elements would include "incarnate men [sic] (patient and nurse) meeting (being and becoming) in a goal-directed (nurturing well-being and more-being) intersubjective transaction (being with and doing with) occurring in time and space (measured and as lived by patient and nurse) in a world of men [sic] and things" (p. 18). Thus they readily afford to the environment a subjective and intersubjective nature ("as lived") and also an objective quality ("world of men and things") that must be reckoned with.

Included within the nursing situation is the effect of other human beings on both the nurse and the nursed. The participants' network of significant others influences the immediate nurse-patient situation. Paterson and Zderad (1988) state that the current lived nursing dialogue is "always colored by the patient's current mode of interpersonal relating" (p. 32). This statement further supports the inclusion of past and future elements in the here-and-now.

"Things" are also a significant part of the nursing situation within the metatheory. Not only does nursing dialogue take place in a "real world of men [*sic*] and things" (Paterson & Zderad, 1988, p. 32), but these ordinary things often take on a different significance in the nursing situation because of their connection to the health-illness quality of life and because of the different ways of being in the situation as nurse and patient. For example, because of a health-illness situation, the patient may at times attribute great significance to ordinary things previously taken for granted, such as being able to use a knife or fork. Likewise, the nurse's familiar things include machines and instruments and use of space in ways that are not familiar to patients. Both the individual and the shared meanings of the things that are in the situation are highly significant within humanistic nursing. For example, the humanistic nurse might take special precaution to avoid "medicalizing" familiar things within the patient's world such as food and drink. Judicious use of both medical and lay terminology is needed in humanistic nursing practice.

All-at-Once

All-at-once is a pivotal concept within the metatheory. It is the primary way in which the theorists convey both the paradoxical nature of human reality and the complex reality of the nursing world. The many paradoxical qualities of humans include the fact that, while all persons are unique, they are also similar. Another important paradox is that the individual's capacities include virtue and vice, spiritual and animal qualities, that are experienced all-at-once. Paterson and Zderad (1988) state that "human existence in the world calls for an enduring with our virtues and vices, our energy and our laziness, our altruism and our selfishness, in a word with our humanness" (p. 55). To deny either polarity as possibilities within ourselves or others results in a milieu of blame instead of one of responsibility and fosters a sense of powerlessness instead of well-being.

The use of the term *all-at-once* to communicate the complexity of the nursing situation is also common. This use underscores human existence as "never completely fathomable" (Paterson & Zderad, 1988, p. 8) and difficult to convey in words by use of strictly scientific processes of inquiry. As for the nursing situation, Paterson and Zderad (1988) use the term *multifarious multiplicities* to convey the complex web of occurrences that take place on a daily basis in everyday nursing situations. Nursing situations are "loaded with all kinds of incomparable data" (p. 96). Thus *all-at-once*, more than any

other term, describes the "what" of the nursing situation and is used
to describe its complexity. In fact, according to the theorists, a hallmark of nursing skill is the ability to balance these multifarious
multiplicities as they occur in the health world.

Finally, with regard to nurses' relating, Paterson and Zderad (1988)
use the notion of all-at-once to refer to the dual nature of nursing's
engagement in the worlds of "I-Thou" and "I-It." They state that

> the "all-at-once" is equated by [us] to Buber's "I-Thou" and "I-It"
> occurring simultaneously and not only in sequence as he expressed it.
> These two ways that man [sic] can relate to and come to know his [or
> her] world and himself [or herself] demand sequential expres-
> sion.... However, the responsible authentic nurse in the nursing arena
> lives them "all-at-once." (p. 110).

The nursing world thus mirrors the essential tension between these
two modes of relating and reflects a resolution of the tension in the
all-at-once experience that is the lived nursing act.

Community

The nurse-patient relationship can be defined as a form of community given Paterson and Zderad's (1988) definition of *community* as
"two or more persons struggling toward a common center" (p. 121).
Nonetheless, community is also portrayed as an element within
which this relation unfolds.

When it is experienced as a "between" phenomenon, it is more
readily experienced than explained. Paterson and Zderad's view of
community values differences and does not seek conformity. In the
experience of community, "discovered differences in similar realities
do not compete, one does not negate the other. . . . Differences can
make visible the greater realities of each" (p. 73).

Complementary Synthesis

This notion is highly related to the term *all-at-once*. It again refers
to the fact that nursing's reality is a multiple one in which the nurse
must traverse both the objective scientific world and the subjective
and intersubjective realms of nursing situations. The tension between
these realms is lived out in the nursing act. They state, "Doing with

and being with the patient calls for a complementary synthesis by the nurse of these two forms of human dialogue, 'I-It' and 'I-Thou.' Both are inherent in humanistic nursing, for it is a dialogue lived in the objective and intersubjective realms of the real world" (Paterson & Zderad, 1988, p. 36).

This concept is also seen in Paterson and Zderad's process of inquiry. Complementary syntheses occur in both Phases 4 and 5 of nursology. When used as part of the inquiry process, it refers to a process of attending to realities other than one's own "angular view." It thus is a form of communicating and connecting self and others and self and world. Thus the process of complementary synthesis characterizes both nursing situations and the process of nursology.

45

General Theory of Nursing

The second phase of theorizing, that of relating the explicated concepts, is illustrated by Paterson and Zderad's (1988) "theory of nursing" (p. 111). They propose relationships among their phenomenologically derived concepts. They state, "A human nurse nurses through a clinical process of I-Thou I-It all-at-once to comfort" (p. 111). Although the concepts arose from psychiatric mental health nursing, the theorists assert that they are applicable across all nursing contexts. This affirmation illustrates a movement from the "many to the paradoxical one" (p. 74) whereby their particular conception of nursing is held to be meaningful to "the many or to all" (p. 75).

The specific form of the nursing relationship proposed by Paterson and Zderad is that of the "I-Thou, I-It, all-at once" (p. 111). This relation can be described as a reformulation of Buber's (1953) "I-Thou" relationship. The reformulation is necessary to portray the unique aspects of relating within nursing situations. Specifically, the need to include some objectifying features of relating (i.e., looking at) in nursing while maintaining the foundational orientation to the subjectivity of the recipient of nursing care, to whom they refer as "the nursed" (Paterson & Zderad, 1978), seems to underlie this reformulation.

A noted Buber scholar (Manheim, 1974) pointed out that Buber understood that not all relationships at all times must reflect the ideal

I-Thou relation. According to Manheim (1974), in some "fruitful" (p. 38) relationships, relations of "imbalance" are the appropriate norm. These "unbalanced" (p. 38) relationships do not contain "complete reciprocity" (p. 37). Using as examples of these unbalanced relationships the teacher-pupil and the patient-therapist relationship, Manheim suggests that a "genuine Thou relationship, for instance, can hover between teacher and pupil" (p. 38). The mutuality is incomplete because the pupil (or patient) "cannot exercise the same participation in the mutual situation, except if it were in a transfer to a friendship. . . . Buber believes that, whenever an aim is to be accomplished, mutuality cannot be complete" (p. 38).

With regard to the outcomes of this relating, Paterson and Zderad (1988) posit that of "comfort" (p. 99). This is defined as "an umbrella concept under which all the other terms—growth, health, freedom and openness—could be sheltered" (p. 99). The chief dimension of relating, according to Paterson and Zderad's general theory of nursing, is presence. Presence is really what enables comfort. They state, "Through her [the nurse's] presence it is possible for other persons to be all they can be [i.e., be comfortable] in crisis situations of their worlds" (p. 56). Thus a relational statement between presence and comfort is proposed within the general theory of nursing.

What theoretical explanation is given to account for this proposed relationship? Paterson and Zderad (1988) draw an explanation of this relationship from existential philosophy, primarily the work of Buber and Marcel, who maintain "that it is through his [sic] relations with other men [sic] that a man [sic] becomes, that his [sic] unique individuality is actualized" (p. 16). Paraphrasing Buber (1965, cited in their 1988 work), Paterson and Zderad state that knowledge of oneself as an individual comes through experiencing oneself as "this particular unique here-and-now person and other than that there-and-now person . . . to know myself as me is to see myself in relation to and distant from other selves" (p. 16). They conclude the discussion by posing that the possibility for "self-confirmation exists in any intersubjective situation" (p. 16) but that availability and presence immediately precede choice, which is "a response to possibility" (p. 16) and through which people become more. Therefore the two major processes that underlie humanistic nursing are choice and presence. While these processes are separated for the purposes of discussion, in the lived nursing situation, they are inextricably interwoven. Together they explain the proposed link between presence and comfort, which is the central tenet of Paterson and Zderad's general theory of nursing.

46

Clinical Example

Paterson and Zderad (1978) describe the process of nursing as "quality caring based in the concept of community," which presupposes adequate knowledge and skill. They state that, from the simplest greeting of a patient to the most advanced resuscitation, nurses act as "imaginative artists" (1978) calling forth the actualities of patients by being open to the unique possibilities in the situation. This calling forth can be seen as a form of assessment and planning that takes place with the patient. The "intervention" phase is always occurring because assessment is ongoing; nonetheless, for purposes of understanding, this phase is similar to the point in which the envisioned potentials are brought forth and realized. This realization might take the form of an increased feeling of well-being, more-being, comfort, or growth. Thus "intervention" is accomplished by presence. Nurses help patients make choices from within the realities of their situations by sharing their knowledge and experience and nurturing a patient's responsible choosing. The nurse and the nursed together search for the meaning in the health-illness situation. Clinical nursing can therefore be seen as comfort promotion by means of a process of presencing.

One specific approach to comfort promotion that has been described by Zderad (1978) is the process of listening to others and living past events through with them. This allows the experience to be reinterpreted by the patient and facilitates the development of a new

perspective on the experience. Zderad speaks of this process as one
that deals with the effects of the past and future on the "here-and-
now" (p. 68). Other specific comfort promoting strategies have been
elucidated by Paterson and Zderad (1988, pp. 99-100) and have been
enlivened by a detailed clinical example from psychiatric nursing in
their major text (pp. 113-119). Many of these aspects of humanistic
nursing practice theory can be discerned in the following illustration,
which comes from the writer's nursing experience within a primary
health care context in an urban setting.

Example of Humanistic Nursing Practice

Jack was an African American man in his early 40s who was
referred by a community health nurse to our primary nursing care
practice for ongoing health care. Community health nurses staffed
our hospital's walk-in referral service. Jack had made only sporadic
health care visits to various medical providers across the 20-year
period that followed a lengthy hospitalization in his early 20s for
meningitis secondary to tuberculosis. He lived alone and was supported by a meager welfare allotment. He described a profound
distrust and fear of hospitals and doctors and prided himself in a
fierce independence that had enabled him to live independently
despite significant memory loss related to the earlier meningitis.
Nonetheless, certain symptoms would prompt Jack to seek health
care.

Jack's first visit to our practice was one such occasion. His symptom
of concern at the time was a cough. When listening to Jack's description of his concern, the nurse became aware of Jack's terror regarding
the cough, which seemed out of proportion to the severity of the
clinical picture. When Jack was invited to explore his feelings and
perceptions related to the symptom, he readily revealed fear of a
recurrence of tuberculosis. He was also reliving his fears of being
hospitalized for an extended time and held the past hospitalization
of 20 years before very close to the current time. For example, he
worried about disclosing the etiology of his "memory problem"
to anyone for fear they would avoid him due to fears of contagion.
This fear had contributed to the development of an interpersonal

relating style that encouraged distance and evasion rather than friendship or intimacy. Significant losses had accompanied his prior illness experience. His wife had divorced him during the course of his lengthy hospitalization and had withheld visitation privileges of their only son. Jack's mother, who had been his major source of nurturance throughout the 20 years following his lengthy hospitalization, had recently died. Jack's ruggedly independent way of being in the world was severely threatened as he experienced frightening symptoms and tried to face them alone. Jack's call was heard by the nurse, who responded with an invitation to further dialogue.

During the first visit with Jack, the nurse focused on his concerns related to recurrence and began to explore with him the significance of the illness experience of 20 years ago. These issues were addressed by the engagement of the nurse and Jack in a presencing process that wove together the health history, physical examination, and narrative accounts of Jack's current concern and past illness experiences. Jack responded to the nurse's call to explore both his current concerns and his past illness experience; Jack's well-being was restored when his fears were acknowledged and addressed. Jack left the visit feeling hopeful about coming to a greater understanding of what he termed his "memory problem" during future planned visits to the nursing service.

Jack's hope was lived out through the experience of more-being that can be discerned in his life over the next 4 years. During this time Jack remained a continuing client of the nursing service and maintained a primary health care relationship with the nurse with whom he had initially connected. Within this relationship across the years, limits and possibilities of living with chronic memory impairment were explored. Jack elected to participate in both a vocational rehabilitation program and a high school equivalency program, during which he confronted the limits of his analytic ability. Never able to pass a required math class, Jack worked through a choice to disclose his past history to the instructor so that alternate learning experiences could be planned. Jack was ultimately able to secure a more stable financial status for himself by qualifying for medical disability instead of general welfare and by using his vocational skills for part-time work. He proudly reported to the nurse that he was happy now to pay for his office calls to the nursing service!

Across this 4-year time period, the more-being of the nurse also grew steadily. The ongoing relationship with Jack and others within the context of an autonomous nursing group practice was the fountainhead of much learning about dependence, independence, and interdependence. This learning endures as a guiding insight for the nurse's ongoing clinical scholarship.

47

Scholarship Related to the Model

Review of the scholarship related to humanistic nursing practice theory reveals that the work is commonly cited in discussions of qualitative methods, philosophies of nursing science, ethical aspects of nursing science, and summaries of major theoretical perspectives in nursing. Also, many researchers continue to refer to humanistic nursing practice theory and/or the process of nursology as they discuss their findings. This is particularly noted in research in the areas of caring and presence (Brown, 1986; Drew, 1986), dialogue and mutuality in relationship (Baer & Lowery, 1987; Rigdon, Clayton, & Dimond, 1987), humanism and nursing, and empathy and in research related to common existentialist themes such as loneliness (Mahon, 1982) and commitment. A few studies have used the metatheory as a guide for the study proper; only these few studies are included in the research bibliography. Thus humanistic nursing has awakened new understandings of the nursing situation and continues to inspire new ways of thinking about nursing. As a metatheory, it continues to hold promise for inviting further theoretical formulations.

48

Future Direction of Humanistic Nursing Practice Theory

Paterson and Zderad's (1988) work underscores two of the essential tensions within the nurse-patient relationship: namely, the need to balance the purely human elements of the encounter with the professional dimensions of the relationship and the related issue of boundaries within the relationship as a function of its purposiveness. The importance of this aspect of their work will continue to be recognized by scholars of the nurse-patient relationship. Also, Paterson and Zderad's work will likely provide direction for fruitful systematic ethical inquiry.

Ethical Considerations

The nature of the nurse-patient relationship in light of its purposiveness has recently been discussed as having a critical ethical dimension in, for example, the work of Gadow (1985). Gadow states that nursing care requires "attending to the 'objectness' of persons without reducing them to the moral status of objects" (pp. 33-34). The issue has also been discussed in the recent work of Bishop and Scudder (1990). Scudder, in earlier work with Mickunas (1985, cited in Bishop & Scudder, 1990), posits a necessary reformulation of

Buber's (1953) "I-Thou" relationship when it is used to describe relations between nurses and patients. Scudder and Mickunas do so in a manner similar to that of Paterson and Zderad (1976, 1988). Scudder and Mickunas (1985, cited in Bishop & Scudder, 1990) state, "Such relationships between nurse and patient could neither be described as I-Thou or as I-It but could be described as I-It (Thou)" (p. 148). Such relationships are ones in which "a person is recognized as a person, even when limited time, the need for routine precision, or the patient care situation requires impersonal treatment" (Bishop & Scudder, 1990, p. 148). It is not known if Paterson and Zderad's (1976, 1988) work influenced Gadow or Bishop and Scudder despite the similarities with which they reformulated Buber's thought for use in nursing relationships. Gadow's work and its similarity to their own work is pointed out by Bishop and Scudder (1990, pp. 154, 156). These independent working styles typify the lack of connectedness among nurse ethicists and nurse theorists in the area of the nurse-patient relationship as well as in other domains of inquiry within nursing (Reed, 1989; Sarter, 1988). As the ethical nature of theorizing is increasingly realized in nursing (Reed, 1989; Yeo, 1989), Paterson and Zderad's humanistic nursing practice theory will be recognized for its strengths in this regard and for its consonance with the ethical positions put forward by Gadow (1985) and Bishop and Scudder (1990).

Current Resources

Because Paterson and Zderad are both retired from nursing, it seems particularly important to name those scholars currently engaged in work arising from humanistic nursing practice theory. Paterson and Zderad (personal communication, July 1991) identify the following as currently engaged in such work:

- Sumiko Fujiki (psychiatric mental health nursing educator), 600 New Stine Road, Apt. 22, Bakersfield, CA 93309-2970, telephone 805-664-3111 (work) and 805-397-1699 (home)
- Doris R. Hines (clinical nurse specialist in adult health and researcher), RR#1, Box 341, Agency, MS 64401, telephone 816-271-7111 (page through operator), 816-271-7707 (office), and 816-253-9443 (home)

Those listed here have expressed their willingness to serve as resources for future development of humanistic nursing practice theory.

The writer is also interested in applications of humanistic nursing practice theory in nonpsychiatric nursing settings, in particular in adult primary health care contexts. She can be reached at Oakland University School of Nursing, Rochester, MI 49309-4401, telephone 313-370-4076 (office) and 313-549-6398 (home).

Glossary

All-at-once
"Awareness of living many concepts, emotions, desires, values in a particular instance dispels narrow singularity of purpose and complements wisdom" (Paterson, 1978, p. 51).

Between
Mutual presence of the nurse-nursed; "the basic relation in which and through which nursing can occur" (Paterson & Zderad, 1988, p. 22); the realm of intersubjective experience.

Choice
"Response to possibility" (Paterson & Zderad, 1988, p. 16).

Clinical
"Aware presence in the health situation" (Paterson, 1978, p. 51).

Comfort
"Persons being all they can be in particular life situations" (Paterson, 1978, p. 51).

Complementary synthesis
Seeing through multiple realities to a unified insight.

Empathy
"Imaginative moving towards oneness with another, sharing his [or her] being in a situation, resulting in an insightful knowledge of his [or her] perspective" (Paterson, 1978, p. 51).

More-being
The *becoming* aspect of the being-becoming polarity.

Multifarious multiplicities
The complex nature of the nursing situation with its diverse concerns.

Noetic locus
Source of knowing; refers to the synthesis of knowledge that occurs within humans.

Nursology
Phenomenological method of inquiry into nursing phenomena aimed toward developing nursing theory.

Nurturance
"Promoting growth through relating" (Paterson, 1978, p. 51).

Phenomenology
A descriptive method of inquiry into the nature of phenomena *as experienced.*

Presence
"Being with" another as compared with "seeming-to-be"; existential relating of one being-as-being to another being-as-being.

Transaction
A descriptor highlighting the two-way nature of relating; the relating goes both ways between participants.

Well-being
The being aspect of the being-becoming polarity.

References

American Nurses' Association. (1980). *Nursing: A social policy statement.* Kansas City, MO: Author.

Baer, E. D., & Lowery, B. J. (1987). Patient and situational factors that affect nursing students' like or dislike of caring for patients. *Nursing Research, 36*(5), 298-302.

Benner, P., & Wrubel, J. (1989). *The primacy of caring.* New York: Addison-Wesley.

Bishop, A. H., & Scudder, J. R. (1990). *The practical, moral, and personal sense of nursing: A phenomenological philosophy of practice.* Albany: State University of New York Press.

Brown, L. (1986). The experience of care: Patient perspectives. *Topics in Clinical Nursing, 8*(2), 56-62.

Buber, M. (1953). I and Thou. In W. Herberg (Ed.), *The writings of Martin Buber* (pp. 43-62). New York: World.

Drew, M. (1986). Exclusion and confirmation: A phenomenology of patient's experiences with caregivers. *Image: Journal of Nursing Scholarship, 18*(2), 39-43.

Fawcett, J. (1980). A framework for analysis and evaluation of conceptual models. *Nurse Educator, 5*(6), 10-14.

Fawcett, J. (1984). *Analysis and evaluation of conceptual models of nursing.* Philadelphia: F. A. Davis.

Flaskerud, J. H., & Halloran, E. J. (1980). Areas of agreement in nursing theory. *Advances in Nursing Science, 3*(1), 1-7.

Gadow, S. A. (1985). Nurse and patient: The caring relationship. In A. H. Bishop & J. Scudder (Eds.), *Caring, curing, coping* (pp. 31-43). University: University of Alabama Press.

Guigan, C. (1986). Existentialist ethics. In J. P. Demarco & R. M. Fox (Eds.), *New directions in ethics* (pp. 73-91). New York: Routledge & Kegan Paul.

Leininger, M. M. (1985). *Qualitative research methods in nursing.* Orlando, FL: Grune & Stratton.

Mahon, N. E. (1982). The relationship of self-disclosure, interpersonal dependency, and life changes to loneliness in young adults. *Nursing Research, 31*(6), 343-347.

Manheim, W. (1974). *Martin Buber.* New York: Twayne.

Newman, M. A. (1983). The continuing revolution: A history of nursing science. In N. L. Chaska (Ed.), *The nursing profession: A time to speak* (pp. 385-393). New York: McGraw-Hill.

Parse, R. R. (1987). *Nursing science: Major paradigms, theories and critiques.* Philadelphia: W. B. Saunders.

Paterson, J. G. (1971). From a philosophy of clinical nursing to a method of nursology. *Nursing Research, 20*(2), 143-146.

Paterson, J. G. (1978). The tortuous way toward nursing theory. In *Theory development: What, why, how?* (NLN Publication No. 15-1708, pp. 49-65). New York: National League for Nursing.

Paterson, J. G., & Zderad, L. T. (1976). *Humanistic nursing.* New York: John Wiley.

Paterson, J. G., & Zderad, L. T. (Speakers). (1978). *Humanistic nursing practice theory* [Audio cassette, taped from the Second Annual Nurse Educator Conference]. New York. New York: Concept Media.

Paterson, J. G., & Zderad, L. T. (1988). *Humanistic nursing* (NLN Publication No. 41-2218, 2nd ed.). New York: National League for Nursing.

Reed, P. G. (1989). Nursing theorizing as an ethical endeavor. *Advances in Nursing Science, 11*(3), 1-9.

Rigdon, I. S., Clayton, B. C., & Dimond, M. (1987). Toward a theory of helpfulness for the elderly bereaved: An invitation to a new life. *Advances in Nursing Science, 9*(2), 32-43.

Sarter, B. (1988). Philosophical sources of nursing theory. *Nursing Science Quarterly, 1,* 52-59.

Smith, J. A. (1981). The idea of health: A philosophic inquiry. *Advances in Nursing Science, 3*(3), 43-50.

Stevens, B. J. (1990). *Nursing theory analysis, application, evaluation* (3rd ed.). Glenview, IL: Scott Foresman/Little, Brown.

White, M. (1983). *The age of analysis.* Boston: Houghton Mifflin.

Yeo, M. (1989). Integration of nursing theory and nursing ethics. *Advances in Nursing Science, 11*(3), 33-43.

Zbilut, J. P. (1980). Holistic nursing: The transcendental factor. *Nursing Forum, 19*(1), 45-49.

Zderad, L. T. (1969). Empathic nursing: Realization of a human capacity. *Nursing Clinics of North America, 4,* 655-662.

Zderad, L. T. (1978). From here and now to theory: Reflections on "how." *Theory development: What, why, how?* (NLN Publication No. 15-1708, pp. 35-48). New York: National League for Nursing.

Bibliography

Published Works of Paterson and Zderad

Paterson, J. G. (1971). From a philosophy of clinical nursing to a method of nursology. *Nursing Research, 20*(2), 143-146.

Paterson, J. G. (1978). The tortuous way toward nursing theory. In *Theory development: What, why, how?* (NLN Publication No. 15-1708, pp. 49-65). New York: National League for Nursing.

Paterson, J. G., & Zderad, L. T. (1970). All together through complementary syntheses the worlds of the many. *Image, 4*(3), 13-16.

Paterson, J. G., & Zderad, L. T. (1976). *Humanistic nursing.* New York: John Wiley.

Paterson, J. G., & Zderad, L. T. (1988). *Humanistic nursing* (NLN Publication No. 41-2218). New York: National League for Nursing.

Zderad, L. T. (1969). Empathic nursing: Realization of a human capacity. *Nursing Clinics of North America, 4,* 655-662.

Zderad, L. T. (1970). Empathy: From cliché to construct. In *Proceedings of the Third Nursing Theory Conference* (pp. 46-75). Lawrence: University of Kansas Medical Center, Department of Nursing.

Zderad, L. T. (1978). From here and now to theory: Reflections on "how." *Theory development: What, why, how?* (NLN Publication No. 15-1708, pp. 35-48). New York: National League for Nursing.

Summary, Critique, and Analysis

Brouse, S. H., & Laffrey, S. C. (1989). Paterson & Zderad's humanistic nursing framework. In J. J. Fitzpatrick & A. H. Whall (Eds.), *Conceptual models of nursing: Analysis and application* (2nd ed., pp. 205-225). Norwalk, CT: Appleton-Lange.

Kleinman, S. (1986). Humanistic nursing: The phenomenological theory of Paterson & Zderad. In P. Winstead-Fry (Ed.), *Case studies in nursing theory* (NLN Publication No. 15-2152, pp. 167-195). New York: National League for Nursing.

Meleis, A. F. (1991). *Theoretical nursing: Development and progress.* New York: J. B. Lippincott.

Praeger, S. G., & Hogarth, C. R. (1990). Josephine E. Paterson and Loretta T. Zderad. In J. B. George (Ed.), *Nursing theories: The base for professional practice* (3rd ed., pp. 287-299). Norwalk, CT: Appleton-Lange.

Stevens, B. J. (1990). *Nursing theory analysis, application, evaluation* (3rd ed.). Glenview, IL: Scott Foresman/Little, Brown.

General Commentary

Boyd, C. O. (1990). Critical appraisal of developing nursing research methods. *Nursing Science Quarterly, 3*(1), 42-43.

Cohen, M. Z. (1987). A historical overview of the phenomenologic movement. *Image: Journal of Nursing Scholarship, 19*(1), 31-34.

Munhall, P. L., & Oiler, C. J. (1986). *Nursing research: A qualitative perspective.* Norwalk, CT: Appleton-Century-Crofts.

Oiler, C. J. (1986). Qualitative methods: Phenomenology. In P. Moccia (Ed.), *New approaches to theory development* (NLN Publication No. 15-1992, pp. 75-103). New York: National League for Nursing.

Sarter, B. (1987). Evolutionary idealism: A philosophical foundation for holistic nursing theory. *Advances in Nursing Science, 9*(2), 1-9.

Taylor, S. G. (1985). Rights and responsibilities: Nurse-patient relationships. *Image: Journal of Nursing Scholarship, 17*(1), 9-13.

Watson, J. (1981). Nursing's scientific quest. *Nursing Outlook, 29,* 413-416.

Research

Hinds, P. S. (1988). The relationship of nurses' caring behaviors with hopefulness and health care outcomes in adolescents. *Archives of Psychiatric Nursing, 2*(1), 21-29.

Hines, D. R. (1991). *The development of the measurement of presence scale.* Unpublished doctoral dissertation, Texas Woman's University.

Kleinman, S. (1986). Humanistic nursing: The phenomenological theory of Paterson & Zderad. In P. Winstead-Fry (Ed.), *Case studies in nursing theory* (NLN Publication No. 15-2152, pp. 167-195). New York: National League for Nursing.

Pettigrew, J. M. (1988). *A phenomenological study of the nurse's presence with persons experiencing suffering.* Unpublished doctoral dissertation, Texas Woman's University.

PART VIII

Madeleine Leininger

Cultural Care Diversity and Universality Theory

CHERYL L. REYNOLDS

MADELEINE LEININGER

Biographical Sketch of the Nurse Theorist Madeleine Leininger, PhD, RN, CTN, LHD, FAAN

Born: July 6, 1924, Sutton, Nebraska

Current Position: Professor of Nursing and Anthropology, Wayne State University, Detroit, Michigan

Education: Diploma at St. Anthony's School of Nursing, Denver, Colorado, 1948

BS Biological Science, Benedictine College, Atchison, Kansas, 1950

MSN Catholic University of America, Washington, DC, 1954

PhD Anthropology, University of Washington, Seattle, Washington, 1965

Fellow, American Academy of Nursing

Honorary Doctor of Humane Letters, Benedictine College, 1975

Honorary Doctor of Science: University of Indianapolis, Indianapolis, Indiana

Honorary Doctor of Nursing Science: University of Kuopio, Kuopio, Finland (the only woman nurse scientist and anthropologist to receive this degree)

Editor, *Journal of Transcultural Nursing*

Founder, transcultural nursing field and Transcultural Nursing Society

President, International Association of Human Caring

Recipient of numerous awards and honors

Foreword

This section provides an overview of basic information about *Culture Care Diversity and Universality: A Theory of Nursing*. Undoubtedly, nursing students as well as interested colleagues will be eager to learn about a theory that is growing in relevance and usefulness worldwide.

In a world that is rapidly becoming multicultural, it is imperative that nurses consider theories that help them discover relevant dimensions of nursing. It is timely that nursing students study theories that make them think about the care of people from diverse cultures in relation to health, human care, and illness. The theory of culture care focuses on generating knowledge related to the nursing care of people who value their cultural heritage and lifeways. The theory has great significance because nurses are realizing that today, and even more in the near future, they need knowledge to guide them in their decisions and actions as they care for clients of different cultures.

As a culture care theorist, I have devoted a lifetime of creative thinking to developing the theory that could be used in all cultures to study and discover culture care differences (the diversities) and similarities (the universals) about transcultural human care. Accordingly, the theory with research findings is viewed not only as highly relevant but also as a powerful and meaningful theory to understand human beings of diverse cultures. The theory, and findings from the use of the theory, will remain important well into the 21st century because of increased multiculturalism worldwide.

Currently, nurses are traveling and working in many foreign cultures. However, they often realize, by cultural shock or in other ways, that people differ in the way they view professional nursing and client care needs. Nurses are almost forced to consider the role of cultural factors in client care.

The culture care theory has helped many nurses focus on the diverse cultural factors that influence client behavior and well-being. Because culture is holistic and comprehensive, the nurse discovers important *emic* (local) views and *etic* (outsider's) views to develop nursing care practices. Data from the culture care theory will also assist nurses to avoid cultural imposition and other unfavorable nursing care practices. Most important, the theory with concomitant research findings often becomes a "blueprint" to guide nursing decisions, actions, and outcomes for quality-based nursing care practices. The theory also supports the work of transcultural nursing specialists or generalists as they use culture-specific knowledge generated from the theory. The theory and transcultural nursing have been evolving together for 3 decades, bringing many new benefits to nurses and clients.

The authors of this section begin with an overview of the theory of culture care with a focus on the origin and the development of the theory over time. They provide highlights of the theory using the well-known sunrise model to depict and study the components of the theory in Western and non-Western cultures. It has always been exciting to see nurses who use the theory greatly expand their thinking as they realize different cultural factors that influence illness, wellness, and ways that clients maintain their wellness or become ill. The authors present fundamental perspectives of the theory to help students discover new facts, insights, meanings, and expressions about culture care that can change nursing practices significantly in providing culture-congruent care as the goal of the theory. Students will find the content fascinating and different as they shift from traditional medical model symptoms and disease orientations to cultural ways of knowing.

The next section is actually a shorthand version of Leininger's comprehensive and definitive work about her theory, *Culture Care Diversity and Universality: A Theory of Nursing*, published by the National League for Nursing in 1991. (The reader is encouraged to read the 1991 book to gain more in-depth insights about the theory and the ethnonursing research method.) Leininger's book contains several research studies and findings of nearly 30 cultures to guide nurses' thinking for Leininger's three models of nursing practice. Some very practical ways to use the research findings from many different cultures are discussed with the transcultural nursing research studies of different cultures.

Finally, one must commend editors Chris McQuiston and Adele Webb for their genuine desire to facilitate student learning about nursing theorists and to emphasize the critical importance of nursing theories to advance nursing knowledge.

MADELEINE LEININGER, RN, CTN, PhD, LHD, DS, FAAN
Professor of Nursing and Anthropology
Colleges of Nursing and Liberal Arts
Wayne State University, Detroit, Michigan

49

Origin of Leininger's Theory

CHERYL L. REYNOLDS

Through clinical practice with disturbed children while developing the role of the clinical specialist in child psychiatric nursing, Leininger became aware that cultural differences between patients and nurses made a difference in health outcomes. Children of diverse cultures reacted to the interventions of nurses differently. Thus Leininger credits children with pointing out that culture was the link to understanding the nursing care of persons from different backgrounds. This discovery led her to study cultural differences in the perceptions of care in 1954 and doctoral work in cultural anthropology in 1959 (Leininger, 1980, 1988a).

Leininger (1988a) was concerned with "ways that care and nursing practice could accurately describe and reflect nursing knowledge" (p. 152). This search, coupled with the discovery of culture as the missing link in nursing theory, set the stage for Leininger to determine that "care and culture were inextricably linked together and could not be separated in nursing care actions and decisions" (p. 153).

Doctoral study in anthropology and a background in nursing provided Leininger with expertise in two major disciplines—both of which support the concept of holism and have as their object knowledge of human phenomena (Leininger, 1970). With an understanding of how anthropology could contribute to nursing knowledge and how nursing could contribute to anthropological knowledge, Leininger began to look at the practice and discipline of nursing in a new way.

She became interested in questions about "the role of caring and curing in human evolution and survival of the species" (Leininger, 1980, p. 137). Through observation she determined that medical practice was oriented toward curing while nursing was oriented toward "caring acts and processes focusing on multiple factors influencing wellness and illness" (Leininger, 1980, p. 137). The result of reflecting on this difference was Leininger's conclusion that patterns of human caring and curing could be identified if anthropological and nursing perspectives were blended.

The combined nursing and anthropological inquiry into care and cure phenomena provided her with the knowledge base to develop concepts, hypotheses, and other building blocks for the theory of cultural care. Leininger (1988a) writes,

> It took time and in-depth study to link culture and care into a meaningful relationship. The theory of cultural care diversity and universality was difficult to formulate because there was so much to understand about cultures in the world and nursing's perspectives of cultural phenomena. (p. 153)

Because so few nurses were prepared in both anthropology and nursing, Leininger tackled much of this inquiry and theory development on her own (Leininger, 1980, 1984a, 1988a, 1989a, 1991b). Her recognition that there was a lack of nurses prepared for such a challenge and her beliefs that "patients have a *right* to have their sociocultural backgrounds understood" (Leininger, 1970, pp. 45-46) led her to develop courses and programs in what came to be known as transcultural (or crosscultural) nursing (Leininger, 1984b).

Leininger (1991) writes that she is frequently asked what has most influenced her theoretical thinking. To these queries she replies,

> I would have to answer, rather candidly, that there was no one person or philosophic school of thought, or ideology, *per se*, that directly influenced my thinking. I developed the theory by working on the potential interrelationships of *culture* and *care* through creative think-

ing and by philosophizing from my past professional nursing experiences and anthropological insights. (p. 20)

Ideas and themes related to the development and refinement of the theory of culture care are found in virtually all of her publications. As a prolific writer, Leininger has authored articles, book chapters, and books focusing on a number of subjects—most of which are related through ideas about cultural care. Topics for which Leininger is most well known are the theory of culture care, care and caring concepts, transcultural nursing concepts, and qualitative research methods.

Evolution of the Theory

Components of the theory of culture care diversity and universality and the sunrise model have been under development for over 3 decades. Leininger recently commented that she knows of at least 10 versions of her model. Although there are many versions of the model, there are fewer publications that address the theory as a whole. Two major articles that present Leininger's theory of cultural care were published in 1985 and 1988. A book outlining the theory and its research applications was published in 1991. Thus rigorous preparatory work in concept analysis and model development have been Leininger's focus in preparation for the presentation of the ideas in theory form.

Concept Development

Development of the concepts of care and caring was a necessary first step in the evolution of Leininger's theory. Therefore more of her publications have been directed toward describing aspects of these concepts than have been directed toward describing either the sunrise model or the theory of culture care. Understanding the history of Leininger's ideas pertaining to the concepts of care and caring is crucial to understanding her model and theory.

As early as 1970, Leininger identified the words *care* and *caring* in a major publication as important nursing elements. These components of nursing were chosen by Leininger (1970) for discussion in a book chapter describing the nature of nursing and how nursing and anthropology could complement each other. *Care* was first defined as a noun that implied "the provision of personalized and necessary services to help man maintain his health state or recover from illness" (p. 30). *Caring* was the verb counterpart to the noun and Leininger believed it implied "a feeling of compassion, interest, and concern for people" (p. 30). This publication not only signaled Leininger's focus on care in nursing but also on the importance of the separation of the concepts "care" and "caring" for fuller understanding. This separation remains a theme throughout the rest of Leininger's writings to the present day. Definitions of these concepts have continued to evolve over time.

By the mid 1970s, Leininger had begun the development of ideas about the dichotomy between caring and curing. Caring was viewed as the most critical component of curing consequences (Leininger, 1977). By 1984, Leininger had expanded this idea to maintain that there could be no curing without caring but that caring could take place without curing. This theme also remains prevalent in Leininger's writings to date.

In the late 1970s, Leininger focused on the differences between caring in a generic and professional sense. Generic care/caring was defined as "those assistive, supportive, or facilitative acts toward or for another individual or group with evident or anticipated needs to ameliorate or improve a human condition or lifeway" (Leininger, 1981b, p. 9). Professional caring was seen as "those cognitive and culturally learned action behaviors, techniques, processes, or patterns that enable (or help) an individual, family, or community to improve or maintain a favorably healthy condition or lifeway" (p. 9). Further, professional nursing care was also defined. It was viewed as "those cognitively learned humanistic and scientific modes of helping or enabling an individual, family, or community to receive personalized services" (p. 9).

Leininger's focus on distinguishing between care/caring as known from the perspective of lay people of the culture with that known by professionals reflects her background in anthropology. In cultural anthropology, a prominent theme is the importance of understanding differences between an emic and an etic view. *Emic* "refers to the language expressions, perceptions, beliefs, and practices of individuals or groups of a particular culture in regard to certain phenomena" (Leininger, 1984c, p. 135). *Etic* "refers to the *universal* language expressions, beliefs, and practices in regard to certain phenomena that pertain to several cultures or groups" (Leininger, 1984c, p. 134). This anthropological theme, then, is a logical basis for Leininger's differentiation between generic and professional care.

In early definitions of generic and professional care, it was only professional care that included the idea that the behaviors, acts, or processes were learned. By the late 1980s, Leininger had further developed the concept of generic care by identifying the concept of generic care knowledge. The concept was defined as referring "to the *epistemological and theoretically derived sources that characterize the fundamental nature of the human care phenomenon*" (Leininger, 1988b, p. 16). The concept of professional care knowledge was also developed at this time. It referred to "the *application of generic knowledge, by the use of learned professional knowledge about care, in creative and practical ways to alleviate a human condition or to sustain health caring practices*" (Leininger, 1988b, p. 17).

By the early 1980s, Leininger had become known as a leading proponent of the idea that nursing was synonymous with caring. This was evidenced in such statements as "caring is the central, unique, dominant, and unifying focus of nursing" (Leininger, 1984c, p. 92) and "caring is nursing" (Leininger, 1984c, p. 83). These themes remain prominent in Leininger's writings to date.

Paralleling concerns emerging in nursing about the value of, and contrast between, subjective and objective knowledge, Leininger (1981c) found it useful to distinguish between humanistic caring and scientific caring. She proposed that humanistic caring be given as much attention as scientific aspects of caring. Humanistic caring was characterized as "*the subjective feelings, experiences, and interactional behaviors between two or more persons (or groups)* in which assistive or enabling acts are performed generally without prior sets of verified or tested knowledge" (p. 101). Scientific caring differed in that it was thought to be "*tested activities and judgments in assisting an individual or group,* based upon verified and quantified knowledge related to specific variables" (p. 101).

The identification of care diversities and care universals was another concern of Leininger. She defined transcultural nursing as comparative caring (Leininger, 1981a). To compare caring, it was important that nurses learn culturally congruent care/caring ideas and analyze the similarities and differences in care/caring between or among cultures. This theme remains prominent in Leininger's writings and is the basis for the title of her theory, culture care diversity and universality.

Culture care diversity "refers to the variabilities and/or differences in meanings, patterns, values, lifeways, or symbols of care within or between collectivities that are related to assistive, supportive, and facilitative, or enabling human care expressions" (Leininger, 1991a, p. 47). Cultural care universality

> refers to the common, similar, or dominant uniform care meanings, patterns, values, lifeways, or symbols that are manifest among many cultures and reflect assistive, supportive, facilitative, or enabling ways to help people, another individual, or group that are derived from a specific culture to improve or ameliorate a human condition or lifeway. (Leininger, 1991a, p. 47)

Leininger further developed the concepts of care and caring by describing ethnocaring and cultural care. Ethnocaring referred "to *emic* cognitive assistive, facilitative, or enabling acts or decisions that are valued and practiced to help individuals, families, or groups" (Leininger, 1984c, p. 135). Cultural care was defined as "the subjectively and objectively learned and transmitted values, beliefs, and patterned lifeways that assist, support, facilitate, or enable another individual or group to maintain their well-being and health, to improve their human condition and lifeway, or to deal with illness, handicaps, or death" (Leininger, 1991a, p. 47). The concepts of "ethnocaring" and "cultural care" are very closely related and at times may be used interchangeably.

Other concepts that Leininger clarified by adding the prefix ethno- are ethnohealth, ethnonursing, and ethnohistory (Leininger, 1984c, 1991a). The term *cultural* is used as an adjective in many of Leininger's concepts. Examples are cultural care diversity, cultural care universality, cultural care accommodation, cultural care preservation, cultural care repatterning, and new cultural care practices.

Leininger developed the concepts of care and caring by analyzing them within new contexts and in the face of new trends emerging in the disciplines of both anthropology and nursing. A recent example of this is Leininger's (1990a) concern with ethical culture care and her description of four contextual spheres of ethical and moral care (personal or individual, professional or group, institutional or community, and cultural or societal). Leininger wants nurses to understand that ethical and moral aspects "are *culturally constituted and expressed* within meaningful living contexts" (p. 64).

Model Development

Leininger is well known for the sunrise model (depicted later in this section). This model first appeared in a major publication in 1984 in the book *Care: The Essence of Nursing and Health.* A few prominent early models contributing to the development of the sunrise model are reviewed here.

In 1976, Leininger presented what she called a transcultural health model. It was described as a "structural functional culture-based model" in that it included major social and cultural factors influencing health care systems. The model was designed to provide a guide for the study and analysis of the major variables found within different cultures in order to obtain a "transcultural health care perspective of health-illness systems" (Leininger, 1976, p. 17).

The 1976 model consisted of two major components: levels of analysis and major domains of study and analysis. Four major levels of analysis and corresponding domains of study were suggested. Level I was analysis of social structure features and the domains associated with the level were political, economic, social (including kinship), cultural (including religion), technological, educational, demographic, and environment factors. Level II was analysis of cultural values and health care. The domains associated with this level of analysis were dominant cultural values and health care values. Level III was analysis of health care systems and typologies. Major domains of study associated with this level were folk and professional health systems. Level IV analysis focused on roles and functions of health professionals. Domains of study were role responsibility and functions.

In 1978, Leininger presented another model building on the 1976 work for use in studying transcultural and ethnocaring concepts. The 1978 model, published in Leininger's (1981b) *Caring: An Essential Human Need,* contained three phases:

I. Major sources of ethnocaring
II. Classification of ethnocaring and nursing care constructs
III. Analysis and testing of constructs and use of findings

In Phase I analysis, the general ethnography of lifeways, major social structure features, cultural values, and health illness caring system ("including beliefs, values, norms, and role caring practices") are examined (p. 13). Phase II involves learning and classifying care concepts. Phase III consists of analysis of major ethnocaring constructs, theoretical formulations, research testing of the theory, analysis of ethnocaring research data, and determining nursing interventions based on research findings (Leininger, 1981b).

In 1979, Leininger offered what she called a "multilevel conceptual model for caring" (Leininger, 1981c, p. 99). This model was developed to "conceptualize and analyze the scope, nature, and structures of caring phenomenon [sic]" (Leininger, 1981c, p. 99). Once again, the model contains levels of analysis corresponding to levels of abstraction. It depicts six levels of caring phenomena: those of the individual, family or social group, the institution or system, specific culture, the societal focus, and the worldwide or multicultural focus. Worldwide and societal levels represent the highest level of abstraction, specific culture and institutional levels represent the middle level of abstraction, and family or social group and individual focus represent the lowest level of abstraction. Leininger (1981c) maintains that "the interplay and interrelationships among *all* levels of the model are important for a complete analysis of caring" (p. 100).

In 1980, Leininger described a "taxonomy model to study types of care phenomenon" (Leininger, 1981d, p. 137). In this article, Leininger (1981d) referred to the 1978 model (described above) as helping nurses "conceptualize, order, and study types of caring phenomenon" (p. 137). Leininger's contribution to the further development of the model in this work is the proposal of a suggested taxonomy of care/caring. The taxonomy of care/caring constructs presented in 1980 builds on Phase II of the 1978 model. Leininger's taxonomy is categorized as follows:

    I. Universal care types and attributes
   II. Cultural specific care types and attributes
  III. Transcultural emic-etic care relationships
  IV. Health professional and nonprofessional care attributes
   V. Social structure and individual group/care types and relationships
  VI. Transcultural nursing care by specific cultures

VII. Interdisciplinary care types

VIII. Other types of care and relation to cure types (Leininger, 1981d, p. 142)

Since 1984, Leininger has consistently represented her model as the Leininger sunrise model. The model has been variously described as a theoretic and conceptual model that depicts transcultural dimensions for "culturologic interviews, assessments, and therapy goals" (Leininger, 1984c, p. 137), a "differential conceptual theoretical and research method to study diversity and universality of care phenomena" (Leininger, 1985b, p. 44), "a conceptual picture to depict components of the theory to study how these components influence care and health status of individuals, families, groups and sociocultural institutions" (Leininger, 1988a, p. 156), and "a valuable cognitive map to guide researchers" (Leininger, 1991a, p. 53).

Leininger (1991a) explains that the model assists readers to keep "in mind the total gestalt of diverse influences to describe and explain care with health and well being outcomes" (p. 50). As such, it serves as a safeguard against viewing salient cultural dimensions as fragmented parts.

The model is likened by Leininger to a culture because it "has wholeness and interrelatedness with the nature of the full connections to be studied in relation to human care" (1991a, p. 50). It is designed to help nurses "envision a cultural world of different life forces or influencers on human conditions which need to be considered to discover human care in its fullest ways" (Leininger, 1991a, p. 50).

Theory Development

Numerous premises, assumptions, and hypotheses describing the nature of cultural care have been presented over the years by Leininger. Two major articles and one book fully address her theory; the articles were published in 1985 and 1988, the book in 1991.

In the 1985 article, Leininger (1985a) presents what she calls a general theory statement. She writes, "With the theory, I predict that different cultures perceive, know, and practice care in different ways, yet there are some commonalities about care among all the cultures in the world" (p. 4). This is the core of the theory of care diversity and universality from a transcultural viewpoint. Moreover, she states that the theory

> explains and predicts human care patterns of cultures and nursing care practices. It can explain and predict factors that influence care, health, and nursing care. Folk, professional, and nursing care values, beliefs, and practices as well as institutional norms, can be identified and explained by the theory. (p. 210)

In the 1985 description, the theory is referred to as "the theory of transcultural care diversity and universality" (Leininger, 1985a, p. 209). In the 1988 article, Leininger (1988a) refers to the work as "the nursing theory of cultural care diversity and universality" (p. 152). The word transcultural has been replaced with cultural in the latest publications.

Leininger's 1985 representation of the theory contained a description of 10 concepts, 13 assumptions, and 14 relational statements. The 1988 version contained 8 assumptions, 15 definitions, and no explicit relational statements. Most of the changes in the latter publication reflect a synthesis or reformulation of elements found in the 1985 work. The 1991 version of the theory contained definitions of 18 concepts, 13 assumptions, and no explicit relational statements.

It should be noted that Leininger prefers the use of the word construct instead of concept in discussing components of her theory and research findings. She writes, "Construct is a much broader and more inclusive term than concept, for it has many implicit and explicit meanings that have to be teased out in research processing" (Leininger, 1991a, p. 63).

Leininger maintains that care is the central concept for nursing theory and research. In promoting this idea she questions the very foundation that many nurses accept as the basis for their discipline and profession. For example, Leininger questions the themes of focus for nursing enquiry presented by Donaldson and Crowley (1978) and also states that "the four proclaimed concepts of health, nursing, person, and environment . . . seem no longer acceptable" (Leininger, 1991a, p. 59). She states that care is the major metaparadigm or core nursing concept, believing that there are numerous inadequacies with the concepts of health, nursing, person, and environment as major dimensions of nursing.

Leininger (1988a) does not believe that the concepts of nursing and person (adopted by other nurse theorists as core concepts) can help to explain nursing. She maintains that "one cannot explain nor predict the same phenomenon one is studying" and "nursing is the phenomenon to be explained" (p. 154). The concept of person "is not sufficient to explain nursing as it fails to account for groups, families, social institutions, and cultures" (p. 154), and many non-Western cultures do not believe in or focus on the concept of person (Leininger, 1991). Leininger acknowledges the importance of the concepts of environment and health to nursing but notes that these concepts are not unique to nursing as they are studied by other disciplines.

Another area in which Leininger differs from many nurses is in her definition of theory. In 1988, Leininger (1988a) presented a definition of theory as "sets of interrelated knowledge with meanings and experiences that describe, explain, predict, or account for some phenomenon (or domain of inquiry) through an open, creative, and naturalistic discovery process" (p. 154). The theory of cultural care fits this definition.

Leininger's definition varies from the classic characterization of theory. It was designed by Leininger to encourage research and the discovery of care phenomena that might be stifled by rigid adherence to other scientific methods. Leininger promotes the use of qualitative research methods in explaining and predicting care phenomena.

Future Theory Development

Leininger (1988b) predicts a greater interest in her theory in the future as a result of market forces affecting nursing such as desire for personalized care services and the promotion of quality care as a product. The theory is thought to be "the broadest and most wholistic guide to study human beings with their lifeways, cultural values and beliefs, symbols, material and nonmaterial forms, and living contexts" (Leininger, 1988a, p. 155).

Future market and societal forces combined with a broad view make the theory desirable and potentially applicable to a wide range of cultures, problems, and nursing situations. As the theory is used by nurses in practice and in research it will be further refined.

Future work might focus on the area of further outlining relationships between components of the theory. For example, Tripp-Reimer and Dougherty (1985) believe that "assumptions on which the model are based are not separated from the theoretical statements" (p. 79).

Leininger continues to refine and develop the theory through application in research examining care values and practices of differing cultural groups. Numerous nurses in the United States and around the world are contributing to these efforts.

Summary

The theory of cultural care diversity and universality developed by Madeleine Leininger has its roots in both anthropology and nursing. She maintains that culture and care are inextricably linked and that care/caring is the central concern of nurses. The goal of her theoretical works is to provide culturally congruent nursing care.

Leininger has been involved in concept, model, and theory development for over three decades. As a result, the concept of care has been analyzed in many different ways in her writings. Examples of this analysis are the definition and comparison of the terms care and caring, generic and professional care, and humanistic care and scientific care. Numerous early models have led to the well-known Leininger sunrise model currently in use.

The theory of culture care diversity and universality has as its core the idea that there are differences and similarities in care among all cultures of the world. The theory is different from the model in that the model only depicts components of the theory to provide a conceptual picture. The theory was originally known as the theory of transcultural diversity and universality but more recently the prefix trans- has been dropped. Concept, model, and theory development efforts are continuing.

50

Assumptive Premises of the Theory

MADELEINE M. LEININGER

Making assumptive premises about a theory is important; indeed, they can be considered as the basic "givens" of a theory. Initially, I wondered what could be the relationship of nursing care to culture, and I came to believe that care was dependent on culture and that culture could not survive without care. Hence culture was critical and essential to understand people and nursing.

I am continually examining assumptions about the theory and how it could generate fresh knowledge in nursing. The assumptions below (Leininger, 1991a, pp. 44-45) came from thinking inductively and deductively and from readings and experiences in nursing and anthropology. They have been refined over the past three decades, but they are major ideas that guided my deliberations in developing the theory of cultural care.

1. Care is the essence of nursing and a distinct, dominant, central, and unifying focus.
2. Care (caring) is essential for well-being, health, healing, growth, survival, and facing handicaps or death.

3. Culture care is the broadest holistic means to know, explain, interpret, and predict nursing care phenomena to guide nursing care practices.

4. Nursing is a transcultural humanistic and scientific care discipline and profession with the central purpose to serve human beings worldwide.

5. Care (caring) is essential to curing and healing, for there can be no curing without caring.

6. Culture care concepts, meanings, expressions, patterns, processes, and structural forms of care have different (diversity) and similar (toward commonalities or universalities) characteristics among all cultures of the world.

7. Every human culture has generic (lay, folk, or indigenous) care knowledge and practices and usually professional care knowledge and practices, which vary transculturally.

8. Cultural care values, beliefs, and practices are influenced by and tend to be embedded in world view, language, religion (or spiritual), kinship (social), politics (or legal), education, economic, technology, ethnohistory, and environmental context of a particular culture.

9. Beneficial, healthy, and satisfying culturally-based nursing care contributes to the well-being of individuals, families, groups, and communities within their environmental context.

10. Culturally congruent nursing care can only occur when culture care values, expressions, or patterns are known and used appropriately and meaningfully by the nurse with individuals or groups.

11. Culture care differences and similarities between professional caregivers and clients (with their generic needs) exist in human cultures worldwide.

12. Clients who show signs of culture conflicts, noncompliance, stresses, and ethical or moral concerns need nursing care that is culturally-based.

13. The qualitative paradigm with naturalistic inquiry modes provides the essential means to discover human care transculturally.

SOURCE: From *Culture Care Diversity and Universality: A Theory of Nursing*, by M. Leininger, 1991, New York: National League for Nursing. Reprinted by permission.

These assumptive premises guided and stimulated my thinking as I systematically developed and studied the theory of culture care with the ethnonursing, ethnoscience, and ethnographic methods. The assumptions served as a springboard for my theoretical understandings, hunches, and predictions about culture care.

Orientational Definitions of the Theory

To develop fully the theory of culture care, I realized that I had to have *orientational concepts* or *constructs*. Thus I developed the idea of orientational definitions (or ballpark ideas), which was in contrast to *operational definitions* (a very tightly constructed ballpark idea).

In the early 1980s, a small group of nurse leaders proposed four nursing concepts: nursing, person, health, and environment (Fawcett, 1984, 1989; Fitzpatrick & Whall, 1989). In my work, I had already focused on care as central to nursing and on culture and environmental context as critical to nursing, yet the concept of care was missing from their concepts, and culture was never identified. I found some of the concepts inadequate to explain, predict, and know nursing. First, I felt nursing could not be explained in terms of nursing itself; a theorist needs to use different ideas to discover the nature of a phenomenon. Second, from a social science perspective, *person* has a specific definition—someone with a particular status and social role. Hence it would be inappropriate to focus only on the person as central to nursing because nurses function with families, groups, communities, and institutions.

I believed the concept of "environment" could be important to nursing because nurses function in many different kinds of environments, but I did not view it as central. In the development of the theory, I had already defined and used the term *environmental context*, a much broader concept. I saw this term refer to the totality of human existence in different kinds of sociocultural and psychophysical environments. Thus environment had a much broader meaning and referred to holism—or the totality of human living.

The concept of "health" is important, but I found it limiting as defined by the theorists. From my transcultural studies, I had discovered that well-being and other phenomena were closely related to or used interchangeably with health.

Today, it is encouraging to witness the increased focus on human "care" and "caring" and to see more nurses study and value care as the central and most important phenomenon of nursing (Gaut, 1981; Leininger, 1981a, 1981b, 1984a, 1984b, 1984c, 1988a, 1988b, 1988c, 1988d, 1990a, 1990b, 1991a, 1991b; Ray, 1981; Valentine, 1988; Watson, 1985). In fact, there has been a groundswell of interest in human care as the central focus of nursing education and practice in the past decade. The focus on human care with culture has stimulated many nurses to obtain a more complete and holistic view of nursing.

Another unique feature in developing the culture care theory was mainly the use of an inductive research method called ethnonursing to define and discover culture care. The theory was developed from the qualitative paradigm or perspective in order to tease out the meanings, understanding, characteristics, and attributes of culture care from the people's local viewpoints or the emic views (Leininger, 1978, 1985b), a markedly different approach from the traditional quantitative paradigm in which researchers focus on testing hypotheses and specific variables that are predetermined and interesting mainly to the researcher and not necessarily to those being studied. With the qualitative paradigm, the researcher uses "orientational" rather than "operational" definitions. The latter definitions are used with the "quantitative paradigm." Orientational definitions facilitate an open discovery way to uncover phenomena or a broad domain of inquiry. This approach in theory development and study is important because it permits the local people's viewpoints, ideas, and experiences to come forth and because it contrasts sharply with "etic" or the researcher's viewpoints and helps the research to enter the informant's world. Orientational definitions might change according to what the reseacher discovers. I also used the term *construct*, which refers to many embedded ideas or concepts "within" a term, whereas *concept* is a single idea or phenomenon.

The major orientational definitions for the theory are as follows (Leininger, 1991a, pp. 46-47):

1. *Care* (noun) refers to abstract and concrete phenomena related to assisting, supporting, or enabling experiences or behaviors toward or for others with evident or anticipated needs to ameliorate or improve a human condition or lifeway.

2. *Caring* (gerund) refers to actions and activities directed toward assisting, supporting, or enabling another individual or group with evident or anticipated needs to ameliorate or improve a human condition or lifeway or to face death.

3. *Culture* refers to the learned, shared, and transmitted values, beliefs, norms, and lifeways of a particular group that guides their thinking, decisions, and actions in patterned ways.

4. *Culture care* refers to the cognitively learned and transmitted values, beliefs, and patterned lifeways that assist, support, facilitate, or enable another individual or group to maintain their well-being or health, to improve their human condition and lifeway, or to deal with illness, handicaps, or death.

5. *Health* refers to a state of well-being that is culturally defined, valued, and practiced, and that reflects the ability of individuals (or groups) to perform their daily role activities in culturally expressed, beneficial, and patterned lifeways.

6. *Environmental context* refers to the totality of an event, situation, or particular experiences that give meaning to human expressions, interpretations, and social interactions in particular physical, ecological, sociopolitical, and/or cultural settings.

7. *Cultural care diversity* refers to the variabilities and/or differences in meanings, patterns, values, lifeways, or symbols of care within or between collectivities that are related to assistive, supportive, or enabling human care expressions.

8. *Cultural care universality* refers to the common, similar, or dominant uniform care meanings, patterns, values, lifeways, or symbols that are manifest among many cultures and reflect assistive, supportive, facilitative, or enabling ways to help people. (The term *universality* is not used in an absolute way nor as a fixed statistical finding.)

9. *Generic folk or lay system* refers to culturally learned and transmitted, indigenous (or traditional), folk (home-based) knowledge and skills used to provide assistive, supportive, enabling, or facilitative acts toward or for another individual, group, or institution with evident or anticipated needs to ameliorate or improve a human lifeway, health condition (or well-being), or to deal with handicaps and death situations.

10. *Professional system(s)* refers to formal and cognitively learned professional knowledge and practice skills that are taught in professional institutions to a number of multidisciplinary personnel in order to serve consumers seeking health services.

11. *Cultural care preservation or maintenance* refers to those assistive, supportive, facilitative, or enabling professional actions and decisions that help people of a particular culture to retain and/or preserve relevant care values so that they can maintain their well-being, recover from illness, or face handicaps and/or death.

12. *Culture care accommodation or negotiation* refers to those assistive, supportive, facilitative, or enabling creative professional actions and decisions that help people of a designated culture to adapt to, or to negotiate with, others for a beneficial or satisfying health outcome with professional care providers.

13. *Cultural care repatterning or restructuring* refers to those assistive, supportive, facilitative, or enabling professional actions and decisions that help clients reorder, change, or modify their lifeways for new, different, or more beneficial health care patterns while respecting the client's cultural values and beliefs and providing a better (or healthier) lifeway than before.

14. *Cultural congruent (nursing) care* refers to those cognitively based assistive, supportive, facilitative, or enabling acts or decisions that are tailor-made to fit with an individual's, group's, or institution's cultural values, beliefs, and lifeways in order to provide meaningful, beneficial, and satisfying health care, or well-being services.

SOURCE: From *Culture Care Diversity and Universality: A Theory of Nursing*, by M. Leininger, 1991, New York: National League for Nursing. Reprinted by permission.

Other Orientational Definitions
(Leininger, 1991a)

1. *Nursing* refers to a learned humanistic and scientific profession and discipline that is focused on human care phenomena and activities in order to assist, support, facilitate, or enable individuals or groups to maintain or regain their well-being (or health) in culturally meaningful and beneficial ways, or to help people face handicaps or death.

2. *Worldview* refers to the way people tend to look out on the world or their universe to form a picture or a value stance about their life or world around them.

3. *Cultural and social structure dimensions* refer to the dynamic patterns and features of interrelated structural and organizational factors of a particular culture (subculture or society), which includes religious, kinship (social), political (and legal), economic, educational, technologic, and cultural values, and how these factors may be interrelated and function to influence human behavior in different environmental contexts.

4. *Ethnohistory* refers to those past facts, events, instances, and experiences of individuals, groups, cultures, and institutions that are primarily people-centered (ethno) and that describe, explain, and

interpret human lifeways within particular cultural contexts and space-time referents.

SOURCE: From *Culture Care Diversity and Universality: A Theory of Nursing*, by M. Leininger, 1991, New York: National League for Nursing. Reprinted by permission.

The above orientational definitions serve as guideposts to discover phenomena bearing upon culture care. These definitions orient the theorist and researcher to explore general ideas under study with the ethnonursing research method—a method explicitly designed to study culture care theory (Leininger, 1991a). The ethnonursing method was developed to tease out culture care meanings, expressions, and patterns bearing upon nursing because culture care was usually lodged or embedded in the social structure and language uses. Quantitative methods are extremely difficult to use to study covert and complex culture care meanings and expressions such as compassion, hope, empathy, and many other constructs. A researcher could study culture care from both quantitative and qualitative paradigms; however, one must remember *not* to mix the paradigms as this would be violating the philosophy, purposes, and goals of each paradigm (Leininger, 1990b, 1991a; Lincoln & Guba, 1985).

Essential Features of the Culture Care Theory

Because a researcher needs to discover and explicate meanings, expressions, and patterns of culture care from different cultures, I needed an inductive theory and thus defined theory as *patterns or sets of interrelated concepts, constructs, expressions, meanings, and experiences that describe, explain, predict, and account for some phenomena or domain of inquiry through an open, creative, and naturalistic discovery process* (Leininger, 1991a, p. 34). This definition of a theory would facilitate studying culture care using a naturalistic discovery process and lead to in-depth descriptions as well as ways to understand, explain, interpret, and even predict nursing phenomena through patterns and themes. My theory definition is similar to Steven's (1979) and Watson's (1985), which focus on discovery describing and interpreting phenomena as fully as possible. An inductive-based theory allows for thick descriptive data from informants, situations, events, instances, and groups and from environmental contexts to be uncovered by the researcher. Teasing out covert and complex phenomena requires considerable attention to the people's values and lifeways. Making interpretations from informants' ideas are important, as is documenting the context being studied. Thus these broad and open definitions were essential to tap unknown areas, to get data directly from the people to understand culture care phenomena, and to examine the assumptive premises of the theory.

In developing the theory of culture care, I wanted to consider what is universal and diverse about culture care worldwide. A broad theoretical perspective was essential to study cultural care variations and similarities among and between cultures of the world. The theory was, therefore, very broad in scope, with a worldwide perspective. I was curious if there were patterns, meanings, and practices of care that were universal or common because this knowledge would help nurses as they cared for people in different cultures. At the same time, I was curious about what was diverse or different about care. Discovering the universals (or commonalities) and differences (diversities) was essential to establish a foundation of nursing knowledge. Nurses could use findings from the theory in practical ways to improve or provide nursing care that was meaningful and culturally sensitive to the client's needs. Such discoveries would be an entirely new breakthrough in nursing and provide new knowledge to nurses.

The theory was envisioned and developed so that it could be used in our Western world, such as the United States, Canada, and Europe, and also in non-Western cultures, such as China, Korea, South Africa, and other places. Comparative data about human care was essential to provide differential care to clients and to make decisions and actions about the nursing care that fit clients' needs. Over time, the theory focused on where nursing was practiced or needed to be practiced in the future based on the people's needs and desires. Thus the theory was designed to have very useful and practical outcomes and to be used to provide culturally sensitive and competent care.

The *purpose* of culture care theory was to discover, through open naturalistic inquiry, culture care diversities and universality in order to generate nursing knowledge for the discipline and profession of nursing. The *goal* of the theory was ultimately to provide "culturally congruent nursing care" in order to improve nursing care to people of different or similar cultures. The latter meant helping clients, through culturally based care, to recover favorably from illness or to prevent conditions that would limit the client's health or well-being. The goal was, therefore, to provide "culturally congruent" and "culturally specific" nursing care that would lead to health or well-being. Nursing care needed to be tailored to or to fit the clients' cultural values, beliefs, and lifeways. Providing culturally congruent care to individuals, families, groups, or cultures meant that nursing care actions and decisions needed to be beneficial, satisfying, and/or meaningful to the sick, well, or disabled and to help the dying person. I theorized that if nursing care was not culturally congruent a host of conflicts and problems would occur that would delay recovery, prevent wellness, or could even lead to unexpected death. For example, the idea of "protective care" to the elderly in the community could have unfavorable consequences if protective care of the elderly was not valued by that culture.

In theorizing further about culture care, I held to the belief that humanistic care was important and was different from scientific and technical care. Humanistic care was a central and a distinct feature to characterize and identify nursing as a profession and discipline. The term *essence* in nursing meant that which makes nursing "that it is" and is an essential feature of how it becomes manifest and expressed to others. "Nursing was held to be caring" and "caring was essential and a dominant feature of nursing" (Leininger, 1981a, 1984a, 1988a). Moreover, nursing needed to be known to consumers and the public at large from both scientific and humanistic perspectives. Discovering differences and similarities between scientific and humanistic viewpoints was a research goal. From my clinical and research experiences, I had already discovered some of the meanings and patterns of care as being compassion, presence, enabling, and many other caring expressions. These discoveries revealed that there is still much more to learn about caring. Competent care is what people seek and expect when ill, but it is also needed to maintain their state of wellness.

I had several predictions about culture care that greatly stimulated my thinking. I predicted that nurses could discover largely unknown, covert, or taken-for-granted features about nursing care modes as they studied different cultures in the world in-depth. New insights about culture care could transform nursing education and practice in the future. This body of new knowledge would be viewed as the "new nursing and discipline knowledge" to guide nurses' actions, decisions, and judgments. Such knowledge was predicted to lead to very different practices from the present-day medical disease and symptoms model. How different cultures perceived and knew of care from their viewpoint and cultural needs was important new knowledge. It was this largely hidden and unknown culture care knowledge that would lead nurses to develop many different kinds of care practices and new understandings that would benefit clients. Such care patterns and practices were *mainly "rooted" or grounded in culture values, language, and social structures.* Nurses could no longer treat all clients alike because of cultural variabilities and different care expectations. Cultural diversities and similarities of knowledge of Western and non-Western cultures would lead nurses to value the importance of culture-specific care.

From the beginning I theorized that care was an "essential human need" to help people keep healthy, grow, and function (Leininger, 1980, 1981a, 1981c). Human beings in any culture had to learn about caring attitudes and practices in order to survive in the past and today. Most important, human caring was learned and transmitted to others. *Being human was to be caring, and caring was culturally based.* Caring for others or self required using culturally learned and transmitted values of care, primarily from one's family or cultural group. Healthy people, I held, had learned good caring patterns that kept them well or healthy. In contrast, unhealthy patterns of caring led to illness, disability, and even death. I also held there were *"caring cultures"* where people in organizational structures knew how to care for people. Where beneficial caring patterns and experiences existed, there were healthy caring people. In contrast, noncaring patterns and cultures, I predicted, would lead to illness, death, or a host of unhealthy conditions (Leininger, 1988a, 1991a). Moreover, the well-being of individuals, families, and specific cultures would be threatened by noncaring expressions, resulting in cultural violence, destruction, and death. Caring patterns were held to be essential to keep people well and to live satisfying and meaningful lives.

These ideas led me to theorize about differences between generic and professional caring. I conceptualized that there were two kinds of caring that existed in every culture and that needed to be discovered as they had not been identified for their comparative uses in nursing (Leininger, 1970, 1978, 1981a, 1991a). *Generic care* was the oldest form and basic expression of human caring essential for the growth, health, and survival of *Homo sapiens.* Generic care as the foundational prototype of care included local home remedies and folk care.

It was predicted that all families or households had some forms of generic or basic caring that was used by family members or by special caregivers. These generic caring behaviors or expectations needed to be identified for their efficacy or beneficial outcomes and used with professional care practices where indicated. If beneficial generic care were not practiced, one could predict "noncaring" outcomes, such as poor recovery from illness, failure to stay well, and other problems. It would be helpful for nurses to know some families with special caregiving and care-recipient practices in home and institutional hospital care. Hence generic care was a new construct conceptualized as important to the theory of culture care and especially in relationship to professional care practices.

Professional care was conceptualized to be different from generic care in that professional care was defined as cognitively learned, practiced, and transmitted knowledge learned through formal and informal professional education nursing schools (Leininger, 1991a, p. 34). When nursing students entered nursing, they were taught about professional nursing techniques, practices, and related topics that constituted fundamentals of nursing. Students were expected to learn what constituted professional care or nursing care practices. In some nursing schools, nursing care was often about procedures and practices or ways to handle medical diseases and symptoms. Professional nursing content was often directed toward carrying out aseptic medical techniques, or the "right ways" to be an effective, competent, or skilled nurse in "psychomotor" nursing practices. Professional care also included learning about communication techniques, interpersonal relationships, ethical aspects, and other content held important by nursing leaders. Professional nursing did not include ideas about folk care since it was largely unrecognized and not valued as useful to nursing. With the advent of transcultural nursing, professional and generic care began to be valued and studied.

In theorizing about generic and professional care, I predicted that generic care as naturalistic local, folk, and familiar home care practices would differ considerably from professional care due to cultural factors. If professional and generic care practices did not reasonably fit together, this would influence client recovery, health, and wellbeing. To provide culturally congruent care, professional and generic care needed to be considered to facilitate meaningful care practices. Thus the ultimate goal was to link and synthesize generic and professional care knowledge to benefit the client. But before this could occur, nurse researchers needed to explicate and know the differences and similarities between the two types of care. This would be extremely important to provide culturally congruent care, which I held was essential for quality nursing care practices. I speculated that world-view, social structure, language, ethnohistory, and environmental context as defined above would greatly influence both generic and professional care beliefs and practices. Cultural values, religious beliefs, economic concerns, attitudes about technology, kinship ties, educational interests, and worldview would impact on caring methods and, ultimately, the health or well-being of clients. Knowledge of generic and professional care of individuals, families, groups, institutions, and communities was essential to provide professional nursing care.

To help nurses visualize components of the theory influencing human care, I developed the sunrise model (see Figure 50.1), a depiction of the components and conceptual areas of the theory that need to be considered in the discovery of factors that influenced generic and professional care practices, which develop culturally congruent nursing care. The model symbolically portrays a rising sun. If nurses systematically examined the conceptual components in the model, they would discover human care and the influence on the health and well-being of individuals, families, communities, and institutions and become enlightened by these findings. The model conceptually depicts the worldview, religion, kinship, cultural values, economics, technology, language, ethnohistory, and environmental factors that are predicted to explain and influence culture care. Thus it serves as a cognitive orientation to obtain a complete, holistic, and comprehensive way to examine the theory. Discovering the meanings, and expressive factors of culture care and its potential influence on care and the health or well-being of clients is crucial to the theory. The sunrise model is truly a holistic model that the nurse researcher needs to use as a guide to study the theoretical predictions or hunches made by the theorist. If these different factors were not studied, the nurse would have only partial, fragmented, and inadequate knowledge about culture care. With the use of the sunrise model, the nurse assesses all aspects, including generic folk and professional systems, which give clues to theoretical ways of developing culturally congruent nursing care. Courses in transcultural nursing, anthropology, and health sciences help the nurse researcher to identify and understand the different components depicted in the sunrise model and focus on the tenets of the theory.

The sunrise model reflects my theory about nursing not only as an intellectual discipline but as a practice profession. Accordingly, I

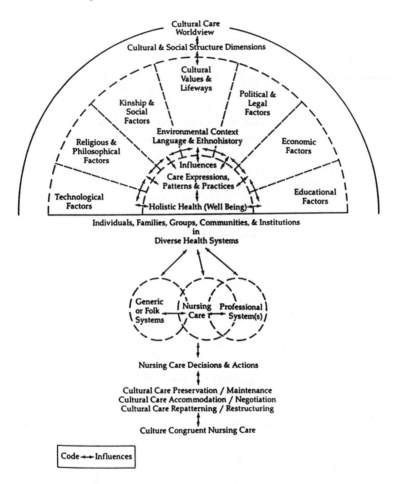

Figure 50.1. Leininger's sunrise model to depict theory of cultural care diversity and universality.
SOURCE: From *Culture Care Diversity and Universality: A Theory of Nursing*, by M. Leininger, 1991, New York: National League for Nursing. Reprinted by permission.

theorize that there are "three modes of action or decision" to guide nurses in providing culturally congruent care: (a) *cultural care preservation and/or maintenance,* (b) *cultural care accommodation and/or negotiation,* and (c) *cultural care repatterning and restructuring* (Leininger, 1988a, 1991a). These three modes could lead to the goal of the theory, which is to provide culturally congruent nursing care. The nurse would consider data obtained from the informant, from observations, and from the study of all components in the sunrise model to identify which care mode (or modes) would best fit and benefit the client's needs. Data from the sunrise model would guide the nurse to develop creative and appropriate ways to examine the three action or decision modes. From the use of grounded, culturally-based people data, cultural patterns, and culture-specific ideas for congruent nursing care practices would emerge. The wealth of data from the individual or family about their worldview, social structure factors, environmental context, and other aspects should reveal fresh and informative modes to guide nursing care practices.

In general, I held with the theory of culture care that there would be some similarities (the commonalities or universalities) along with the differences (diversities) among cultures with regard to culture care meanings, patterns, expressions, functions (uses), structural features, and practices (Leininger, 1988a, 1991b). These similarities and differences needed to be teased out and made known in order to arrive at a holistic perspective of human care with specific cultures. I also postulated that specific care expressions or patterns such as presence, respect, support, enabling, compassion, and many other care constructs could be powerful factors for the nurse to use to help people remain well or healthy (Leininger, 1981a, 1984a, 1991a). I called these care constructs the "golden nuggets" that needed to be fully discovered, valued, and used in order to provide therapeutic and meaningful nursing care practices to culturally diverse clients. These golden nuggets were essential for nurses to help people recover from illnesses, to remain well, or to face dying in a culturally congruent and satisfying way. I predicted that where specific caring meanings and patterns were known and used in nursing, health ways would prevail; if noncaring expressions existed, one would find unfavorable, unhealthy care practices. These culture care constructs were, indeed, the *essence* of what nursing is or should be and were the means to help nurses provide meaningful quality nursing care. Even today these powerful care constructs of different cultures are slowly being discovered and understood to guide professional nursing education care practices. Nursing with a culture care focus can influence the outcome of professional care practices. Thus culture care theory was a new, comprehensive means to discover embedded care phenomena and to use the knowledge to transform nursing education and practice. Culture care knowledge was much needed to provide specific and differential nursing care practices and to shift current nursing practices from dominant medical emphases to a nursing perspective.

In studying and examining the theory, the *ethnonursing qualitative paradigm research method* proved to be most helpful to tease out and understand culture data and its meanings within nursing contexts. The ethnonursing method has helped nurse researchers (a) explicate nursing phenomena about culture care; (b) get emic-grounded data through inductive and naturalistic approaches rather than focusing on the researcher's etic (outsider's) knowledge and interpretations; (c) use different enabling inquiry guides to probe for embedded meanings, interpretations, and relationships among different components of the theory; (d) discover specific details related to the care constructs and ideas related to the theory; (e) identify highly creative ways that nurses can use culture care knowledge in client care; (f) show ways that nurses can get close to culture-specific ideas about human care; and (g) discover ways to blend professional and generic care knowledge for the benefit of clients from diverse cultures.

Research Findings

The seven major research studies presented in the *Culture Care Diversity and Universality* theory publication (Leininger, 1991, pp. 73-119) demonstrate the importance of the ethnonursing method and the theory with research findings by Bohay, Gates, Leininger, Rosenbaum, Spangler, Stasiak, and Wenger. I have studied a number of cultures and found culture-specific care values, meanings, and actions from 23 cultures as generated from the theory (Leininger, 1991a, pp. 119-134). These findings are already providing new insights to the practice of nursing.

Because the theory is being used extensively around the world to study multicultural and culture care phenomena, one can predict that it will spread even more in the future. Currently, the theory is being used by nurses in Finland, Sweden, the Middle East, Africa, Japan, Canada, Australia, Europe, Korea, China, South America, Russia, Tibet, and several places in the Pacific Islands. In addition, some nonnurses and other professionals are finding the theory relevant to their work by modifying some terms of the theory to fit their discipline uses. Organizational theorists and administrators are excited about the theory because it gives them a broad framework to understand the diverse factors impacting their areas of interest. Corporate executives have told the theorist how much it helped them to study broad areas they needed to include in assessing their administrative goals and caring ethos.

Nurse theorists and researchers will continue to realize the critical importance of the theory as one of the most comprehensive, holistic means to discover human care phenomena. Nurses are realizing the actual and potentially powerful role of culture care that influences nursing practice and education. Culture care as a theoretical synthesis construct also has practical uses to discover, understand, and make decisions about nursing practices, especially with the use of the sunrise model. The theory is being taught in schools of nursing and used as a major conceptual guide for nursing curricula. Culture care provides the "golden nuggets" and many other rich insights for advancing nursing's discipline knowledge. Growing multiculturalism will make it imperative for nurses to function in diverse cultures. Transcultural care research knowledge based on culture care and health will guide nursing decisions and actions. The future for this culture care theory looks exceedingly promising for the discipline and profession of nursing. The next section reveals some exciting implications for the use of culture care theory in clinical nursing practices and education.

51

The Theory of Culture Care:
Implications for Nursing

CHERYL L. REYNOLDS

The broad scope of the theory of culture care diversity and universality as proposed by Madeleine Leininger makes it useful in many nursing settings and situations. Contributions of the theory to the profession and discipline of nursing can be found in practice, administration, education, and research.

Nursing Practice

Leininger has very clearly described the way her theory applies to nursing practice. The goal of the theory is to provide culturally congruent nursing care to persons of diverse cultures (Leininger, 1988a). Discovering cultural care/caring beliefs, values, and practices and analyzing the similarities and differences of these beliefs between and among cultures will help nurses attain this goal.

Leininger states that it is important for the nurse to understand the patient's view of illness. This includes "how the patient knows and understands his illness, how he desires to be helped, and the ways health personnel can help him" (Leininger, 1969, p. 2). The Leininger sunrise model portrayed in the book *Care: The Essence of Nursing and Health* is described as a model for culturologic interviews, assessments, and therapy goals (Leininger, 1984a). Thus the model can help nurses develop questions for the assessment of client cultural beliefs related to health and illness. Leininger has also developed a videotape demonstrating major components, techniques, and skills in doing a cultural care assessment of an American-Polish informant.

Few nurse theorists have clearly identified theory-based modes of nursing action that help practitioners understand how to intervene with clients based on their theory. Leininger has clearly stated ways that nurses can provide culturally congruent care. The dominant modes to guide nursing decisions and actions based on the theory of cultural care are (a) cultural care preservation or maintenance, (b) cultural care accommodation or negotiation, and (c) cultural care repatterning or restructuring (Leininger, 1988a).

Cultural care preservation "refers to those assistive, supporting, facilitative, or enabling professional actions and decisions that help people of a particular culture to retain and/or preserve relevant care values so that they can maintain their well-being, recover from illness, or face handicaps and/or death" (Leininger, 1991a, p. 46). Cultural care accommodation "refers to those assistive, supporting, facilitative, or enabling creative professional actions and decisions that help people of a designated culture to adapt to, or to negotiate with, others for a beneficial or satisfying health outcome with professional careproviders" (Leininger, 1991, p. 48). Cultural care repatterning

> refers to those assistive, supporting, facilitative, or enabling professional actions and decisions that help a client(s) reorder, change, or greatly modify their lifeways for new, different, and beneficial health care pattern while respecting the client(s) [*sic*] cultural values and beliefs and still providing a beneficial or healthier lifeway than before the changes were coestablished with the client(s). (Leininger, 1991a, p. 49)

In an earlier publication, Leininger (1984b) identified another mode of nursing action: new cultural care practices. New cultural care practices refer "to the cognitive action of incorporating different or new assistive or facilitative actions designed to be beneficial to the client" (p. 135). This way of acting to promote culturally congruent care has not been addressed in later publications.

It should be noted that Leininger does not characterize her modes of nursing actions as interventions. She maintains that nursing intervention is a Western professional nursing culture-bound term that may communicate to some clients "ideas of cultural interferences and imposition practices" (Leininger, 1991a, p. 55). Moreover, Leininger does not use the terminology "nursing problems" because "all too often the client may not have a problem, or the problem may not be seen as relevant to the people by the nurse" (Leininger, 1991a, p. 55). Leininger is well known as the founder of the transcultural nursing movement in the United States. The motto of the Transcultural Nursing Society is a quote from Leininger that reads "That the cultural needs of people in the world will be met by nurses prepared in transcultural nursing."

Transcultural nursing is comparative caring (Leininger, 1981a). It is a "formal area of study and practice of diverse cultures in the world with respect to their care, health and illness values, beliefs, and practices in order to provide culture specific or universal nursing care that is congruent with the client, family, or community's cultural values and lifeways" (Leininger, 1989a, p. 4). Nurses can become certified in this specialty area.

Transcultural nursing is different from international nursing. The term *transcultural* was deliberately chosen by Leininger because it refers to world cultures whether or not they are nationalized, whereas international nursing refers to nationalized cultures only (Leininger, 1991a).

A recent article applying Leininger's theory to intensive care unit (ICU) nursing practice was published by Kloosterman (1991). The phenomena of sensory alteration frequently encountered in the ICU was described by Kloosterman as resulting from culturally incongruent nursing care. Clients unfamiliar with the culture of nursing in the ICU became confused when their normal and familiar care patterns were altered.

Leininger has long been concerned with cultural imposition and ethnocentrism on the part of nurses in their daily practice. Awareness of Leininger's theory will help nurses to avoid this problem. Although not all transcultural nurses use Leininger's theory as a guide for practice, the Transcultural Nursing Society promotes culturally congruent nursing care in their publications and yearly conferences.

Nursing Administration

The theory of culture care diversity and universality can be used to analyze the culture of nursing or the culture of an organization just as it can be used in assessment of the individual client. Leininger (1988b) writes that "nurses seldom pause to reflect on how the culture of nursing can influence care practices and attitudes" (p. 21). The culture of nursing is defined as "those identifiable and inferred normative patterns, values, beliefs, and practices that characterize the profession of nursing over time" (Leininger, 1986, pp. 2-3). This knowledge could be especially important for nurse administrators.

Identifying nurses as members of a cultural group means that it is useful to "examine nurses' cultural values, meanings, and experiences of care so that they can be understood in caregiving experiences" (Leininger, 1986, p. 3). Through analysis of the culture of nursing, Leininger has identified care facilitation and resistance factors inherent in the culture.

Leininger (1986) defines care facilitation as "those factors, forces, or conditions that tend to enhance or enable nurses to discover the full meanings and uses of care in their thinking and work" (p. 2). Care resistance is "those factors, forces, or conditions that tend to limit or curtail nurses in the full discovery of the meanings and uses of care" (p. 2).

In describing other ways her theory can be useful in administration, Leininger (1988b) writes that "from an institutional perspective, it provides a theoretical framework to study how institutions use, interpret, and predict goals that fit with the communities they serve" (p. 25). She maintains that "one can predict the health of an institution by its care beliefs, values, and practices" (p. 25). A list of areas of inquiry for nursing service administrators consistent with her theory have been outlined by Leininger (1988b).

Leininger's theory is applicable to the study of organizations and institutions in part because she does not define the singular person as one of the key concepts in the theory. There are many reasons behind Leininger's purposeful omission of this concept, but the main one useful for nursing administrators is that she recognizes that a definition of person "fails to account for groups, families, social institutions, and cultures" (Leininger, 1988a, p. 154).

The theory of culture care diversity and universality is also useful to administrators who are concerned that their institutions deliver quality care to clients of multicultural populations. Nursing administrators with such concerns could use the theory concepts, tenets, and modes of nursing action as means of facilitating the delivery of this care within the organization.

Nursing Education

Leininger has developed and taught undergraduate and graduate courses in transcultural nursing at the University of Colorado, the University of Washington, the University of Utah, and Wayne State University; the latter three offer doctoral programs in transcultural nursing or with a transcultural nursing emphasis that she developed. These courses and curricula were developed consistent with the theory of cultural care diversity and universality.

By 1980, about 20% of nursing programs accredited by the National League for Nursing incorporated cultural concepts and principles into the undergraduate program (Leininger, 1989b) and by 1991, 15% of graduate nursing programs in the United States had transcultural nursing courses. In 1991, the Transcultural Nursing Society listed five graduate programs in transcultural nursing in the United States and three additional universities where the faculty members are prepared in transcultural nursing and are developing courses on the subject. It is unknown how many nursing programs use Leininger's theory as the basis of their cultural diversity curricula.

Because the theory has direct applicability to nursing practice and research, and because of recent societal and worldwide trends toward increasing travel and respecting cultural diversity, the theory of culture care diversity and universality is useful for nurse educators. In 1986, the American Nurses' Association Council on Cultural Diversity in Nursing Practice stated that "one way to promote an appreciation of various cultures is to develop and implement nursing school curricula that incorporate practice-related concepts of cultural diversity" (p. 1). They also maintain that "nursing education programs must include content in the curriculum pertaining to culturally diverse groups if nurses are to be prepared to provide safe, effective care acceptable to all consumers" (p. 2).

Research

Application of the theory and model in research was published by Leininger in the study of "Southern Rural Black and White American Lifeways With Focus on Care and Health Phenomena" (1984b, 1985) and a study of "Culture Care of the Gadsup Akuna of the Eastern Highlands of New Guinea" (1991b). Leininger reports that she has also collected and analyzed culture values and culture care themes from 54 cultures. To date, she has identified well over 175 care/caring constructs (Leininger, 1991a).

Leininger lists cultural values and culture care meanings and action modes for 23 cultural groups in her book *Culture Care Diversity and Universality: A Theory of Nursing*. The findings include studies of the following cultural groups: Anglo American, Mexican American, Haitian American, African American, North American Indian, Gadsup Akuna, Filipino American, Japanese American, Vietnamese American, Southeast Indian American, Chinese American, Arab American Muslim, old order Amish Americans, Appalachian culture, Polish American culture, German American culture, Italian American, Greek American, Jewish American, Lithuanian American, Swedish American, Finnish American, and Danish American.

Numerous graduate and doctoral students have used Leininger's theory as a basis for their research. However, many of these studies are unpublished. Published studies include Wenger and Wenger's (1988) study of old order Amish, Gates's (1988) study of caring behaviors experienced by couples during a hysterectomy, Monsma's (1988) study of children of battered women, Rosenbaum's (1988) study of mental health care needs of Soviet-Jewish immigrants, and Luna's (1989) study of transcultural nursing care of Arab Muslims. Research reported in Leininger's 1991 book, *Culture Care Diversity and Universality: A Theory of Nursing*, includes Bohay's study of culture care meanings and experiences of pregnancy and childbirth of Ukrainians, Gates's study of dying in hospital and hospice contexts, Rosenbaum's study of Greek Canadian widows, Spangler's study of Filipino and Anglo American nurses, Stasiak's study of Mexican American urbanites, and Wenger's study of old order Amish. In addition, Rosenbaum (1990, 1991a, 1991b) has published a number of articles outlining many dimensions of cultural care and health of Greek Canadian widows.

A review of qualitative research literature published in six major refereed nursing journals spanning the period 1985-1990 uncovered no research studies that used the theory of cultural care as a theoretical framework (Reynolds, 1991). This finding reflects trends such as the general lack of identification of well-organized nursing theoretical frameworks in qualitative research.

With the advent of the *Journal of Transcultural Nursing*, researchers using Leininger's theory have another vehicle for the publication of their work. This journal may promote an increase in the publication of research that uses her theory. Other sources that frequently include research using Leininger's theory are the National Care Conference proceedings.

Future plans in the area of research are to continue examining commonalities, patterns, and themes derived from the many researchers using the theory as a basis for building on knowledge gained from research in the development of additional studies. After review of her work in 1988, Leininger (1988b) concluded that

there are no universal or worldwide ethnocare concepts, but there are some recurrent care concepts such as (1) concern for, (2) attention to, (3) respect for, and (4) helping. More diversity in human care forms, meanings, processes and uses was found than universalities or similarities. (p. 29)

This finding remains true to the present day (Leininger, 1991a).

Leininger (1991a) provides a list of additional findings gleaned from studies using her theory. The results are the following:

- Care meanings and practices are difficult to ascertain because they are embedded in social structure.
- Cultural context and care values influence the expression and meaning of care.
- To understand care meanings and uses often requires knowledge of the culture.
- High technology nursing practices in Western cultures increase the distance between clients and nurses.
- Generic care is little understood and valued by nurses and other health providers.

- Key and general informants for the studies have expressed positive feelings about the research.
- Clients believe that their ideas, beliefs, and lifeways must be understood by health providers before clients can be helped appropriately.

SOURCE: From *Culture Care Diversity and Universality: A Theory of Nursing*, by M. Leininger, 1991, New York: National League for Nursing. Reprinted by permission.

Implications of the research for further development of the theory also continues to be discussed. Leininger is focusing on these efforts by inviting selected researchers known to be using her theory to confer and examine research and theory issues. The results of a recent culture care theory invitational conference have yet to be published.

Summary

The theory of culture care diversity and universality proposed by Madeleine Leininger is a useful guide for nursing practice, administration, education, and research. Two reasons why the theory is applicable to a wide range of nursing settings and situations are that the theory is broad in scope and it does not depend on a definition of singular person as the object of the theory.

Leininger has clearly identified three major modes of nursing action for nursing practice: dimensions of the culture of nursing, described care facilitation, and resistance factors within the culture. Numerous undergraduate courses and curricula have been developed by Leininger, and she has undertaken and directed a wide variety of research projects exploring aspects of culture care. Through these contributions, Leininger has demonstrated the applicability of her theory to the profession and discipline of nursing.

References

American Nurses' Association. (1986). *Cultural diversity in the nursing curriculum: A guide for implementation*. Kansas City, MO: Author.

Bohay, I. Z. (1991). Culture care meanings and experiences of pregnancy and childbirth of Ukrainians. In M. M. Leininger (Ed.), *Culture care diversity and universality: A theory of nursing*. New York: National League for Nursing.

Donaldson, S. K., & Crowley, D. M. (1978). The discipline of nursing. *Nursing Outlook, 26*(2), 113-120.

Fawcett, J. (1984). The metaparadigm to nursing: Present status and future refinements. *Image, 16*(34), 84-86.

Fawcett, J. (1989). *Analysis and evaluation of conceptual models of nursing*. Philadelphia: F. A. Davis.

Fitzpatrick, J., & Whall, A. (1989). *Conceptual models of nursing: Analysis and application*. Bowie, MD: Brady.

Gates, M. (1988). Caring behaviors experienced by couples during a hysterectomy. In M. M. Leininger (Ed.), *Care: Discovery and uses in clinical and community nursing*. Detroit, MI: Wayne State University Press.

Gates, M. (1991). Culture care theory for study of dying patients in hospital and hospice contexts. In M. M. Leininger (Ed.), *Culture care diversity and universality: A theory of nursing*. New York: National League for Nursing.

Gaut, D. (1981). Conceptual analysis of caring: Research method. In M. M. Leininger (Ed.), *Caring: An essential human need* (pp. 17-44). Thorofare, NJ: Charles B. Slack.

Kloosterman, N. D. (1991). Cultural care: The missing link in severe sensory alteration. *Nursing Science Quarterly, 4*(3), 119-122.

Leininger, M. M. (1969). Ethnoscience: A promising research approach to improve nursing practice. *Image, 3*(l), 2-8.

411

Leininger, M. M. (1970). *Nursing and anthropology: Two worlds to blend.* New York: John Wiley.

Leininger, M. M. (1976). Towards conceptualization of transcultural health care systems: Concepts and a model. In M. M. Leininger (Ed.), *Transcultural health care issues and conditions.* Philadelphia: F. A. Davis.

Leininger, M. M. (1977). Caring: The essence and central focus of nursing. In *The phenomenon of caring: Part V.* Kansas City, MO: American Nurses' Foundation.

Leininger, M. M. (1978). *Transcultural nursing: Concepts, theories and practices.* New York: John Wiley.

Leininger, M. M. (1980, October). Caring: A central focus of nursing and health care services. *Nursing and Health Care,* 135-176.

Leininger, M. M. (1981a). *Caring: An essential human need.* Thorofare, NJ: Charles B. Slack.

Leininger, M. M. (1981b). The phenomenon of caring: Importance, research questions and theoretical considerations. In M. M. Leininger (Ed.), *Caring: An essential human need.* Thorofare, NJ: Charles B. Slack.

Leininger, M. M. (1981c). Cross-cultural hypothetical functions of caring and nursing care. In M. M. Leininger (Ed.), *Caring: An essential human need.* Thorofare, NJ: Charles B. Slack.

Leininger, M. M. (1981d). Some philosophical, historical, taxonomic aspects of nursing and caring in American culture. In M. M. Leininger (Ed.), *Caring: An essential human need.* Thorofare, NJ: Charles B. Slack.

Leininger, M. M. (1984a). *Care: The essence of nursing and health.* Thorofare, NJ: Charles B. Slack.

Leininger, M. M. (1984b). Transcultural nursing: An overview. *Nursing Outlook,* 32(2), 72-73.

Leininger, M. M. (1984c). Southern rural black and white American lifeways with focus on care and health phenomena. In M. M. Leininger (Ed.), *Care: The essence of nursing and health.* Thorofare, NJ: Charles B. Slack.

Leininger, M. M. (1984d). Caring is nursing: Understanding the meaning, importance, and issues. In M. M. Leininger (Ed.), *Care: The essence of nursing and health.* Thorofare, NJ: Charles B. Slack.

Leininger, M. M. (1985a). Transcultural care diversity and universality: A theory of nursing. *Nursing and Health Care,* 6(4), 209-212.

Leininger, M. M. (1985b). Ethnography and ethnonursing: Models and modes of qualitative data analysis. In M. M. Leininger (Ed.), *Qualitative research methods in nursing* (pp. 33-32). Orlando, FL: Grune and Stratton.

Leininger, M. M. (1985c). Southern rural black and white American lifeways with focus on care and health phenomena. In M. M. Leininger (Ed.), *Qualitative research methods in nursing.* Orlando, FL: Grune & Stratton.

Leininger, M. M. (1986). Care facilitation and resistance factors in the culture of nursing. *Topics in Clinical Nursing,* 8(2), 1-12.

Leininger, M. M. (1988a). Leininger's theory of nursing: Cultural care diversity and universality. *Nursing Science Quarterly,* 1(4), 152-160.

Leininger, M. M. (1988b). History, issues, and trends in the discovery and uses of care in nursing. In M. M. Leininger (Ed.), *Care: Discovery and uses in clinical and community nursing.* Detroit: Wayne State University Press.

Leininger, M. M. (1988c). Cultural care theory and administration. In B. Henry, C. Arndt, M. Di Vincent, & A. Mariner-Tomey (Eds.), *Dimensions of nursing administration*. Boston: Blackwell Scientific.

Leininger, M. M. (1988d). Leininger's theory of transcultural nursing: Culture care diversity and universality. *Nursing Science Quarterly, 2*(4), 11-20.

Leininger, M. M. (1989a). Transcultural nurse specialists and generalists: New practitioners in nursing. *Journal of Transcultural Nursing, 1*(1), 4-16.

Leininger, M. M. (1989b). Transcultural nursing: Quo vadis (where goeth the field)? *Journal of Transcultural Nursing, 1*(l), 33-45.

Leininger, M. M. (1990a). Culture: the conspicuous missing link to understanding ethical and moral dimensions of human care. In M. M. Leininger (Ed.), *Ethical and moral dimensions of care*. Detroit, MI: Wayne State University Press.

Leininger, M. M. (1990b). Ethnomethods: The philosophic and epistemic bases to explicate transcultural nursing knowledge. *Journal of Transcultural Nursing, 1*(2), 40-51.

Leininger, M. M. (1991a). *Culture care diversity and universality: A theory of nursing.* New York: National League for Nursing.

Leininger, M. M. (1991b). Culture care of the Gadsup Akuna of the Eastern highlands of New Guinea. In M. M. Leininger (Ed.), *Culture care diversity and universality: A theory of nursing*. New York: National League for Nursing.

Leininger, M. M. (1993). Culture care theory: The comparative global theory to advance human care nursing knowledge and practice. In D. Gaut (Ed.), *A global agenda for caring* (pp. 3-18). New York: National League for Nursing.

Lincoln, Y., & Guba, E. (1985). *Qualitative research methods in nursing*. Orlando, FL: Grune & Stratton.

Luna, L. (1989). Transcultural nursing care of Arab Muslims. *Journal of Transcultural Nursing, 1*(1), 22-26.

Monsma, J. (1988) Children of battered women: Perceptions, actions, and nursing care implications. In M. M. Leininger (Ed.), *Care: Discovery and uses in clinical and community nursing*. Detroit, MI: Wayne State University Press.

Rosenbaum, J. (1988). Mental health care needs of Soviet-Jewish immigrants. In M. M. Leininger (Ed.), *Care: Discovery and uses in clinical and community nursing*. Detroit, MI: Wayne State University Press.

Rosenbaum, J. (1990). Cultural care of older Greek Canadian widows within Leininger's theory of culture care. *Journal of Transcultural Nursing, 2*(1), 37-47.

Rosenbaum, J. (1991a). Culture care theory and Greek Canadian widows. In M. M. Leininger (Ed.), *Culture care diversity and universality: A theory of nursing*. New York: National League for Nursing.

Rosenbaum, J. (1991b). Widowhood grief: A cultural perspective. *Canadian Journal of Nursing Research, 23*(2), 61-76.

Rosenbaum, J. (1991c). The health meanings and practices of older Greek Canadian widows. *Journal of Advanced Nursing, 16*, 1320-1327.

Reynolds, C. (1991). *The relationship between theory and qualitative research*. Unpublished manuscript.

Spangler, Z. (1991). Culture care of Philippine and Anglo-American nurses in a hospital context. In M. M. Leininger (Ed.), *Culture care diversity and universality: A theory of nursing*. New York: National League for Nursing.

Stasiak, D. B. (1991). Culture care theory with Mexican-Americans in an urban context. In M. M. Leininger (Ed.), *Culture care diversity and universality: A theory of nursing*. New York: National League for Nursing.

Steven, B. J. (1979). *Nursing theory: Analysis, application evaluation*. Boston: Little, Brown.

Tripp-Reimer, T., & Dougherty, M. C. (1985). Cross-cultural nursing research. In H. Werley & J. Fitzpatrick (Eds.), *Annual review of nursing research* (Vol. 3, pp. 77-104). New York: Springer.

Valentine, K. (1988). Advancing care and ethics in health management: An evaluation strategy. In M. M. Leininger (Ed.), *Care: Discovery of uses in clinical and community nursing* (pp. 151-168). Detroit, MI: Wayne State University Press.

Watson, J. (1985). *Nursing: Human science and human care: A theory for nursing*. Norwalk, CT: Appleton-Century-Crofts.

Wenger, A. F. Z., & Wenger, M. (1988). Community and family care patterns of the Old Order Amish. In M. M. Leininger (Ed.), *Care: Discovery and uses in clinical and community nursing*. Detroit, MI: Wayne State University Press.

Wenger, A. F. (1991). The culture care theory and the old order Amish. In M. M. Leininger (Ed.), *Culture care diversity and universality: A theory of nursing*. New York: National League for Nursing.

PART IX

Florence Nightingale

An Environmental Adaptation Theory

LOUISE C. SELANDERS

Biographical Sketch of the Nurse Theorist:
Florence Nightingale

Born: May 12, 1820 in Florence, Italy
Education: Privately educated in the classical mode with
    emphasis on languages, literature, philosophy, history,
    and mathematics
Nursing education briefly obtained at Kaiserswerth in
    Germany during 1850 and 1851
Achievements: Superintendency of the London Institution
    for the Care of Sick Gentlewomen in Distressed
    Circumstances; Superintendent of English nurses in
    the Crimean conflict; reform of English Army Medical
    School; establishment of military statistics;
    establishment of formalized nursing education at St.
    Thomas' Hospital, London; reform of hygienic
    standards for India; publication of more than 200
    books and monographs
Awards: Order of Merit
Died: August 13, 1910 in London. Consistent with
    Nightingale's wishes, she was buried in the family plot
    in East Wellow. There are no direct descendents of the
    Nightingale family.

Foreword

Florence Nightingale's name and reputation clearly symbolize the nursing profession. Few would doubt the claim that any other name is as well known as hers to modern nurses. Yet, if asked, few would be able to offer much information about Nightingale's life, particularly beyond the Crimean War. Even fewer could add anything at all about Nightingale and nursing theory.

This section by Louise C. Selanders corrects this deficiency by combining a succinct but well-crafted summary of Florence Nightingale's life and legacy with an interpretive and useful analysis of her nursing theory and its meaning. The comparison to the American Nurses' Association's most recent *Standards of Nursing Practice* is particularly relevant. This analysis effectively demonstrates that Nightingale's theory serves uniquely and brilliantly as a model for current practice.

Selanders also reminds the reader, appropriately, that Nightingale's greatest contributions stem not from the Crimean War experience but from her postwar activities, her prodigious writings, and especially her determination to create nursing as a profession. In the concluding section, "The Legacy of Florence Nightingale," the author effectively reminds us of the enormous debt the current nursing profession owes to Florence Nightingale—a fact that is often forgotten.

This section, then, is a tribute to Florence Nightingale. It is also a tribute to Louise Selanders. As the careful reader will note, Selanders has only recently completed her dissertation for Western Michigan

University: "An Analysis of the Utilization of Power by Florence Nightingale 1856-1872." During the years of research and writing, the author steeped herself in the life, spiritual nature, dreams, and legacy of the remarkable Florence Nightingale. As Selanders states in the Preface, this book is dedicated, "to Florence Nightingale, who has driven, delighted, mystified, and, at times, consumed me."

For those of us who have studied Nightingale in depth, and for the general reader alike, this section is a true testament to what can be learned from a total commitment to a study of an individual such as Nightingale. We thank the author for sharing the fruits of her labors. In short, both the subject and the author remind us, appropriately, to never forget that "learning the lessons which [Florence Nightingale] offered provides nursing with a wealth of possibility—and a lasting legacy."

RAYMOND G. HEBERT

Preface

The study of Florence Nightingale represents the study of a unique woman in a unique position of power and prestige. One of her many accomplishments included the development of the philosophical base of modern Western secular nursing. The purpose of this section is to provide the reader with an overview of Nightingale's perceptions of nursing and to demonstrate how this view remains applicable in today's high-tech world.

Florence Nightingale was a prolific writer. At least 12,000 letters, monographs, and books remain available to those wishing to research her life and thoughts in depth. Numerous biographies, drawn from these primary sources, also exist. Therefore Nightingale should not remain a mystery to those practicing nursing; neither should she be shrouded in myth and fiction. Rather, Nightingale should emerge as a complete human being with strengths and weaknesses, likes and dislikes, accomplishments and failures.

To assist the reader in sorting out the myth and the reality surrounding Nightingale, the initial section describes her life and times. However, space dictates that this be only a brief overview. Consequently, the reader is encouraged to read Nightingale from the primary sources. Of greatest interest to nurses may be *Notes on Nursing: What It Is and Is Not* (1859/1946) and *Sick Nursing and Health Nursing* (1893/1949), which together describe the nucleus of her thoughts regarding the profession.

The reader is encouraged to apply cultural context when reading the concepts and assumptions of Nightingale. Nineteenth-century England represented a world that was vastly different from today's society in the United States. Gender and class dictated the expectations for and goals of the population. Much less was known of the world in which they lived.

Finally, the reader is encouraged to remember that the development of the philosophical base of nursing and nursing education represents only a portion of the accomplishments that Nightingale achieved in her lifetime. Nursing came under the larger umbrella of improving public well-being and standards of hygiene and sanitation. If more people felt and worked as passionately as Nightingale did about improving their world, what a magnificent showcase of accomplishment it would be.

I would like to acknowledge and thank Ray Hebert for his comments and discussion. His insight has continued to make this project worthwhile. I would also like to thank the students of the Michigan State University College of Nursing who have provided a continual source of stimulation and encouragement. It is my intent that this section provide them with a valuable resource and the stimulus to study modern nursing from its origin. Finally, I want to acknowledge Nightingale herself, who has driven, delighted, mystified, and, at times, consumed me.

LOUISE C. SELANDERS

52

The Life and Times
of Florence Nightingale

The Philosophical Development
of Nightingale

During a life that spanned slightly more than 90 years, Florence Nightingale gained recognition for her accomplishments in sanitary and social reform. Her most recognized achievement was the establishment of the principles for modern nursing education and practice. Nightingale's life demonstrated continuing development of the principles that directed her toward goal achievement.

Early Life and Education

The life of Florence Nightingale was one of privilege associated with family wealth set in pre-Victorian and Victorian England. Born May 12, 1820 in Florence, Italy, she was named for the city of her birth.

Miss Nightingale was the second daughter and last child of William Edward and Frances Smith Nightingale. Both parents were of wealthy backgrounds that allowed them to provide an upper-class standard of living for their children. This included frequent travel, a classical education, and social prominence. As a result, Miss Nightingale became well traveled and known for her linguistic and mathematical skills. She also was conversant in history, economics, and the arts (Palmer, 1977).

The original family name was Shore. Upon the impending inheritance of the family estate of Lea Hurst in Derbyshire from his mother's uncle, William assumed the name of Nightingale to fulfill the terms of the will (Keen, 1982). Lea Hurst was considered too small by Victorian standards (15 bedrooms); it was cold and difficult for entertaining. Consequently, the second family estate of Embley Park in Hampshire in southern England was purchased.

Befitting the English gentry lifestyle, the Nightingale family lived a life of convenience. Time spent at the two estates, combined with extensive annual stays in London, provided the environment of Nightingale's childhood. The family entertained frequently, was considered socially prominent, and introduced Florence and her sister, Parthenope, to politicians, social reformers, and intellectuals of the period. At age 19, Florence and her sister were presented at court (Woodham-Smith, 1953).

Nightingale's parents were diverse in their beliefs and values. Her father was university educated and a supporter of Parliamentary reform (Allen, 1981). He valued education and saw to it that his daughters were tutored in the classics, an advantage not offered many women.

Encouraged by her father, Florence became a capable student, excelling in her studies and demonstrating a real thirst for knowledge. She maintained a close relationship with her father that continued until his death in 1874 (Cook, 1913).

Nightingale's mother was the antithesis of her father. Considered to be very beautiful and an expert at entertaining, Fanny was primarily interested in maintaining social stature and seeing that her daughters married well. Throughout her life, Fanny maintained a close relationship with Parthenope, who seemed to share her mother's goals and ambitions.

Fanny was never supportive of Florence's nursing efforts. Nursing was not considered a suitable occupation for a young lady of stature. Nightingale's mother did not seem to understand her younger daughter's need for independence, either as a child or later as an adult.

In Florence, one is able to see a mixture of the characteristics of her parents. Her father taught her to be scholarly and to use educated arguments; from her mother she learned drive and ambition.

Despite the privilege and travel of Nightingale's early life, these years were marked by periods of depression, illness, family discord, and disenchantment with her lifestyle. Nightingale perceived a need to be productive and useful and did not find entertaining or the rigors of society to be fulfilling. At an early age, she began to care for the family pets. Soon she was called to care for servants on the family estates who were ill or had been injured.

As early as 1844, at the age of 24, Miss Nightingale determined that her profession should be nursing (Cook, 1913). This decision brought family turmoil, not only because Florence wanted to work but also because of the prevailing reputation of secular nurses. They were felt to be uneducated women of questionable character who sought refuge caring for patients in private homes and hospitals in order to receive room and board. Nurses were stereotyped in the literature by characters such as the drunken Betsy Prig and Sairy Gamp in Charles Dickens's (1843/1986) *Martin Chuzzlewit.*

Miss Nightingale attempted, on several occasions, to receive formalized training in nursing. In 1850, and again in 1851, she was able to spend brief periods at Kaiserswerth on the Rhine in Germany, a Protestant institution that trained Deaconesses in child care and nursing. These two periods represent the only formalized nursing training received by Nightingale (Cook, 1913; Woodham-Smith, 1953).

Nursing in London

In 1853, Miss Nightingale negotiated and obtained the position of Superintendent of Nurses at the Institution for the Care of Sick Gentlewomen in Distressed Circumstances located in London (Vicinus & Nergaard, 1990; Woodham-Smith, 1953). Although she received no pay for this position and became responsible for her own expenses, this employment situation represented the first time she was able to display her skills in nursing and nursing administration.

Miss Nightingale brought about an upgrade in the standards of the nurses and nursing care, expecting that care be based on compassion, observation, and knowledge (Woodham-Smith, 1953). She also designed changes in the building that improved efficiency. These changes included a dumbwaiter to carry trays to and from the basement, hot and cold running water on all floors, and a system of patient call lights. Feeling that her job was complete after a year, she was seeking employment elsewhere when she was called into government service during the Crimean War (Woodham-Smith, 1953).

The Crimean War

By any standard, the Crimean War was neither a well-planned nor a productive conflict. It was fought primarily between Russia and Turkey to gain control over the port of Constantinople, the Eastern Mediterranean, and the overland route to the Eastern trading areas. Great Britain and France entered the war on the side of Turkey in 1854 (Seaman, 1956).

The British were based at Scutari in Turkey, although the fighting occurred in Southern Russia on the Crimean Peninsula. As a result of this location, the wounded and sick had to be transported by ship across the Black Sea nearly 300 miles (Goldie, 1987). The mortality rate approached 60% for the sick and wounded who survived the trip to the Barrack Hospital (Baly, 1988). The British public was alerted to these conditions by the news reporting of correspondent William Howard Russell for the *London Times* (Goldie, 1987).

A public outcry over the plight of the British soldier caused the British government to seek resolution of this problem. It was during this time that the Secretary for War, Sir Sidney Herbert, contacted Miss Nightingale and requested that she and a group of women travel to the Crimea to provide nursing services (Adams & Foster, 1981). Nightingale departed for Turkey with 38 women on October 21, 1854, disembarking at Scutari on November 4 (Cook, 1913).

During the next 21 months, despite resistance from the medical establishment, Nightingale worked to establish hygienic standards in the care of the wounded (Cope, 1958). She insisted that soldiers be bathed, their wounds dressed, and unspoiled food be fed to the sick. A pure water supply was established. As a result of Nightingale's efforts, the mortality rate declined to approximately 2% (Kalisch & Kalisch, 1986).

It should be noted that throughout Nightingale's life she remained absolutely opposed to the notion of germ theory, even though recent discoveries had provided evidence to the contrary (Baly, 1988; Vicinus & Nergaard, 1990). Although many of her reforms proved effective because of the reduction of contagion, she maintained that it was the general introduction of hygienic standards that brought about the improved conditions.

Nightingale returned to England in 1856 at the conclusion of the war. She was sick and exhausted after nearly dying from a bout of Crimean Fever—probably typhus (Veith, 1990). Much to her amazement and dismay, she was a heroine, a status she both disliked and shunned.

The Productive Years

Following her return from the Crimea, Miss Nightingale began her most productive period relative to establishing reform and creating change (Selanders, 1992). By 1872 she had reformed the Army Medical School, established the importance of accurate record-keeping and the need for governmental statistics, developed new systems of purveyance for wartime conditions, and helped to establish standards of hygiene and public health in India. However, her most enduring change was the establishment of formalized secular nursing education.

Miss Nightingale selected St. Thomas' Hospital in London as the site for the Nightingale School. This effort was supported by the Nightingale Fund, monies given by the grateful British public for the service she had rendered in the Crimea. The school opened in 1860 with approximately 10 students (Baly, 1988).

As a result of Nightingale's influence, she was able to define the nature of nursing clearly and how nursing was distinctly different from, but not subservient to, medicine. This effort began the establishment of nursing as a profession with a sound and specific educational base (Nightingale, 1859/1946; 1893/1949).

Nightingale wrote prolifically. *Notes on Nursing: What It Is and Is Not,* her best known work, was first published in 1859. Designed as a general reference for all persons who might care for another and not as a nursing text, it remains perhaps the most widely known and read volume of nursing literature.

The Later Years

Following the creation of her major reforms and the establishment of the Nightingale School at St. Thomas', Nightingale's health declined and she rarely left her apartment on South Street in London (Veith, 1990). However, she did continue to write, receive visitors, and offer advice in those areas in which she was considered an expert.

It has been hypothesized that her invalid state allowed her to continue to be productive without social pressures (Pickering, 1974). Individuals sought Nightingale's advice without demanding her appearance at social functions.

In 1893, a speech that clearly defined Nightingale's beliefs regarding the nature of nursing was delivered for her at the Chicago Exposition (Nightingale, 1893/1949). Her influence on nursing education continued as schools modeled after her philosophy began in the United States, Canada, Europe, and in most of Britain's imperial possessions, including Australia.

In 1907, in recognition of her contributions to the British nation, the first Order of Merit given to a woman was bestowed upon Florence Nightingale. Three years later, at the age of 90, she died in her sleep at her apartment on South Street in London.

Spirituality and Florence Nightingale

Devotion to God became prevalent in Nightingale's writings at an early age (Calabria, 1990; Cook, 1913; Widerquist, 1992). Throughout her life, Nightingale recorded a series of four experiences in which God called her into His service. The first occurred just prior to her 17th birthday. These experiences seemed to give purpose and direction to her life.

Nightingale's family had roots in both the Church of England (similar to the Episcopal Church in the United States) and in the Unitarian Church. However, Nightingale became critical of established religion stating, "the most frightful crimes which the world has ever seen have been perpetuated 'to please God' " (Calabria, 1990, p. 68). Consequently, she rarely practiced organized religion in her adult years, preferring to believe in a Supreme Being who was perfect and eternal (Widerquist, 1992). She also believed that God developed laws that governed the order of the universe. She later applied these laws to nursing, stating that nursing must place the patient in the best possible condition for Nature [God] to act (Nightingale, 1859/1946).

Certain elements of Nightingale's religious beliefs can be seen in her philosophical development. Central to her value system were her work ethic and the potential for the perfection of humankind. These philosophical beliefs played heavily in the development of a basis for nursing practice.

While Nightingale was superintendent of the Institution for Gentlewomen in London, a requirement existed that patients must be members of the Church of England in order to receive care. Nightingale rapidly removed this requirement, stating that religious affiliation should not be a requirement for receiving health care.

A similar situation existed when Nightingale began to determine the requirements for those who would enter nursing education. At the time that the Nightingale School was being developed, nursing education of a sort did exist. Virtually all schools of nursing were in religious institutions, such as Kaiserswerth, and religious affiliation was required for admission.

Nightingale believed that education should be open to women of all beliefs, just as all patients should be cared for regardless of their religious beliefs. Consequently, there was no religious affiliation requirement for admission to the Nightingale School. Although Nightingale is credited as being the founder of modern Western nursing education, more correctly she should be credited as the founder of modern Western secular nursing.

The Cultural Context of the Nightingalean Era

To appreciate the accomplishments of Florence Nightingale fully, it is necessary to understand the age in which she lived and the cultural expectations of the period. During the Victorian era, England had a classed culture with great differences in the expectations of the education, productivity, and social behavior between the rich and the poor. This period followed the Industrial Revolution. Consequently, the cities had seen great population influxes and the proliferation of manufacturing.

Many new scientific discoveries, including Jenner's smallpox immunization and Priestley's isolation of oxygen, established the basis for medical innovation (Williams, 1987). Church reform gave greater religious freedom of choice (Schultz, 1992). In general, the time offered a more open society than had previous centuries.

Although reform marked the character of the 19th century, it should be remembered that British society was clearly restricted by gender. Women of social prominence were not expected to contribute in any significant fashion to society. Although many could read, educational opportunities were severely restricted for women when compared to their male counterparts. Nightingale's reforms are all the more impressive because of the conditions under which they occurred. Only a woman of single-minded purpose and resolve could have brought about such change.

Origins of the Model

On Nightingale's return from the Crimea in 1856, she perceived a great need for change. During the next 15 years she brought major reform to the British Army and its medical education system as well as establishing the philosophical base for modern nursing education and practice. The changes brought to nursing constitute her most enduring reform.

The watershed event that greatly influenced Nightingale's perception of nursing was her experience in the Crimea. Although she had been aware of the need for hygienic care in England, the Crimea served to magnify the need for sanitary reform.

An integral component of creating this change was the development of a formalized standard for the education of nurses. Although nursing education was not her first priority on returning from the Crimea, it became something that literally occupied the remainder of her life.

The Nightingale Fund

The Nightingale Fund consisted of monies donated by a grateful British public to be put at Nightingale's disposal and used in whatever manner she saw fit. The entirety of this fund was used to establish the Nightingale School at St. Thomas' Hospital in London.

The Nightingale Fund established the school of nursing as financially independent from the hospital. This financial independence allowed Nightingale, with the authority of the school's governing body, to establish curricula and hire a matron. The matron was responsible for the day-to-day running of the school without major influence being exerted by the medical community.

The Fund also provided publicity for nursing. This publicity helped begin the process in which nursing was established as a legitimate educational opportunity for women. As a result, the image of nursing was improved and the profession eventually opened to all classes of women (Baly, 1988).

Philosophical Assumptions

Assumptions are ideas that are implicit and assumed to be true without empirical testing (Walker & Avant, 1988). The following assumptions provide insight into Nightingale's values and beliefs. Understanding the assumptions helps to provide a focus for studying the nursing model.

Nightingale did not specifically identify the ideas that formed the basis of her understanding of nursing. Rather, the assumptions were drawn from her books and monographs. Nightingale's belief in God, a strong work ethic, and the functional ability and value of women underlie these assumptions.

Nursing Is a Calling

The context of "calling" in this instance had religious overtones. Nightingale's deeply religious beliefs in the existence of "natural laws" reinforced her perceived nature of nursing. She felt that these laws could be discovered and used to help people improve their health and existence.

To Nightingale, a "calling" was consuming in terms of time and commitment. Therefore nursing was more than an occupation, something that one could not put aside even for short periods of time.

Nightingale also believed that the work of nursing was so important that it should be thought of as though it were a religious vow. Nightingale herself declined marriage on several occasions, stating that she could not carry out the rigorous demands of her chosen work and meet the requirements of family life.

Nursing Is an Art and a Science

Nightingale described the profession as an art and a science in her remarks at the Chicago Exposition (1893/1949). Her concept of nursing as a science was reflected in her mandate that nurses be formally educated. Her own practice demonstrated a grasp of statistics, logic, and laws of health and health practices.

The art of nursing, however, gave the profession both freedom and depth. This aspect allowed and mandated that the nurse act in a creative and proactive fashion. The art of nursing also permitted the nurse to function as an advocate for the patient.

Mankind Can Achieve Perfection

Nightingale believed that people could control the outcomes of their lives. Therefore they could pursue perfection. As related to health care, this meant that people could pursue perfect health. The role of the nurse was to try to provide the environment in which this perfect health could be achieved.

The manner in which perfection could be achieved was through the understanding of Nature's laws. Nightingale believed that each generation moved toward a logical understanding of these universal laws. Ultimately, these laws would be understood and readily used by people to benefit their existence.

Nursing Requires a Specific Educational Base

The idea that nurses required specific education was revolutionary in 19th-century England. Nightingale's focus on providing nursing education underscored her belief in the value of educating women in general.

Nightingale emphasized the need to blend a mixture of theoretical and clinical experiences as part of the educational package, stating, "Neither can it [nursing] be taught by lectures or by books [alone] although these are valuable accessories, if used as such: otherwise what is in the book stays in the book" (Nightingale, 1893/1949, p. 24).

Nursing Is Distinct and Separate From Medicine

Although the physician and the nurse may deal with the same client population, nursing is not to be viewed as subservient to medicine; rather, nursing is aimed at discovering the natural laws that will assist in putting the patient in the best possible condition so that nature can effect a cure.

Nightingale frequently said that nursing was particularly well suited for women. This idea appears to be tied to the gender expectations of the 19th century. Given Nightingale's progressive nature, it is unlikely she would uphold this restriction in today's social environment.

Nightingale's ability, determination, and articulation of the philosophical basis of nursing have endured. Most of her broad beliefs and values continue to hold true in nursing practice a century after they were written.

53

Nightingale's
Theory of Nursing

Each discipline identifies certain phenomena that help to define the nature of the discipline. These concepts remain constant even though a number of different conceptual models or theories may be built around the designated phenomena. These concepts are known as the metaparadigm of a discipline.

The metaparadigm provides a general and consistent perspective for a discipline to develop and to make comparisons among its several conceptual models (Fawcett, 1984). In nursing, the common phenomena around which the discipline has been built are person, environment, health, and nursing (Fawcett, 1984; Fitzpatrick & Whall, 1983; Torres, 1990).

Nightingale did not specifically write in terms of a metaparadigm, nursing theory, or a conceptual model. However, she has been credited with developing the first conceptual model of nursing. Nightingale was a prolific writer. Today, more than 150 monographs and books and over 12,000 letters provide us with a rich legacy of her thoughts and ideas. All of the necessary elements for the description of a nursing theory are present in these documents.

Person

Person is the recipient of nursing care. In the case of Nightingale, person was generally viewed as being an individual, although families occasionally were the focus of nursing care. Individuals were usually called "patients" in Nightingale's writings.

On multiple occasions Nightingale made it clear in her writings that nurses were to care for patients, not diseases. She agreed with a physician who stated, "I do not treat pneumonia, I treat the person who has pneumonia" (Nightingale, 1893/1949, p. 24).

People were viewed as multidimensional; that is, they were composed of biological, psychological, social, and spiritual elements. The interrelationship of these components encompassed holism.

The biological component of people was addressed in relation to the cure and prevention of disease. People were seen as having reparative powers and nursing should assist these powers as the means of returning people to health. However, illness also could be prevented through the provision of the proper environment in which people should live.

The psychological component was composed of things that defined thought processes, self-concept, feelings, and intellect. In *Notes on Nursing* (1893/1946), Nightingale warned about the lack of variety and the degree of monotony found in most patient's environments. She also stated that the lack of variety could impede healing and may actually cause psychological disease processes.

The social element of people consisted of interactions within society. Nightingale appears to have addressed this concept less directly than the other elements; however, she was aware that patients should not be isolated from others. Nightingale did advise against the practices of idle chatter and offering advice to patients.

The spiritual element of people referred to the value systems that assisted them in making decisions determining right from wrong. Religion, while an important component to many people, was not to be interpreted as the equivalent of spirituality.

Spirituality is a difficult element to assess as it relates to Nightingale's beliefs. Nightingale's spirituality was intricately tied to her religious belief system but not to a specific religion. She also felt strongly about the inherent value of people and appeared to assume

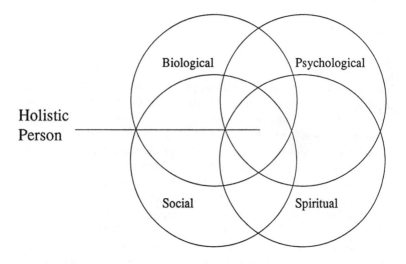

Figure 53.1. Multidimensional holistic person.

that the spiritual nature of patients was an assumed element rather than a prerequisite for care.

Tied directly to the concept of spirituality was the belief that people were in control of their own destiny. This control was created by making choices in life. The ultimate goal was to move toward perfection (Widerquist, 1992).

The dichotomy of this belief system was that Nightingale was also heavily influenced by the cultural standards of 19th-century England, which established rigid rules of social behaviors. Therefore, despite the perceived ability of being able to make choices in life, people were expected to obey the cultural norms established by society.

The interaction of these biological, psychological, social, and spiritual elements defines Nightingale's concept of holism. The classical definition of holism states that interacting wholes are more than the sum of their parts (Torres, 1990). Holism implies that an insult to any one of the components effects the entire person to some degree. Therefore, people cannot experience a physiological illness such as heart disease without it also affecting their psychological, social, and spiritual components.

This perspective of holism is seen in Figure 53.1. All of the elements appear to have equal value.

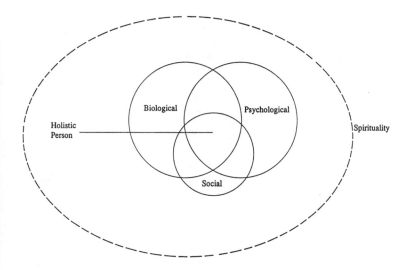

Figure 53.2. Nightingale's conception of holism.

Nightingale's view of holism appears to be less symmetrical than the classical model. Clearly, she did appear to pay more attention to the physical and psychological components than to the other elements of holistic beings. She particularly offers advice in *Notes on Nursing* about various types of physiological care including diet, activity, warmth, light, and care of excrements. Psychological care was also stressed by assuring that patients had variety, an appropriate balance of stimuli and quiet, and that the nurse's behavior did not in any way detract from the patient's environment.

Figure 53.2 more accurately depicts the representation of a holistic individual from Nightingale's perspective. Physiological and psychological needs are seen as predominant, with social needs apparently having less impact on well-being. Spirituality is assumed and pervasive.

Environment

Environment is the core concept in Nightingale's model of nursing. It was her contention that the environment could be altered in such a way as to improve conditions so that nature could act to cure the

TABLE 53.1 Nightingale's Major Environmental Elements

Element
Ventilation
Light
Clean water
Warmth
Noise control
Management of wastes and odors

patient. The environment consisted of those physical attributes that could be altered and thus improve the patient's well-being.

Nightingale specifically defined elements of the environment that she felt should be monitored and improved when necessary. The most important environmental concerns were ventilation and clean air, followed by clean water. Additional needs that Nightingale identified as critical were provision for warmth, control of noise, provision for light, and adequate management of wastes and odors (see Table 53.1).

These needs represented chronic problems in Victorian England. The air, especially in the cities, was choked by smoke from burning coal, the chief source of heat. Because sanitation was not always well understood, water supplies were frequently contaminated by human and animal wastes.

Nightingale highlighted these needs as important from a common-sense approach to sanitation. If a clean environment was available to patients, experience told Nightingale that the ability of a patient to survive and eventually recover from disease improved.

In the 1940s, Maslow developed his needs theory in which he identified human needs necessary for human survival. Needs were ordered according to survival priority. Maslow further postulated that lower-level needs had to be met before being able to move to a higher level of need attainment.

Maslow's first-level needs are physiological and included food, air, water, temperature, elimination, and rest. Second-level needs address safety and security issues. Third-level needs are those of social affiliation (Kozier, Erb, & Olivieri, 1991).

A direct comparison can be drawn between Nightingale's perception of human needs within the environment and Maslow's human needs theory. Both address the primary physiological needs, followed by psychological and social needs. Nightingale's perceptions were drawn from empirical observation, and Maslow's theory adds substantiation to her conceptualization.

Nightingale also saw the environment as having external and internal components. She appeared to be as concerned about elements that entered the body—food, water, and medications—as those that directly affected the external body—temperature, bedding, and ventilation (Nightingale, 1859/1946).

Notes on Nursing, Nightingale's most famous publication, was written for the express purpose of informing the general public about how to maintain hygienic conditions within the home and in an illness situation, not as a textbook for nurses. In the preface to *Notes on Nursing*, Nightingale (1859/1946) writes,

> The following notes are by no means intended as a rule of thought by which nurses can teach themselves to nurse, still less as a manual to teach nurses to nurse. They are meant simply to give hints of thought to women who have personal charge of the health of others. Every woman, or at least almost every woman, in England has, at one time or another of her life, charge of the personal health of somebody, whether child or invalid—in other words, every woman is a nurse.
> (p. 1)

Nightingale did not mean to imply by stating that "every woman was a nurse" that nurses did not require specialized education. Rather, she was stating that nursing is a nurturing art that requires knowledge of sanitary procedures—in essence, how to alter the environment safely. These thoughts were outlined in her 13 canons found in *Notes on Nursing*.

Health

Nightingale (1859/1949) stated that health is "not only to be well, but to be able to use well every power we have to use" (p. 26). Her definition is similar to the World Health Organization's (1947) definition of health that states, "Health is a state of complete physical, mental and social well-being, not merely the absence of disease or infirmity" (p. 29).

TABLE 53.2 A Comparison of Modern Practice Concepts and
Nightingale's Canons for Health

Practice Concept	Canons
Physical environment	Ventilation and warming
	Light
	Cleanliness of rooms and walls
	Health of houses
Comfort and safety	Noise
	Bed and bedding
	Personal cleanliness
Psychological environment	Variety
	Chattering hopes and advices
Nutrition	Taking food
	What food?
Continuity of care	Petty management
	Observation of the sick

Nightingale's view of health separates the concepts of health and wellness. Wellness is an absolute state that may be more accurately described as being one end of the wellness-illness continuum. Although it might be difficult to define parameters that would place an individual on this continuum, it would be theoretically possible to do this. Therefore, one would be more or less well, depending on a variety of measurable factors.

Health, however, connotes a relative state. When defined as "being the best one can be at any given point in time," it allows an individual to be healthy even if not well. This statement relates to "using every power we have to use" (Nightingale, 1859/1949, p. 26).

By Nightingale's definition of health, an individual dying of cancer could still be in a healthy state, providing issues such as coping mechanisms, support systems, pain management, and grief support were provided. Yet this individual could hardly be considered well.

Nightingale's view of health included the idea that health was promoted by discovering the Natural Laws that govern health. By altering the environment according to Nightingale's canons, the Natural Laws would be fulfilled and therefore, health would be promoted. Table 53.2 compares modern practice concepts with her canons for health.

Nightingale (1893/1949) defined disease as "Nature's way of getting rid of the effects of conditions which have interfered with health" (p. 26). These conditions usually related to the effects of "dirt, drink [impure water], diet, damp, draughts [drafts], [and] drains [improper sewage disposal]" (p. 31).

Disease was also defined as a "reparative process" (Nightingale, 1893/1946, p. 5). Viewing disease as "dys-ease," that is, lack of comfort, assists the reader in understanding Nightingale's viewpoint of health and illness. It is helpful to remember that during Nightingale's lifetime the vast majority of illnesses and deaths were caused by infectious disease. Therefore, common symptoms would include fever, vomiting, nausea, diarrhea, and cough.

Each of these symptoms causes a level of discomfort or "dys-ease." However, they are therapeutic in the sense that each indicates a problem that exists within the body. Fever, for instance, only becomes nontherapeutic when not controlled. In most instances, it does appear to be a natural way of ridding the body of the effects of illness. Therefore, in this context fever would be reparative.

Nursing

Nightingale viewed nursing as both an art and a science. The purpose of nursing was to "put the patient in the best possible condition for nature to act upon him" (Nightingale, 1859/1946, p. 6). Nursing was carried out by altering the environment in such a fashion as to implement the natural laws of health.

Nursing was viewed by Nightingale in both a general and specific context. In the general sense nursing was something carried out by women (as previously quoted from *Notes on Nursing*). Women who provided care in a family setting but had no formal training in nursing practiced "health nursing" or "general nursing."

Nightingale believed that women generally were poorly educated in how to care for their family's needs. When condemning the high mortality rate of infants she said,

Is all this premature suffering and death necessary? Or did Nature intend mothers to always be accompanied by doctors? Or is it better to learn the piano-forte than to learn the laws which subserve the preservation of offspring? (Nightingale, 1893/1949, p. 7)

In a specific sense, Nightingale envisioned "nursing proper" as that which was practiced only by women who had been educated as nurses (Nightingale, 1893/1949). This philosophical stance caused her to see the need for formalized nursing education and to work to establish the Nightingale School at St. Thomas' Hospital.

Nightingale's writings related to nursing care suggested that this care be carried out in a manner similar to what is now known as the "nursing process," even though Nightingale was not familiar with this terminology. Client observation was particularly important to the nursing process. It was a skill that she felt should be taught in an organized fashion to educated nurses.

Following observations, Nightingale felt that documentation of the observations should be made in detailed fashion. Organized record keeping resulted in the first nurses' notes. Emphasis was given to the environmental factors that the nurse was responsible for overseeing and altering, such as noise, light, and warmth.

Nightingale's Model of Nursing

Nightingale's model of nursing describes how a nurse is to implement natural laws. This model describes how these laws allow the concepts of person, environment, health, and nursing to interact.

All nursing must take place in the context of society and environment. While the nurse and the patient may be in the same environment, it is assumed that the alteration of the environment is for the improvement of the health of the patient. Certainly, it is clear that the context of 19th-century England and the social values attached to the period had a profound effect on how Nightingale developed nursing.

Central to the nursing act is the person or patient who is the recipient of nursing care (see Figure 53.3). Nightingale was very explicit that the person, not the disease, was to be nursed. The individual who is the recipient of nursing care may be ill or well, as the maintenance and promotion of health is as important as recovery from disease.

The model is linear. In this form the nurse is the active participant in the relationship. The outcome is the health state of the patient. This

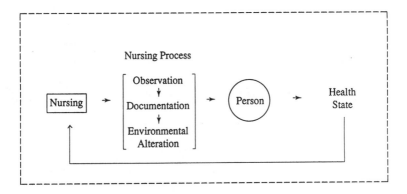

Figure 53.3. Nightingale's model of nursing practice.

combination of process and outcome serves as feedback and indicates whether or not the nurse needs to modify nursing activities.

Nightingale did not see nursing as an event that only took place in the event of illness or injury; rather, she identified that nursing could take place as health promotion and rehabilitation activities as well as in the restorative phase of illness.

Health promotion was a new concept at the time of Nightingale. She carried through with these beliefs by establishing district nursing—a precursor to public health nursing. Its purpose was to promote hygienic practices for the purpose of maintaining health.

Evaluation of Nightingale's Model of Nursing

Nightingale's model of nursing is based on experiential observations made about the relationship of individuals known as patients and their attendant health status. The health of individuals can be altered by manipulating the environment in such a fashion as to create more positive conditions for the patient. The individual who manipulates the environment is the nurse. The nurse would accomplish this manipulation of the environment through knowledge gained by observation and study.

In using observation as the major route to determining the relationship between the client and health, Nightingale employed inductive reasoning, a process by which one moves from a specific set of facts to determine a set of generalizations (Fitzpatrick & Whall, 1983). Nightingale was particularly adept at this method. Her experiences in the Crimea supplied her with the critical set of events and observations. From this experience she was able to identify patterns of change that needed to take place in the environment in order to increase patient well-being.

The model has been in actual practice settings for more than 100 years. Although nurses may not actually recognize that they are practicing nursing according to the Nightingale model, the goal of nursing action is frequently to alter the environment for the purpose of improving patient welfare. This flexibility indicates that it is a generalizable model.

The model is descriptive in nature (Fawcett, 1984). Although Nightingale described certain types of sequelae from patient environmental conditions, she never attempted to describe a causal relationship as to why these sequelae existed. For instance, she described that the lack of light produced rickets in children and thus argued that light must be in the environment, but Nightingale never attempted to explain why a lack of light produced rickets.

Nightingale's theory is also simple. She does not attempt to define complex relationships between the elements of the theory. The simplicity does not seem to detract or reduce the theoretical applicability of the nursing practices that she describes.

Nightingale's theory may be classified as a grand theory (Fawcett, 1984). The theory has very broad terms and is abstract. This causes some difficulty in applying empirical testing to Nightingale's methods because the terms are imprecisely defined.

Perhaps the greatest testament to her concepts of nursing is related to their durability. Although written well over a century ago, they are difficult to dispute and easy to apply even in today's high-tech health care settings.

54

Nightingale
Then and Now

Is the study of Florence Nightingale and her perceptions of nursing merely an exercise in nursing history, or does it have relevance for today's complex, high-tech world? The study of Nightingale proves to be basic to the present study of nursing practice.

Clinical Examples

Nightingale's emphasis was on providing an environment that would allow Nature either to heal or prevent illness. In virtually every modern nursing situation, regardless of the specific setting, the nurse remains responsible for altering the environment to improve it for the benefit of the client.

Case 1

Mr. Wright, a gerontological nurse, has just completed a nursing assessment of Mr. Webster in his apartment. Mr. Webster is 90, lives alone, and has limited mobility. He depends on Social Security as his source of income. His son lives out of state. Although he is supportive of trying to meet his father's needs, he is rarely able to visit.

The apartment has adequate space but is poorly heated. The windows are painted shut and the apartment has a musty odor. The rooms have obviously not been cleaned for a long time. Moldy food is in the refrigerator.

As part of his nursing intervention, Mr. Wright arranges for a neighbor to clean the apartment on a regular basis. A fan is purchased to help with ventilation. Meals-On-Wheels provides at least one warm meal and daily contact with Mr. Webster. Mr. Wright contacted Mr. Webster's son and requested that on his next visit he see that Mr. Webster be provided with warmer clothing in order to try to maintain his body temperature during the upcoming winter.

Case 2

Mrs. Sanchez is caring for Nancy, a 16-year-old primipara who is in the first stage of labor. Having been admitted to the hospital 12 hours previously, Nancy appears tired and close to tears. Her contractions are every 2 to 3 minutes apart, lasting 45 seconds and of moderate intensity. Nancy's mouth appears dry and her lips are cracked. She is sweating profusely. No family or friends are present.

In attempting to make Nancy more comfortable, Mrs. Sanchez encourages Nancy to walk in the hallway. She offers her ice chips, a lollypop, and lip lubricant. When she's in bed, Nancy's lower back is massaged. Mrs. Sanchez bathes Nancy's face and upper extremities and provides peri care. During contractions, Mrs. Sanchez helps Nancy focus her breathing to reduce her discomfort. As a result of these measures Nancy relaxes and is fully dilated within 45 minutes.

In each instance, the nurse manipulated the environment in some manner to benefit the client. In the case of the laboring mother, it is probable that the environment of both the mother and child was improved. The nursing actions are consistent with Nightingale's perception of nursing practice.

Nightingale Today

The real benefit of Florence Nightingale for today's practice is the legacy of values that she conferred upon modern nursing (Selanders,

1990). Much of what is taken for granted today—the clean environment for practice, the defined education, the movement of nursing toward an independent identity—is assumed to be the current standard. The origin of the standard rests with Florence Nightingale. Shealy (1985) has called Nightingale an example of an evolutionary personality because she redefined at least a portion of the universe as it was commonly understood to exist.

Nightingale's perceptions of nursing can be empirically tested as they relate to the modern nursing situation. Skeet (1980) has updated *Notes on Nursing: What It Is and Is Not* using Nightingale's original topic headings. Skeet demonstrated that these headings remain applicable in today's world of practice in *Notes on Nursing: The Science and the Art.*

Dennis and Prescott (1985) undertook a similar task by developing a qualitative database of current nursing practice, using Nightingale's standards, in a contemporary setting. These standards were found to be applicable in modern practice.

Henry, Woods, and Nagelkerk (1990) demonstrated how Nightingale used principles of nursing administration to enhance nursing practice. Further examples exist in clinical studies in which Nightingale has been chosen as the organizing framework.

The strength of Nightingale's work lies partially in the durability of the ideas that she established over a century ago. Although she should be viewed neither as a saint nor seen as invincible, the utility of her principles of practice and education need to be remembered, used, and continually evaluated against the current standard.

Nightingale and Standards of Nursing Practice

Standards of nursing practice are criteria that were developed to allow for the evaluation of care against a known standard. The current criteria were developed by the American Nurses' Association (ANA) and are based on the nursing process (ANA, 1973). If Nightingale's theory is to serve as a model for current practice, then the theory should be able to withstand evaluation against these standards of practice.

Standard 1: Assessment

The collection of data about the health status of the client/patient is systematic and continuous. The data are accessible, communicated, and recorded.

Nightingale originated the concept of organized patient assessment. Further, she established assessment as a standard of nursing practice. In *Notes on Nursing*, she devoted extensive space to the process of observation. In it Nightingale (1859/1946) stated,

> The most important practical lesson that can be given to nurses is to teach them what to observe—how to observe—what symptoms indicate improvement—what the reverse—which are of importance—which are of none—which are the evidence of neglect—and what kind of neglect. All this is what ought to make part, and an essential part, of the training of every nurse. (p. 59)

Nightingale insisted that observations be made of individual patients to allow for individual variation. Routines and preferences of the patients were to be taken into consideration.

Recording of the data was also considered a critical component of nursing function. Record keeping grew out of Nightingale's Crimean experiences. Through thorough data collection and documentation she was able to support her perceived problems with the health care system. On a less global basis, the individual nurse was also expected to be able to write down observations and be able to support conclusions regarding prescribed care.

Standard 2: Nursing Diagnosis

Nursing diagnoses are derived from health status data.

Nightingale was not aware of the terminology of nursing diagnosis. Yet she freely drew conclusions regarding patient status from the data that she collected.

Today, nursing problems are frequently classified by nursing diagnoses. The North American Nursing Diagnosis Association (NANDA) has developed a list of nursing problems—actual, potential, or possible—with which the nurse may need to intervene.

A taxonomy of nursing diagnoses has produced a further ordering of nursing problems. NANDA has approved human response patterns as the accepted taxonomy. These categories include exchanging, communicating, relating, valuing, choosing, moving, perceiving, knowing, and feeling (Kozier et al., 1991).

The problems listed in "Pattern 1: Exchanging" are primarily physiological in nature. This pattern includes such functional categories as air exchange and elimination. Many of these areas were directly or indirectly addressed by Nightingale, such as nursing care for diarrhea, altered nutrition, hypo- and hyperthermia, ineffective airway clearance, and potential for poisoning (Nightingale, 1859/1946).

Standard 3: Planning

The plan of nursing care includes goals derived from the nursing diagnosis.

Standard 4: Planning

The plan of nursing care includes priorities and the prescribed nursing approaches or measures to achieve the goals derived from the nursing diagnoses.

The prioritization of problems indicates that decisions must be made as to how to approach and in what order to approach the problems of a given patient. This ordering of decisions is reflected in Nightingale's prioritization of problems with basic physiological needs being the most important.

During Nightingale's lifetime the primary diseases that caused sudden death were infectious. Common symptoms of fever, diarrhea, vomiting, and dehydration were frequently life threatening. Consequently, these problems required priority intervention. This prioritization is also a reflection of the empirical process by which Nightingale derived her nursing model.

Nightingale's definition of nursing—placing the patient in the best condition for nature to act—implies that the very nature of nursing is goal directed. To achieve the basic goal of nursing, more immediate goals must be designed by the nurse.

Standard 5: Implementation

Nursing actions provide for client/patient participation in health promotion, maintenance, and restoration.

In Nightingale's paper presented at the 1893 Chicago Exposition, she stated,

> Health is not only to be well, but to be able to use well every power we have. . . . Both kinds of nursing [nursing proper and health nursing] are to put us in the best possible conditions for nature to restore or to preserve health—to prevent or to cure disease or injury. . . . Nursing proper is therefore to help the patient suffering from disease to live—just as health nursing is to keep or put the constitution of the healthy child or human being in such a state as to have no disease. (Nightingale, 1893/1949, p. 26)

This definition of health is notable because it represents the first time that levels of health promotion, maintenance, and restoration were identified as being legitimate nursing functions. These functions of nursing remained essentially intact for a century until expanded and refined by reformers such as Virginia Henderson in 1955 (Furukawa & Howe, 1990).

Standard 6: Implementation

The nursing actions assist the client/patient to maximize health capabilities.

The goal of this standard is consistent with Nightingale's interpretation of health: that health is a relative process and involves helping the patient to be the best that he or she can be at any given point in time. Nightingale assumed that much of nursing care was done *to* the patient as opposed to in conjunction *with* the patient. Recipients of health care were not viewed as participants in the process. However, this view is assumed to be cultural and a function of 19th-century ideology.

Standard 7: Evaluation

The client/patient's progress or lack of progress toward goal achievement is determined by the client/patient and the nurse.

As stated above, the patient frequently was not seen as an active participant in care. However, Nightingale did determine that the evaluation of client status was critical to the process of providing adequate care. Only then could it be determined if the care should be continued or altered.

Standard 8: Evaluation

The client/patient's progress or lack of progress toward goal achievement directs reassessment, reordering of priorities, new goal setting, and revision of the plan of nursing care.

This standard implies that the nursing process is circular in nature: As care is given, the assessment process begins again to redetermine the patient status. This process is consistent with the linear model representing Nightingale's practice of nursing. A feedback loop exists that provides the nurse with information about the outcome of care. Care is then altered accordingly.

It is an understatement to say that Nightingale's model of nursing practice is consistent with the *Standards of Nursing Practice* as established by the American Nurses' Association (1973). It is as if Nightingale's documents served as the basis for establishing these standards.

The Legacy of Florence Nightingale

Florence Nightingale is recognized first and foremost as a nurse. She demonstrated skill as a social reformer and in creating change. What, then, is the legacy that has been left to the modern nurse?

Nightingale's skill in nursing was not at the bedside; rather, she was an administrator and reformer. Relative to the reform of nursing, she wrote,

> The whole reform of nursing both at home and abroad has consisted of this: to take the power over nursing out of the hands of the men and put it into the hands of one female trained head and make her responsible for everything being carried out. (cited in Baly, 1981, p. 213)

In seeking to implement these reforms, Nightingale felt that nursing must establish an educational base. The result was the establishment of the Nightingale School and the development of the "Nightingale Model" of nursing education.

The major features of the model emphasized a combination of classroom and clinical experiences. Textbooks specifically designed for nurses were utilized. Nurses taught nurses although lectures by physicians did occur. Nightingale conveyed to the directors of the school her basic wishes in terms of curriculum and practical experience.

However, much of what Nightingale had originally designed was not actually carried out in practice. The most significant alteration of Nightingale's wishes was the apprenticeship system of nursing education that evolved and remained well into the 20th century.

In return for service given for little or no pay the student received a "free" education. The result was that the nursing schools became dependent on training hospitals for financial resources. Consequently, the hospitals began to control training schedules, frequently limiting time and experience in the classroom in favor of the manpower hours that could be garnered at little or no expense to the institution.

Besides issues of training, this situation continued to make nursing more subservient than Nightingale had envisioned. As a result, nursing continues to have problems with image.

A work completed by Etzioni in 1969 concluded that nursing, social work, and teaching were occupations that could never enjoy the same status as medicine and law—the professions. This was due to shorter training and a lack of autonomy. Both of these factors led to a less legitimized status as viewed by other professionals.

Although these arguments may be dated and inaccurate, they underscore the type of image problems with which nursing has had to deal. These arguments also demonstrate that nursing has not done well controlling its own destiny.

Is this the fault of Nightingale? Perhaps. Nightingale demonstrated throughout her lifetime that she was a powerful person and capable of creating change. She also demonstrated that she had the ability to assume leadership roles.

If Nightingale is to be faulted it is from the perspective that she did not appear to empower other nurses to assume the same type of leadership role that she so easily assumed. However, the leadership that she exhibited and the methods that she successfully employed are available for examination.

This point is where the study of Nightingale becomes valuable. Learning the lessons that she offered provides nursing with a wealth of possibility—and a lasting legacy.

References

Adams, E. C., & Foster, W. D. (1981). Heroine of modern progress. In R. G. Hebert (Ed.), *Florence Nightingale: Saint, reformer or rebel?* (pp. 102-107). Malabar, FL: Robert E. Krieger.

Allen, D. R. (1981). Florence Nightingale: Toward a psychohistorical interpretation. In R. G. Hebert (Ed.), *Florence Nightingale: Saint, reformer, or rebel?* (pp. 64-86). Malabar, FL: Robert E. Krieger.

American Nurses' Association. (1973). *Standards of nursing practice.* Kansas City, MO: Author.

Baly, M. E. (1981). Florence Nightingales's influence on nursing today. In R. G. Hebert (Ed.), *Florence Nightingale: Saint, reformer or rebel?* (pp. 210-219). Malabar, FL: Robert E. Krieger.

Baly, M. E. (1988). *Florence Nightingale and the nursing legacy.* New York: Croom Helm.

Calabria, M. D. (1990, Summer). Spiritual insights of Florence Nightingale. *The Quest,* pp. 66-74.

Cook, E. (1913). *The life of Florence Nightingale* (2 vols). London: Macmillan.

Cope, Z. (1958). *Florence Nightingale and the doctors.* London: Museum Press.

Dennis, K. E., & Prescott, P. P. (1985). Florence Nightingale: Yesterday, today and tomorrow. *Advances in Nursing Science, 1*(2), 66-81.

Dickens, C. (1986). *Martin Chuzzlewit.* Suffolk, UK: Richard Clay. (Original work published 1843)

Etzioni, A. (1969). *The semi-professions and their organization.* New York: Free Press.

Fawcett, J. (1984). *Analysis and evaluation of conceptual models of nursing.* Philadelphia, PA: F. A. Davis.

Fitzpatrick, J., & Whall, A. (1983). *Conceptual models of nursing: Analysis and application.* Bowie, MD: Brady.

Furukawa, C., & Howe, J. K. (1990). Virginia Henderson. In J. B. George (Ed.), *Nursing theories: The base for professional nursing practice* (3rd ed., pp. 61-78). Englewood Cliffs, NJ: Appleton & Lange.

Goldie, S. M. (1987). *I have done my duty: Florence Nightingale in the Crimean War, 1854-56.* Manchester, UK: Manchester University Press.

Henry, B., Woods, S., & Nagelkerk, J. (1990). Nightingale's perspective of nursing administration. *Nursing & Health Care, 11*(4), 201-206.

Kalisch, P., & Kalisch, B. (1986). *The advance of American nursing* (2nd ed.). Boston: Little, Brown.

Keen, N. (1982). *Florence Nightingale.* Berby, UK: J. H. Hall.

Kozier, B., Erb, G., & Olivieri, R. (1991). *Fundamentals of nursing: Concepts, process and practice* (4th ed.). Menlo Park, CA: Addison Wesley.

Nightingale, F. (1946). *Notes on nursing: What it is and is not.* London: Churchill Livingstone. (Original work published 1859)

Nightingale, F. (1949). Sick nursing and health nursing. In I. Hampton (Ed.), *Nursing of the sick, 1893* (pp. 24-43). New York: McGraw-Hill. (Original work by Nightingale published 1893).

Palmer, I. S. (1977). Florence Nightingale: Reformer, reactionary, researcher. *Nursing Research, 26*(2), 84-89.

Pickering, G. (1974). *Creative malady: Illness in the lives and minds of Charles Darwin, Florence Nightingale, Mary Baker Eddy, Sigmund Freud, Marcel Proust, and Elizabeth Barrett Browning.* London: Allen & Unwin.

Schultz, H. J. (1992). *British history* (4th ed.). New York: Harper-Perennial.

Seaman, L. C. B. (1956). *From Vienna to Versailles.* London: Coward-McCann.

Selanders, L. C. (1990). An American perspective of the Nightingale legacy. *Nursing Practice, 3*(3), 24-25.

Selanders, L. C. (1992). *An analysis of the utilization of power by Florence Nightingale, 1856-1872* (No. 9310445). Ann Arbor, MI: University Microfilms.

Shealy, M. C. (1985). Florence Nightingale 1820-1910: An evolutionary mind in the context of holism. *Journal of Holistic Nursing, 3*(1), 4-5.

Skeet, M. (1980). *Notes on nursing: The science and the art.* New York: Churchill Livingstone.

Torres, G. (1990). Florence Nightingale. In J. B. George (Ed.), *Nursing theories: The base for professional nursing practice* (3rd ed., pp. 31-42). Englewood Cliffs, NJ: Appleton & Lange.

Veith, S. (1990). The recluse: A retrospective health history of Florence Nightingale. In V. L. Bullough, B. Bullough, & M. P. Stanton (Eds.), *Florence Nightingale and her era: A collection of new scholarship* (pp. 75-79). New York: Garland.

Vicinus, M., & Nergaard, B. (1990). *Ever yours, Florence Nightingale.* Cambridge, MA: Harvard University Press.

Walker, L. O., & Avant, K. C. (1988). *Strategies for theory construction in nursing* (2nd ed.). Englewood Cliffs, NJ: Appleton & Lange.

Widerquist, J. G. (1992). The spirituality of Florence Nightingale. *Nursing Research, 41*(1), 49-55.

Williams, G. (1987). *The age of miracles: Medicine and surgery in the nineteenth century.* Chicago: Academy Chicago Publishers.

Woodham-Smith, C. (1953). *Florence Nightingale, 1820-1910.* New York: Atheneum.

World Health Organization. (1947). [Health definition]. Geneva, Switzerland: Author.

Bibliography

Adams, E. C., & Foster, W. D. (1981). Heroine of modern progress. In R. G. Hebert (Ed.), *Florence Nightingale: Saint, reformer or rebel?* (pp. 102-107). Malabar, FL: Robert E. Krieger.

Agnew, L. R. C. (1958). Florence Nightingale: Statistician. *American Journal of Nursing, 58*(5), 664-665.

Allen, D. R. (1981). Florence Nightingale: Toward a psychohistorical interpretation. In R. G. Hebert (Ed.), *Florence Nightingale: Saint, reformer, or rebel?* (pp. 64-86). Malabar, FL: Robert E. Krieger.

American Nurses' Association. (1973). *Standards of nursing practice.* Kansas City, MO: Author.

Baly, M. E. (1988). *Florence Nightingale and the nursing legacy.* New York: Croom Helm.

Baly, M. E. (1990). Florence Nightingale and the establishment of the first school at St. Thomas's—Myth v. reality. In V. L. Bullough, B. Bullough, & M. P. Stanton (Eds.), *Florence Nightingale and her era: A collection of new scholarship* (pp. 3-22). New York: Garland.

Barritt, E. R. (1973). Florence Nightingale's values and modern nursing education. *Nursing Forum, 12*(1), 6-47.

Bishop, W. J., & Goldie, S. (1962). *A bio-bibliography of Florence Nightingale.* London: Dawsons of Pall Mall.

Bolster, E. (1964). *The sisters of mercy in the Crimean War.* Cork, Ireland: Mercier Press.

Brook, M. J. (1990). Some thoughts and reflections on the life of Florence Nightingale from a twentieth century perspective. In V. L. Bullough, B. Bullough, & M. P. Stanton (Eds.), *Florence Nightingale and her era: A collection of new scholarship* (pp. 153-167). New York: Garland.

Calabria, M. D. (1990, Summer). Spiritual insights of Florence Nightingale. *The Quest,* pp. 66-74.

Cohen, I. B. (1984). Florence Nightingale. *Scientific American, 3,* 128-137.

Cook, E. (1913). *The life of Florence Nightingale* (2 vols). London: Macmillan.

Cope, Z. (1958). *Florence Nightingale and the doctors.* London: Museum Press.

Dennis, K. E., & Prescott, P. P. (1985). Florence Nightingale: Yesterday, today and tomorrow. *Advances in Nursing Science, 1*(2), 66-81.

Dickens, C. (1986). *Martin Chuzzlewit.* Suffolk, UK: Richard Clay. (Original work published 1843)

Etzioni, A. (1969). *The semi-professions and their organization.* New York: Free Press.

Fawcett, J. (1984). *Analysis and evaluation of conceptual models of nursing.* Philadelphia: F. A. Davis.

Fitzpatrick, J., & Whall, A. (1983). *Conceptual models of nursing: Analysis and application.* Bowie, MD: Brady.

Fuld Health Trust. (1990). *The nurse theorists: Portraits of excellence. Florence Nightingale* (Part 1) [VHS videocassette]. Oakland, CA: Studio III.

Furukawa, C., & Howe, J. K. (1990). Virginia Henderson. In J. B. George (Ed.). *Nursing theories: The base for professional nursing practice* (3rd ed., pp. 61-78). Englewood Cliffs, NJ: Appleton & Lange.

Goldie, S. M. (1987). *I have done my duty: Florence Nightingale in the Crimean War, 1854-56.* Manchester, UK: Manchester University Press.

Grier, B., & Grier, M. (1978). Contributions of the passionate statistician. *Research in Nursing and Health, 1*(3), 103-109.

Henry, B., Woods, S., & Nagelkerk, J. (1990). Nightingale's perspective of nursing administration. *Nursing & Health Care, 11*(4), 201-206.

Huxley, E. (1975). *Florence Nightingale.* London: Weidenfeld & Nicholson.

Isler, C. (1981). Florence Nightingale: Rebel with a cause. In R. G. Hebert (Ed.), *Florence Nightingale: Saint, reformer or rebel?* (pp. 176-190). Malabar, FL: Robert E. Krieger.

Kalisch, P., & Kalisch, B. (1983a). Heroine out of focus: Media images of Florence Nightingale—Part I: Popular biographies and stage productions. *Nursing & Health Care,* No. 4, 181-187.

Kalisch, P., & Kalisch, B. (1983b). Heroine out of focus: Media images of Florence Nightingale—Part II: Film, radio, and television dramatizations. *Nursing & Health Care,* No. 5, 270-278.

Kalisch, P., & Kalisch, B. (1986). *The advance of American nursing* (2nd ed.). Boston: Little, Brown.

Keen, N. (1982). *Florence Nightingale.* Berby, UK: J. H. Hall.

Keith, J. M. (1988). Florence Nightingale: Statistician and consultant epidemiologist. *International Nursing Review, 35*(5), 147-150.

Kozier, B., Erb, G., & Olivieri, R. (1991). *Fundamentals of nursing: Concepts, process and practice* (4th ed.). Menlo Park, CA: Addison Wesley.

Monteiro, L. A. (1974). *Letters of Florence Nightingale.* Boston: Boston University Press.

Monteiro, L. A. (1985). Public health nursing then and now: Florence Nightingale on public health nursing. *American Journal of Public Health, 75*(2), 181-186.

Newton, M. (1949). *Florence Nightingale's philosophy of life and education.* Unpublished doctoral dissertation, Stanford University, CA.

Nightingale, F. (1852). *Cassandra.* London: Macmillan.

Nightingale, F. (1946). *Notes on nursing: What it is and is not.* London: Churchill Livingstone. (Original work published 1859)

Nightingale, F. (1949). Sick nursing and health nursing. In I. Hampton (Ed.), *Nursing of the sick, 1893* (pp. 24-43). New York: McGraw-Hill. (Original work published 1893)

Nightingale, F. (1954). Nursing the sick. In L. R. Seymer (Ed.), *Selected writings of Florence Nightingale* (pp. 319-352). New York: Macmillan. (Original work published 1882).

Palmer, I. S. (1977). Florence Nightingale: Reformer, reactionary, researcher. *Nursing Research, 26*(2), 84-89.

Palmer, I. S. (1981). Florence Nightingale and the international origins of modern nursing. *Image, 13,* 28-31.

Palmer, I. S. (1983a). Florence Nightingale and the first organized delivery of nursing services. *American Association of the Colleges of Nursing,* pp. 1-14.

Palmer, I. S. (1983b). Nightingale revisited. *Nursing Outlook, 31*(4), 229-233.

Palmer, I. S. (1983c, August 3). Florence Nightingale: The myth and the reality. *Nursing Times,* pp. 40-42.

Pickering, G. (1974). *Creative malady: Illness in the lives and minds of Charles Darwin, Florence Nightingale, Mary Baker Eddy, Sigmund Freud, Marcel Proust, and Elizabeth Barrett Browning.* London: Allen & Unwin.

Riehl-Sisca, J. (1989). *Conceptual models for nursing practice* (3rd ed.). Englewood Cliffs, NJ: Appleton & Lange.

Schultz, H. J. (1992). *British history* (4th ed.). New York: Harper-Perennial.

Seaman, L. C. B. (1956). *From Vienna to Versailles.* London: Coward-McCann.

Selanders, L. C. (1990). An American perspective of the Nightingale legacy. *Nursing Practice, 3*(3), 24-25.

Selanders, L. C. (1992). *An analysis of the utilization of power by Florence Nightingale, 1856-1872* (No. 9310445). Ann Arbor, MI: University Microfilms.

Shealy, M. C. (1985). Florence Nightingale, 1820-1910: An evolutionary mind in the context of holism. *Journal of Holistic Nursing, 3*(1), 4-5.

Showalter, E. (1981). Florence Nightingale's feminist complaint: Women, religion, and suggestions for thought. *Journal of Women in Culture and Society, 6*(3), 395-412.

Skeet, M. (1980). *Notes on nursing: The science and the art.* New York: Churchill Livingstone.

Strachey, L. (1988). *Eminent Victorians.* New York: Weidenfeld & Nicholson.

Torres, G. (1990). Florence Nightingale. In J. B. George (Ed.), *Nursing theories: The base for professional nursing practice* (pp. 31-42). Englewood Cliffs, NJ: Appleton & Lange.

Veith, S. (1990). The recluse: A retrospective health history of Florence Nightingale. In V. L. Bullough, B. Bullough, & M. P. Stanton (Eds.), *Florence Nightingale and her era: A collection of new scholarship* (pp. 75-79). New York: Garland.

Vicinus, M., & Nergaard, B. (1990). *Ever yours, Florence Nightingale.* Cambridge, MA: Harvard University Press.

Walker, L. O., & Avant, K. C. (1988). *Strategies for theory construction in nursing* (2nd ed.). Englewood Cliffs, NJ: Appleton & Lange.

Widerquist, J. G. (1992). The spirituality of Florence Nightingale. *Nursing Research,* *41*(1), 49-55.

Williams, G. (1987). *The age of miracles: Medicine and surgery in the nineteenth century.* Chicago: Academy Chicago Publishers.

Woodham-Smith, C. (1953). *Florence Nightingale, 1820-1910.* New York: Atheneum.

PART X

Hildegard E. Peplau
Interpersonal Nursing Theory

CHERYL FORCHUK

Biographical Sketch of the Nurse Theorist:
Hildegard E. Peplau, BA, MA, EdD

Born: September 1, 1909
Position: Professor Emerita, Rutgers University, New
    Brunswick, NJ
Registered Nurse: Pottstown, Pennsylvania Hospital School
    of Nursing
BA: (interpersonal psychology) Bennington College,
    Bennington, VT
MA: (teaching and supervision of psychiatric nursing)
    Teachers College, Columbia University, New York, NY
Ed.D: Teachers College, Columbia University, New York, NY
Fellow: American Academy of Nursing
Other: Honorary doctorates from University of Indianapolis,
    Rutgers University, Columbia University, Duke
    University, Boston College, and Alfred University and
    numerous other honors.

Foreword

Theory has become a compelling interest within the nursing profession since the mid-20th century. Many nurses have been focusing on theory, defining what it is, and discussing how it is produced, how it is tested clinically, and how it is generated by various nursing research methods. Since the 1950s several different theoretical frameworks have been published by nurses. These theories have spawned considerable discussions, comparisons, many conferences, publications, as well as major changes in nursing education curricula. Out of this ferment of ideas, a knowledge base called "nursing science" is evolving.

The knowledge that a profession uses in its work is the product of many scholars who research, refine, and build upon their own work and upon theories that their colleagues have published. This section is an illustrative example.

Cheryl Forchuk has devoted years of sustained study to the work that I have published. She has traced it to its roots, reviewed assessments of the work made by other scholars, and subjected the theoretical framework to critical analysis and to considerable research testing in clinical practice of psychiatric nursing. The substance of my published work is put forth in an updated, clearly organized form and in easily readable style. Forchuk has enriched the work by providing many illuminating examples of application in the current practice of nursing.

It is a distinct honor for me to have the remarkable intelligence and sustained effort of Cheryl Forchuk brought to bear upon my work, originally published four decades ago. I am very proud to have been a minor participant in the creative reordering as presented in this section.

The section portrays significant scholarship applied to a theoretical framework that has had a definitive impact on the practice of nursing. It also suggests a model of the kind of careful scrutiny that is central to the knowledge building trend currently in process within the nursing profession.

HILDEGARD E. PEPLAU
Professor Emerita
Rutgers University

Acknowledgment

The ongoing assistance and support of Hildegard Peplau is gratefully acknowledged.

I would also like to acknowledge the loving support from my husband, Gerry Smits; my children, Ian, Robin, and Callista; and my mother, Dorothy Forchuk.

55

Peplau's Theory: Origins

Peplau stated that she began her theory development in response to "the need in the late 1940s to develop 'advanced psychiatric nursing' for graduate programs in psychiatric nursing. The available nursing literature in psychiatric nursing at that time was not in any way adequate for graduate level, university-based psychiatric nursing education programs" (personal correspondence, December 23, 1990). Her original intent was not theory development but "only to convey to the nursing profession ideas [she] thought were important to improve practice" (personal correspondence, July 1989).

Peplau's first book, *Interpersonal Relations in Nursing,* was published in 1952 (Peplau, 1952a) and reissued in 1988 and 1991. That book outlined her conceptual framework for psychodynamic nursing. Peplau's conceptual framework signified the end of a long drought in the development of nursing theory; it was the first published nursing theory development since Nightingale.

Origins of the Theory

Peplau first studied interpersonal relations theory in the 1930s-1940s at Bennington College (personal correspondence, December 23, 1990). This interpersonal focus underpinned her later theory development.

Peplau, strongly influenced by the interpersonal development model of Harry Stack Sullivan (1952), incorporated his theory of personality development and the self system in her work. Peplau, like Sullivan, was also influenced by the early work of symbolic interactionists such as George Herbert Mead (1934). Examples of the influence of symbolic interactionism can be seen in the focus on social influences on personal development and with the idea that communication involves the use of symbols. Other influences include Rollo May's (1950) work on anxiety and the understanding of learning developed by Miller and Dollard (1941).

Peplau's 1952 work was grounded in interpersonal theory and the clinical experiences of herself and students. Peplau stated that "concepts emerged from practice—my own and supervisory review of graduate student nurses beginning in 1948—from actual nurse-patient relationship data" (personal correspondence, August 1989).

Since 1952, Peplau has been a prolific writer. She published a second book in 1964, dictated a series of 20 audiotapes to teach and communicate her theory, and has published more than 80 chapters and articles. Her work has endured over the years and is widely used in clinical practice. Sills (1978) reviewed several prominent nursing journals and found that references to Peplau's work had not only been sustained but actually had increased over the years.

Two recent Canadian surveys (Martin & Kirkpatrick, 1987, 1989) found that in a tertiary care psychiatric hospital, approximately two thirds of the nursing staff used Peplau's theory as a basis for their practice. Similarly, an American survey (Hirschmann, 1989) of mental health nurses in private practice found that approximately half were guided by Peplau's theory.

Although Peplau's theory has been most frequently used by psychiatric or mental health nurses, Peplau believed that psychodynamic nursing transcended all clinical nursing specialties and that all nursing is based on the interpersonal process and relationship that develops between the nurse and client.

56

Assumptions, Concepts, and Propositions of Peplau's Theory

Assumptions are basic beliefs within a given theory that are accepted as true. One must accept the given assumptions of a theory in order to adopt it. The concepts are the major components or building blocks of the theory. Propositions describe the relations among concepts.

Assumptions of the Theory

In Peplau's (1952a) book she identified two "guiding assumptions" that were underpinnings to her framework:

1. The kind of nurse each person becomes makes a substantial difference in what each client will learn as she or he is nursed throughout her or his experience with illness (p. xi).
2. Fostering personality development in the direction of maturity is a function of nursing and nursing education; it requires the use of principles and methods that permit and guide the process of grappling with everyday interpersonal problems or difficulties (p. xi).

Peplau (1989d; personal correspondence, December 1990) also stated as assumptions the following:

3. Nursing can take as its unique focus the reactions of clients to the circumstances of their illnesses or health problems (1989d, p. 28).

4. Because illness provides an opportunity for learning and growth, nursing can assist clients to gain intellectual and interpersonal competencies beyond those that they have at the point of illness by gearing nursing practices to evolving such competencies through nurse-client interactions (1989d, p. 28). Peplau references Gregg (1954) and Mereness (1966) in the development of this fourth assumption.

Additional implicit and explicit assumptions were identified by Forchuk (1991c)[1] (all cited pages are from Peplau, 1952a):

5. Psychodynamic nursing crosses all specialty areas of nursing. It is not synonymous with psychiatric nursing since every nurse-client relationship is an interpersonal situation in which recurring difficulties of everyday life arise (summarized from Peplau's "Introduction").

6. Difficulties in interpersonal relations recur in varying intensities throughout the life of everyone (p. xiv).

7. The need to harness energy that derives from tension and anxiety connected to felt needs to positive means for defining, understanding, and meeting productively the problem at hand is a universal need (p. 26).

8. All human behavior is purposeful and goal-seeking in terms of feelings of satisfaction and/or security (p. 86).

9. The interaction of nurse and client is fruitful when a method of communication that identifies and uses common meanings is at work in the situation (p. 284).

10. The meaning of behavior to the client is the only relevant basis on which nurses can determine needs to be met (p. 226).

11. Each person will behave, during any crisis, in a way that has worked in relation to crises faced in the past (p. 255).

Concepts of the Theory

Peplau's theory focuses on the interpersonal processes and therapeutic relationship that develops between the nurse and client. Figure 56.1 depicts the major concepts of Peplau's theory within this interpersonal perspective.

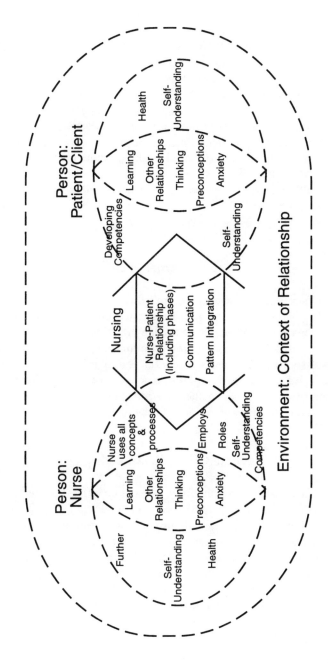

Figure 56.1. Peplau's framework: Major concepts and their interrelationships.

467

The metaparadigm, or core concepts, of nursing includes nursing, person, environment, and health. Peplau's theory defines the concepts of the metaparadigm in the following way:

1. *Nursing* is an educative instrument, a maturing force, that aims to promote health (Peplau, 1952a).
2. *Person* is an individual, developed through interpersonal relationships, that lives in an unstable environment (Peplau, 1952a).
3. *Environment* is physiological, psychological, and social fluidity that may be illness-maintaining or health-promoting (Peplau, 1952a, p. 82, 1973c, 1987a).
4. *Health* is forward movement of personality and other ongoing human processes in the direction of creative and constructive personal and community living (Peplau, 1952a).

Interpersonal Focus

The interpersonal focus of Peplau's theory requires that the nurse attend to the interpersonal processes that occur between nurse and client. This is in sharp contrast to many nursing theories that focus on the client as the unit of attention. Although individual client factors are assessed, the nurse also self-reflects. The focus is the interpersonal process and relationships, not the constituent parts (or individuals). Interpersonal processes include the nurse-client relationship, communication, pattern integration, and the roles of the nurse.

Nurse-Client Relationship

Peplau's interpersonal theory of nursing identifies the therapeutic nurse-client relationship as the crux of nursing. The nurse-client relationship evolves through identifiable, overlapping phases, which include orientation, working, and resolution. The relationship form (see Figure 56.2), developed by Forchuk et al. (1986) and tested by Forchuk and Brown (1989), gives a pictorial overview of the nurse and client behaviors at each phase. The reliability and validity of the form was reported in Forchuk and Brown (1989).

The initial phase of the nurse-client relationship is the orientation phase where the nurse and client come to know each other as persons

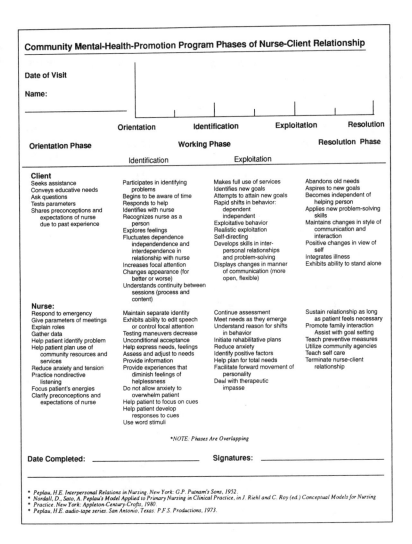

Community Mental-Health-Promotion Program Phases of Nurse-Client Relationship

Date of Visit

Name:

| Orientation | Identification | Exploitation | Resolution |

| Orientation Phase | Working Phase | | Resolution Phase |
| | Identification | Exploitation | |

Client

Seeks assistance	Participates in identifying problems	Makes full use of services	Abandons old needs
Conveys educative needs	Begins to be aware of time	Identifies new goals	Aspires to new goals
Ask questions	Responds to help	Attempts to attain new goals	Becomes independent of helping person
Tests parameters	Identifies with nurse	Rapid shifts in behavior:	Applies new problem-solving skills
Shares preconceptions and expectations of nurse due to past experience	Recognizes nurse as a person	dependent independent	Maintains changes in style of communication and interaction
	Explores feelings	Exploitative behavior	Positive changes in view of self
	Fluctuates dependence independence and interdependence in relationship with nurse	Realistic exploitation Self-directing Develops skills in interpersonal relationships and problem-solving	Integrates illness Exhibits ability to stand alone
	Increases focal attention	Displays changes in manner of communication (more open, flexible)	
	Changes appearance (for better or worse)		
	Understands continuity between sessions (process and content)		

Nurse:

Respond to emergency	Maintain separate identity	Continue assessment	Sustain relationship as long as patient feels necessary
Give parameters of meetings	Exhibits ability to edit speech or control focal attention	Meet needs as they emerge	Promote family interaction
Explain roles	Testing maneuvers decrease	Understand reason for shifts in behavior	Assist with goal setting
Gather data	Unconditional acceptance	Initiate rehabilitative plans	Teach preventive measures
Help patient identify problem	Help express needs, feelings	Reduce anxiety	Utilize community agencies
Help patient plan use of community resources and services	Assess and adjust to needs	Identify positive factors	Teach self care
Reduce anxiety and tension	Provide information	Help plan for total needs	Terminate nurse-client relationship
Practice nondirective listening	Provide experiences that diminish feelings of helplessness	Facilitate forward movement of personality	
Focus patient's energies	Do not allow anxiety to overwhelm patient	Deal with therapeutic impasse	
Clarify preconceptions and expectations of nurse	Help patient to focus on cues		
	Help patient develop responses to cues		
	Use word stimuli		

NOTE: Phases Are Overlapping

Date Completed: _____   Signatures: _____

* Peplau, H.E. Interpersonal Relations in Nursing. New York: G.P. Putnam's Sons, 1952.
* Nordall, D., Sato, A. Peplau's Model Applied to Primary Nursing in Clinical Practice, in J. Riehl and C. Roy (ed.) Conceptual Models for Nursing Practice. New York: Appleton-Century-Crofts, 1980.
* Peplau, H.E. audio-tape series. San Antonio, Texas: P.F.S. Productions, 1973.

Figure 56.2. Relationship Form.
SOURCE: Reprinted with permission from Forchuk and Brown (1989, p. 32).

and the client begins to trust the nurse. The time in the orientation phase can vary from a few minutes of the initial meeting to months of regular sessions.

The second phase of the nurse-client relationship, the working phase, is subdivided into identification and exploitation subphases. In the identification subphase the client begins to identify problems to be worked on within the relationship. The nature of the problems identified can be as diverse as the scope of nursing practice. Examples are identifying inadequate pain management, requests for health teaching regarding breast-feeding, or wanting to discuss unresolved issues related to past sexual abuse. The exploitation subphase occurs as the client makes use of the services of the nurse to work through the identified problems. Often, as initial problems are worked through, further problems are identified by the client.

The nurse does not "solve" the client's problems but, rather, gives the client the opportunity to explore options and possibilities within the context of the relationship. For example, the nurse may provide information on community resources or provide health teaching related to medication, illness, or health promotion if appropriate in the context of the relationship. However, the nurse employing Peplau's theory would resist all temptation related to "advice giving" because this would undermine the roles and responsibilities of the client.

The resolution phase of the relationship occurs between the time the actual problems are resolved and the relationship is terminated. Examples of work that may need to be done in this period are connecting the client to community resources, working through dependency issues in the relationship, learning preventative measures, strengthening social supports, and summarizing the work completed.

The nurse-client relationship does not evolve as a simple linear process. Although the relationship may be predominantly in one phase, reflections of all phases can be seen in each interaction. Every interaction has a beginning (orientation), middle (working), and end (resolution) that reflect the larger pattern of the ongoing nurse-client relationship.

Communication

Communication includes both verbal communication and nonverbal communication. Verbal communication is expressed through language, whereas nonverbal communication is expressed through empathic linkages, gestures, postures, and patterns.

Verbal communication, or language, is important as a reflection of thought processes. This is obvious on the literal content level: For example, the client gives information on pain, on current abilities, or on perceptions of problems. However, in addition to the literal content, there are symbolic meanings, patterns, and underlying assumptions that can be conveyed through the choice of words or phrases. Consider the differences among the following statements: "I have a chronic migraine headache problem and it appears to be starting to flare up," "My head is killing me," and "I'm getting a headache." Different information is conveyed regarding ownership of the headache, possible intellectualizing, and degree of distress. However, one would not make immediate assumptions but, rather, be attentive to emerging patterns and validate these with the client (or better yet encourage the client to note the patterns and validate these with the nurse).

Peplau (1989a) considers the use of verbal communication an essential component of the nurse-client relationship. She states, "The general principle is that anything clients act out with nurses will most probably not be talked about, and that which is not discussed cannot be understood" (p. 197). Talking about issues and concerns gives the client an alternative to acting out these issues.

Peplau (1973d) has described common patterns of word usage that may require corrective action on the part of the nurse, such as the following:

1. Overgeneralization—For example, the client says, "The worst things always happen to me." The nurse would attempt to help the client be more specific by asking for one incident.
2. Inappropriate use of pronouns—A paranoid client may insist "they" are out to get him, and the nurse asks, "Who are they?"
3. The suggestion of automatic knowing through repetition of the phrase "you know"—The nurse conveys the information that "I only know what you tell me about it" and drops such phrases from his or her own language.

This corrective use of language is similar to approaches suggested by cognitive therapists such as Aaron Beck (1976) and Albert Ellis (1962). One difference is that cognitive therapy assumes one is directly changing the thought. Peplau believes one is changing the language, but because thought and language are part of an integral whole, a change in one is reflected in the other.

Nonverbal language is more subtle than verbal language and may at times contradict the verbal message. Consider the example of the person who screams "I am not upset!" In such cases, it is the nonverbal message that tends to be believed. Congruence is an important consideration for the nurse to monitor in his or her own communication. Empathy and caring can be transmitted on a nonverbal level as can feelings such as indifference or hostility.

Most nonverbal communication is culturally influenced, so one must be cautious in transcultural interpretation and use of gestures. For example, does avoiding eye contact suggest dishonesty, shyness, or respect? It can depend on the cultural orientations of the sender and receiver of the message.

A personal example that exemplifies the need for awareness of cultural differences occurred in the author's work with a native Indian client. I had concerns about how the sessions were progressing. The client stated he felt things were going well. I could not identify what it was that was bothering me but thought the problem might be culturally related. The client and I had one session videotaped to be viewed by a cultural anthropologist. The client and I viewed the videotape with the anthropologist and we all noticed the almost comical "dance of the eyes." He was attempting to avoid eye contact as I was attempting to maintain it. We discussed our different interpretations of eye contact (he avoided eye contact in deference to authority and out of respect; I was trying to maintain our open communication through eye contact). We agreed to not impose our rules on each other. However, the client noted that every time he went for a promotion interview he was unsuccessful and that the feedback I had given prior to the tape about "something not seeming quite right" was similar to the feedback he received after the interviews. He decided to use eye contact in job interview/promotion situations. Although I believe his success reflected more than a change in eye contact, that client was convinced that the two promotions he received in the next year were related to his new awareness of this difference in communication. This situation also exemplifies how learning in the nurse-client relationship can be used in other relationships and that both nurse and client learn and grow in the therapeutic relationship.

Similar examples of nonverbal communications that can be interpreted very differently by different people are touching, hugging, smiling, passing flatulence, hand movements, comfortable social distances, crossing legs, gestures, offering food, and gift giving. These can have vastly different cultural meanings to different groups and individuals. Therefore, the nurse needs to be aware of issues related to differences in interpretation of nonverbal communication when providing care to a client from a different cultural group. The nurse, through self-reflection and clinical supervision, also needs to be aware of his or her own personal and cultural nonverbal patterns that might, at times, interfere with the evolving nurse-client relationship.

Pattern Integration

Each individual and each system have customary patterns of interacting with others. Pattern integrations are the products of the interaction of the patterns of more than one individual or system. Peplau (1973c, 1987a) has identified four common pattern integrations: complementary, mutual, antagonistic, and mixed.

A *complementary* pattern integration involves patterns that are different yet fit together like parts of a jigsaw puzzle. The "fit" assists in ensuring the continuity of the single patterns that make up the integration. An example of this integration can be found with the nurse who insists on "helping" clients by doing things they could actually do for themselves. This could range from cutting their meat at dinner to arranging an outpatient appointment. A complementary pattern occurs when this nurse works with a dependent client who prefers that others make all possible decisions. The nurse and client will form a comfortable partnership that will make it difficult for either to change. A similar integration could be perpetuated on a larger systems level if this dyad worked in the context of a hospital that emphasized the accountability of the nurse but not the accountability or involvement in decision making of the client. Similar examples of complementary pattern integrations are anger-withdrawal, domination-submission, and belittling others-belittling self.

A *mutual* pattern integration occurs when two or more interacting individuals/systems display a similar pattern. The multiple use of a single pattern also assists in the continuity of each similar pattern. A classic example from the nursing literature is the mutual-withdrawal pattern first identified by Tudor (1956/1970) as occurring between specific clients and staff on an inpatient psychiatric unit. Unfortunately, examples of this mutual pattern can still be found across nursing specialties: consider the placement of selected, less desirable, medical or surgical patients as far away from the nursing station as possible, or the early discharge of some community clients who give the impression they are not interested in interacting with the nurse, despite their ongoing personal health problems.

Additional examples of mutual pattern integrations are mutual anger, mutual disrespect, and mutual self-denigration. Positive examples could include mutual respect or mutual concern. It is important to consider that the nurse should employ mutual pattern integrations only with those patterns that the nurse and client would want to perpetuate.

Antagonistic pattern integrations include the combination of different individual patterns that do not fit well together. The combination, therefore, creates a discomfort or disharmony that can be used as a motivation toward change. An example given by Peplau (1973c) is that of a client with an angry pattern with a nurse who is using an investigative approach ("Tell me about what's going on") rather than responding with a complementary (e.g., withdrawal) or mutual (e.g., also responding in anger) pattern. Obviously, this is the ideal integration for patterns that require change.

The antagonistic pattern can also occur at an individual or larger systems level. An example of an antagonistic pattern at the larger systems level could occur with a client who feels most comfortable being dependent and letting others "take care" of him or her. An antagonistic pattern would emerge if this client was in a therapeutic environment that encouraged the participation and decision making of all individuals. It would become uncomfortable for the client to maintain dependent behaviors.

An even broader systems example of an antagonistic pattern would be the introduction of a nursing care delivery system that emphasizes the accountability of each nurse (e.g., primary nursing) into a traditional paternalistic hospital system that emphasizes centralized decision making rather than decision making and accountability at the staff level. Thus the nursing care delivery system would create an antagonistic pattern with the larger hospital system. If change is desired, it would be beneficial for the antagonistic pattern integration to occur as frequently as possible and at a variety of personal and larger systems levels.

Other examples of antagonistic pattern integrations are withdrawal-seeking out, dependance-promoting independence, and self-denigration-acceptance of self and others. It needs to be remembered that the inherent incongruence of antagonistic pattern integrations is anxiety producing. The resultant anxiety needs to be harnessed and channeled toward change. However, the anxiety also requires careful monitoring so that it does not become overwhelming. This issue is more fully discussed under the concept of anxiety.

Peplau (1987a) has also identified *mixed* or changing pattern integrations. These include a combination of the earlier identified pattern integrations. For example, a person may respond to another's anger by first getting angry (reflecting a mutual pattern integration) and then withdrawing (reflecting a complementary pattern). Mutual-complementary combinations continue to reinforce individual patterns. Antagonistic pattern integration used in combination with a mutual or complementary integration will lose effectiveness in promoting change because individuals are more likely to respond to patterns that reinforce familiar and comfortable personal patterns.

Roles of the Nurse

The nurse may enact several roles with the client. The roles depend on the needs of the client and the skills and creativity of the nurse. The possible roles will also be influenced by the nurse's position and agency policies. For example, a community nurse in a case management program may include a role related to cutting through red tape (the form filler role?) to ensure that appropriate services are in place for the client. A clinical nurse specialist may include roles that allow the nurse to transcend institutional or agency boundaries. An example is following a client through different hospital and community settings. On the other hand, a staff nurse working a set shift may find more limitations to the type of roles he or she can offer to the client. The nurse needs to be aware of the possibilities and constraints so that accurate information can be conveyed to the client.

Peplau's (1952a) book contains the following examples of roles: stranger, resource person, teacher, leader, surrogate for significant others, counselor, arbitrator, change agent, researcher, and technical expert. Regardless of other roles assumed, the nurse and client always begin the relationship as strangers to each other.

In her 1964 book, Peplau emphasized the importance of the counselor role and stated that this was the primary role to be undertaken by nurses in psychiatric-mental health nursing. Traditionally, psychiatric nurses had focused on surrogate roles, particularly parent surrogate roles, and the result was custodial care that minimized the potential for growth and change. Peplau (1964) stated, "If [nurses] are unable to contribute in a truly corrective manner to the care of mental patients, the traditional nurse-patient relationship will be usurped by those who can; and nurses will be shunted into the role of glorified custodian or superclerk" (p. 7).

The counselor role must be valued as the prime vehicle for the development of the nurse-client relationship. Frequently, this involves individual counseling. Other modes, such as group work, community development, and family systems nursing, are also appropriate. Within these modalities, the group, community, or family would be the "client" rather than the individual constituent members. As in the example of the individual as client, the nurse-client relationship would develop in phases, and the concepts of communication (both verbal and nonverbal), pattern integrations, and roles of the nurse would also be applicable.

Intrapersonal Processes

Although the primary focus within Peplau's theory is on *inter*personal processes, *intra*personal processes of both the client and nurse are also considered. Intrapersonal processes are those that occur within the person rather than between people. There is a strong interrelationship between interpersonal and intrapersonal phenomena: Intrapersonal structures, processes, and changes develop through interpersonal activity. Examples of intrapersonal concepts within Peplau's theory include anxiety, learning, thinking, and competencies. Although each of these is observed on an individual level, these concepts have interpersonal implications.

Anxiety

Anxiety is an energy that emerges in response to a perceived threat. The threat could range from the physical to the metaphysical. Peplau

(1989a) described the sequence of steps in the development of anxiety as holding expectations, expectations not met, discomfort felt, relief behaviors used, and relief behaviors justified (p. 281). The expectations can include things such as beliefs, needs, goals, wishes, and feelings. The relief behaviors also cover a wide range of possibilities: aggression, withdrawal, compulsive behavior, psychosomatic complaints, hallucinations, delusions, sexual activity, risk taking, denial, intellectualizing, drug use, humor, self-reflection, discussion with others, validation, and problem solving to seek the sources of difficulty. Only a few of the relief behaviors can be used.

People (not just clients) generally develop patterns of relief behaviors that they tend to use over and over again. Obviously, some of these patterns are more helpful than others. Anxiety is often a basis for the client to seek assistance from the nurse. At times, problems created through these relief behaviors bring the client to seek the services of the nurse. At other times, the client seeks assistance because he or she finds the relief behaviors inadequate in relieving the anxiety.

Peplau (1989a) describes how the nurse can assist the client to channel anxiety productively. First, the client needs to be aware of and be able to name the anxiety. Then, the client needs to see the connection between the anxiety and the relief behavior. Finally, the client formulates and states expectations. This final part of the process includes an understanding of the connection between held expectations and what actually happened and consideration of factors amenable to control (p. 282). Working through this process usually takes place over time and during several interactions. I have had some experiences with chronic mental health clients where it has taken months for the client to even be aware of and to name the anxiety.

Anxiety has been described by Peplau as existing along a continuum including mild, moderate, severe, and panic. Although it is possible to experience a state of no anxiety (euphoria), this seldom occurs. As human beings we constantly face a barrage of information and other stimuli that pose at least some minor threat to our self-views. Therefore, in most nurse-client encounters, both the nurse and client will be experiencing some anxiety.

As a person's anxiety increases, that person's focus of attention becomes increasingly narrow. At the lower end of the anxiety continuum, this may actually be useful in assisting the person to focus on important details. A common example would be writing an exam without being aware of other people or distractions in the room.

However, at higher levels of anxiety, the focus of attention may become so narrow that the individual only sees small details without being able to see the larger picture. A similar example would be the student who becomes so concerned about one exam item that the allotted time is spent on that item and the exam is not completed. For similar reasons, problem solving may be enhanced at lower levels of anxiety but inhibited as anxiety increases. The nurse and client need to monitor anxiety levels and attempt to keep the levels at the mild to moderate levels.

Peplau (1973a) describes how the nursing approach must take into consideration the current anxiety level of the client. For example, as the client's anxiety is increased, the nurse would need to use increasingly short, concrete sentences so as to be understood. At the severe or panic levels, it would be inappropriate to use sentences with more than two or three words. It may be that even these short sentences will not be understood by the client in panic, and the nurse will need to use presence as a simple nonverbal communication. The nurse also needs to be aware of the impact of anxiety on the client's current problem-solving abilities and learning abilities and adjust accordingly. Generally, at severe or panic levels of anxiety no new learning can take place.

Anxiety can be transmitted interpersonally (Peplau, 1989a). It is for this reason that the nurse needs to monitor his or her own anxiety. The anxious nurse will communicate the anxiety to the client and vice versa. A common situation where this can occur is when the client feels out of control and the nurse fears a physical threat. This situation can easily escalate to a self-fulfilling prophecy (i.e., the client loses control and becomes assaultive). Such situations can more easily be prevented by intervening with the anxiety at lower levels and not allowing one's own anxiety to escalate the situation.

Learning

Peplau has described eight stages in the learning process: (a) to observe, (b) to describe, (c) to analyze, (d) to formulate, (e) to validate, (f) to test, (g) to integrate, and (h) to use (Peplau, 1971b). Each stage in the learning process is also a competency. Therefore, as one's learning increases so do one's competencies.

Different individuals will be at different competency levels within the stages of learning. Even within one individual a wide degree of variation is possible. For example, a person with generally high learning abilities may have a dramatic drop in such abilities when faced with a high anxiety-producing situation.

It is important that the nurse determine the current stage of learning of the client so that appropriate comments can be made to build on the current level and to assist the client to move to the next level. For example, if the client is at the very basic level of only being able to observe but unable to share the observations, the nurse would ask simple questions related to observation. Peplau (1971b) gives examples of basic questions as "What do you see?" and "What is that noise?" As the person responds to these questions, he or she begins movement to the next stage—to describe.

There is an assumption that all people will at least be able to observe on some level, even if they cannot respond. For example, even with a comatose client the nurse could use the assumption of the ability to observe. The nurse in this situation may say "I am now going to wash your face" and recognize the client's ability for some level of observation.

Forchuk and Voorberg (1991), in a program evaluation of a community mental health program based on Peplau's theory, found that clients were able to increase their current stage of learning. For example, upon admission, 60% of the clients with chronic mental illnesses were at the first stage of learning. Only 20% remained at this level after 2 years.

Thinking: Preconceptions and Self-Understanding

Thinking is an internal cognitive process. The thoughts of another person can only be inferred through observation of language and behavior. The concept of thinking may be particularly important for the nurse working with clients experiencing difficulty with their thinking processes. Examples are clients with thought disorders related to chronic mental illnesses such as schizophrenia, clients with developmental handicaps, and clients with organic brain disorders or brain injuries. The section on communication describes both the integral relationship between thought and language and appropriate approaches to assist clients with their thinking through the use of language.

Specific thinking processes of both the nurse and client will affect the evolving nurse-client relationship. These include the preconcep-

tions the nurse and client have of each other and the self-understanding of the nurse and client.

Preconceptions are the initial impressions the nurse and client have
of each other before they know each other. The preconceptions may
be formed through stereotyping, gossip, or past experiences with
persons considered to be similar to the partner in the new dyad.
Forchuk (1992a) found that both the nurses' and clients' preconceptions of each other were highly predictive of progress in the evolving
therapeutic relationship. She also found that these initial impressions
were quite stable, with very little change over the first 6 months of
the relationship. This study underlined the importance of consideration of both nurse and client factors. The nurse needs to be aware of
preconceptions of the client, particularly negative impressions that
may impede progress in the relationship. Similarly, client impressions
should also be explored. If negative preconceptions cannot be worked
through, a therapeutic transfer of the client to another nurse should
be considered.

Self-understanding is also a specific thinking pattern that may
influence the evolving relationship. However, within Peplau's theory,
the concept of self-understanding has an unequal importance for the
nurse and client. Self-understanding is considered to be a critical
attribute of the nurse. Through self-reflection and supervision, the
nurse needs to be constantly aware of how her or his own issues and
behaviors are influencing the relationship. It is expected that the
nurse's self-understanding will grow through therapeutic work with
clients.

Clients may also experience an increase in self-understanding
through the therapeutic relationship. However, an increase in interpersonal and problem-solving competencies is the client-related goal
of the relationship rather than self-understanding. Self-understanding is a helpful side effect of the process of developing these
competencies.

Competencies

Competencies are skills that have evolved through practice. Peplau
(1973b) states that we all have numerous interpersonal and problem-
solving capacities, but to become competencies, these must be developed over time and through practice. The nurse-client relationship

provides a venue for the development of capacities into competencies. For example, learning to share selected experiences verbally may be a capacity that the client has not developed; it may be developed during the time spent with the nurse. Other examples of competencies/capacities are sitting for 5 minutes in the presence of another person, discussing one topic for 5 minutes, learning to trust, describing one's feelings to another person, identifying personal goals, and choosing a strategy to move toward a specific goal. From these examples it can be seen that there are a wide variety of competencies and that which ones develop will vary considerably with different client situations. The specific competencies evolve through the developing relationship.

It is expected that the nurse will also develop competencies through the evolving relationship. These would also be primarily of a problem-solving or interpersonal nature. For example, the nurse may learn how a specific person copes with hallucinations, may learn to remain silent for longer periods of time to allow the client the opportunity to initiate conversation, or may develop increased empathy for a certain life situation. As the nurse's competencies grow, so does his or her ability to help other people in similar situations. However, it is the client's development of competencies, not the nurse's, that is the priority. Parallel to the nurse's development of self-understanding, the nurse's competencies develop as a beneficial side effect of the therapeutic relationship. The client's competencies develop as a goal of the therapeutic relationship.

Although the idea that the client's competencies take priority may seem obvious, it is sometimes forgotten in practice. It often appears more expedient for the nurse to complete an activity (e.g., feeding, making a bed, setting an outpatient appointment, listing alternatives, searching out community resources, summarizing progress) rather than the client. Of course, if this occurs, the nurse develops the competency rather than the client.

Clinical Phenomena

Peplau encourages nurses to be aware of patterns with clinical phenomena. Observing patterns in the development and resolution of specific clinical issues allows learning from one clinical situation to potentially assist in others. This in no way negates the uniqueness of each situation and each client. It recognizes that each person and situation, although unique, can reveal aspects of a larger pattern.

Examples of clinical concepts that Peplau has explored are loneliness and hallucinations. Concepts are defined and operationalized with the identification of critical attributes. This would include the observable behaviors associated with the clinical phenomena. For example, observable signs that a person is having auditory hallucinations might include talking to an unobserved person and describing hearing voices in one's head. The nurse could identify a client with such behavior as having a pattern consistent with auditory hallucinations. Such behaviors may also be consistent with other patterns—for example, the pattern of a peak religious experience. In this section, the clinical concepts of loneliness and hallucinations are briefly described as examples of clinical phenomena.

Loneliness

Peplau (1989c) describes the problem of loneliness. She defines this as "an unnoticed inability to do anything while alone" (p. 256). This is contrasted with lonesomeness (a wish to be with others) and aloneness (being without company). She describes the development of loneliness through difficult early interpersonal relationships.

Peplau (1989c) describes the importance of the nurse being aware of clients' defenses of loneliness; examples include time-oriented complaints (endless days), relating to others in an overly familiar or anonymous manner, planlessness, or overplanning.

The nurse assists the client with loneliness through the establishment of a therapeutic relationship, which will include contact and limit setting. Where appropriate, the nurse and client also plan for potentially positive peer relationships.

Hallucinations

Peplau (1989a) defines hallucinations as consisting of "illusory figures, perceived *as if* they were real" (p. 312). Peplau describes the phases through which hallucinations develop in an attempt to avoid anxiety and mitigate loneliness.

The nurse needs to be aware that the experience of hallucinations seems very real to the client. The nurse will carefully use language that does not reinforce the existence of the hallucinations as being a mutually experienced reality. For example, the nurse might say, "What do the voices you are hearing say?" Peplau (1989a) states that the client needs to learn alternative ways of coping with anxiety and loneliness so that the hallucinations are not needed (pp. 319-324).

In summary, Peplau has identified a wide range of concepts that impact on the practice of the nurse and the evolving nurse-client relationship. These include interpersonal factors, intrapersonal factors, and specific clinical phenomena.

Propositions

Relations between major concepts in Peplau's theory are summarized in Table 56.1, which was originally published in Forchuk (1991c). From this table it can be seen that the concepts are all interrelated, and that a change in one concept generally is reflected by further changes of other concepts. Most critically, the evolving nurse-client relationship moves the client through growth and therefore health.

Note

1. Reprinted with permission of Chestnut House Publications. Copyright 1991.

TABLE 56.1 Concepts and Relations

	NURSING *is related to:*	PERSON *is related to:*	HEALTH *is related to:*	ENVIRONMENT *is related to:*	INTERPERSONAL RELATIONSHIPS (I.P.R.s) *are related to:*
PERSON	Nursing is a process between persons (nurse and patient).				
HEALTH	Health is the goal of nursing.	Health is within the person.			
ENVIRONMENT	Environment provides the context of nursing.	The person is within the environment.	Health is within the person, who in turn is within the environment. The environment can be health promoting or illness maintaining.		
INTERPERSONAL RELATIONSHIPS (I.P.R.s)	I.P.R.s are the crux or essential processes of nursing (critical attribute).	I.P.R.s are participated in by persons.	I.P.R.s contribute to a person's health (antecedent) and a person's health will in turn influence ongoing I.P.R.s (consequence).	The environment forms the context of I.P.R.s (critical attribute).	
COMMUNICATION	Communication occurs in nursing (critical attribute).	Communication occurs between persons.	Communication facilitates health, by contributing to I.P.R.s (intervening).	Communication occurs within the context of the environment, and is part of the environment.	Communication occurs within interpersonal relationships (critical attribute).
PATTERN INTEGRATION	Pattern integrations occur in nursing (critical attribute).	Pattern integration occurs between persons.	Pattern integrations can facilitate health, by contributing to ongoing I.P.R.s (intervening).	Pattern integrations are a part of the environment (critical attribute).	Pattern integrations occur within Interpersonal relationships (critical attribute).

ROLES	Roles are the means for conducting nursing.	Roles are used by the nurse to promote health within the patient.	Roles are used by the nurse to promote health.	Roles are used in the context of the environment.	Roles are used within interpersonal relationships (critical attribute).
THINKING	Thinking occurs in nursing as a prerequisite and critical attribute.	Thinking occurs within persons (critical attribute).	Self-understanding can promote health. Preconceptions can impede or promote health depending on their impact on interpersonal relationships (intervening).	Thinking is a within-person phenomenon occuring in context of the person within the environment.	Self-understanding can promote I.P.R.s. Preconceptions can promote or hinder I.P.R.s and vice versa.
LEARNING	Learning occurs in nursing as a consequence.	Learning occurs within persons (critical attribute).	Learning promotes health.	Learning is a within-person phenomenon occuring in the context of the person within the environment.	Learning occurs within the context of I.P.R.s. The interactions between learning and I.P.R.s can enhance or hinder each other.
COMPETENCIES	Competencies develop as a consequence of nursing (intermediate to promoting health).	Competencies develop within persons.	The development of competencies promotes health.	Competencies are a within-person phenomenon occuring in the context of the person within the environment.	Competencies occur within the context of I.P.R.s and can assist in the development of I.P.R.s.
ANXIETY	Anxiety occurs in nursing (critical attribute).	Anxiety occurs within and between persons (critical attribute).	Anxiety impedes health at severe or panic levels.	Anxiety is a within-person phenomenon occuring in the context of the person within the environment.	Anxiety impedes the developmet of relationships at severe or panic levels.

(continued)

485

TABLE 56.1 (Continued)

	COMMUNICATION is related to:	PATTERN INTEGRATION is related to:	ROLES are related to:	THINKING is related to:	LEARNING is related to:	COMPETENCIES are related to:
PERSON						
HEALTH						
ENVIRONMENT						
INTERPERSONAL RELATIONSHIPS (I.P.R.s)						
COMMUNICATION						
PATTERN INTEGRATION	Pattern Integration and communication occur together in interpersonal relationships.					
ROLES	Roles require communication (prerequisite).	Roles are used by the nurse as part of the pattern integration.				

THINKING	Thinking is mediated through symbols (language). Changes in verbal communication reflect changes in thinking and vice versa.	Thinking occurs within the person and therefore indirectly interacts with pattern integration.	Thinking is required by the nurse in the selection and maintenance of appropriate roles.			
LEARNING	Communication promotes learning, and learning can then promote future communication.	Learning occurs within the person and therefore indirectly interacts with pattern integration.	Learning occurs with successful implementation of nurse roles, particularly the counselor and teacher roles.	Thinking is a prerequisite for learning, and learning, in turn, assists thinking.		
COMPETENCIES	Communication promotes the development of competencies.	Competencies occur within the person and therefore indirectly interact with pattern integration.	Competencies are developed through successful implementation of nurse roles, particularly the couselor and teacher roles.	Competencies are both a prerequesite for thinking, and further developed through thinking.	Competencies are learned by developing skills and capacities.	
ANXIETY	Anxiety impedes communication at severe or panic levels.	Anxiety occurs in the person and therefore indirectly interacts with pattern integration.	Anxiety at severe or panic levels will limit the appropriate roles to be used.	Anxiety impedes thinking when at severe or panic levels.	Anxiety impedes thinking when at severe or panic levels.	Anxiety at severe or panic levels impedes the development of competencies.

SOURCE: Reprinted with permission from "Peplau's Theory: Concepts and Their Relations," by C. Forchuk, 1991c, *Nursing Science Quarterly, 4*(2), 54-60.

57

Application to
Practice and Research

Peplau's theory can be used to guide both practice and research. Surveys of psychiatric nurses in both Canada (Martin & Kirkpatrick, 1987, 1989) and the United States (Hirschmann, 1989) found at least half of the sample used Peplau's theory as a basis for practice. As well, Peplau's theory has been the basis of both quantitative research (e.g., Forchuk, 1992a, 1992b) and qualitative research (e.g., Choiniere, 1991; Forchuk et al., in progress).

Peplau's Theory in Practice

Peplau's theory can be used to guide the nurse in the various aspects of practice. It will be reflected in the focus of the assessment, the planned strategies, and the criteria used to evaluate the nursing care.

Assessment includes attention to the various concepts of the theory. The nurse would therefore focus on the interpersonal process of the relationship. A key consideration would be determining the current phase of the relationship. The nurse would employ various roles and be aware of communication and pattern integrations, particularly those occurring at the nurse-client level and the client-system level. The nurse would use self-reflection and self-awareness as well as observing and understanding phenomena related to the client. The nurse would be aware of the client's current level of learning. This awareness would assist the nurse to give comments and ask questions that can be appropriately understood and used to facilitate growth. The anxiety of both client and self would be monitored and approaches modified in context of the current levels of anxiety.

As an example, consider the situation that I encountered in working with Mrs. Oksana Fivechuk (a pseudonym). Mrs. Fivechuk was a 66-year-old inpatient in a long-term-care facility. She had not responded to a series of medications and treatments over the years. She had a long history of admissions for problems related to schizophrenia. Generally, as soon as her involuntary certificates expired, she would discharge herself against medical advice and refuse all aftercare. Admissions were generally precipitated by acute episodes where she would become extremely paranoid and refuse all medication, food, and drink. Staff were extremely frustrated and felt they were unable to help Mrs. Fivechuk out of this revolving door.

Preconceptions were very important to work through in the initial phase of the relationship. Mrs. Fivechuk had initiated conversation with the nurse because she identified by the nurse's name that they belonged to the same ethnic group. The nurse recognized this as an unusual opportunity because Mrs. Fivechuk generally avoided any interaction with staff.

An early question from Mrs. Fivechuk was "Is your family from the Ukraine, or is that just your husband's name?" What it meant to be from the same ethnic group and the numerous assumptions this entailed were explored early in the relationship.

Mrs. Fivechuk's extreme paranoia was interwoven with her experience of having fled the Ukraine under difficult circumstances. She believed Russian spies were pursuing her, and during periods where her psychosis worsened, she believed almost everyone was entangled in plots to murder her. An example of an early assumption was that the nurse would have experienced similar persecution. This was not the case.

Testing was used extensively by the client for the initial 4 months. Examples were trying to extend the agreed-on time for the duration of the interactions or using the interactions to discuss other people's problems, dropping Russian phrases into the conversation to see if they were understood, and asking the nurse to figure out mathematical questions before allowing medications to be dispensed. Testing was understood as a strategy to establish if the nurse was a trustworthy person. Mrs. Fivechuk gradually accepted that it was appropriate to confide in someone with experiences different from her own.

The nurse also needed to be aware of preconceptions. Examples in this situation were cultural background, age (over 65), gender, diagnosis (schizophrenia), concern about the previous hospitalization pattern, and similarity to previous clients.

A language pattern used by Mrs. Fivechuk was vague use of pronouns. In particular, she would use the pronoun "they." At times, this pronoun would be used in a normally socially acceptable manner. The phrase "you know" was peppered throughout her speech. An example of both is "Well, you know what they say about people who eat too much." The nurse was aware that such phrases could reflect underlying difficulties with thinking patterns and would give responses such as "Who are you referring to when you say that?" or "No, I don't know. Tell me about that." Exploring this particular statement with Mrs. Fivechuk allowed her to describe not eating as a means of avoiding potential poisoning. Later, after numerous questions related to "they," she was able to be more specific about people she did not trust rather than generalizing.

The process and experience of being able to trust another person is essential for the person suffering from paranoia. The nurse helped Mrs. Fivechuk use this trusting relationship to extend acceptance to other staff. Mrs. Fivechuk did not want to participate in group activities on the unit, but she did begin to socialize with two other women on the ward. Gradually, the circle of people that could be trusted grew larger. As Mrs. Fivechuk improved, a community nurse visited her on the ward so that the relationship could be established well before discharge. Mrs. Fivechuk became an active participant in the decision making related to her care and discharge into the community.

To determine the effectiveness of the nursing care provided, the nurse was aware of the passage through various stages of the therapeutic relationship. Critical client indicators included movement toward goals set by the client, including being able to confide in another person and being able to stay out of the hospital for a longer period of time. Other client indicators were the ability to trust some others and remaining hospitalized long enough for some therapeutic work to be accomplished and to physically recover from the lack of food prior to admission. Further client progress was indicated through establishing a separate therapeutic relationship with the community nurse. Both the inpatient and community nurses also experienced growth through examining assumptions about the client.

The developing phases can also be seen in group work. A team of nurses worked with a group of clients with chronic mental health problems through a "ward community group" that focused on day-to-day issues. The clients had a minimum of 2 years' hospitalization with a diagnosis of chronic schizophrenia. Initially, there was a lot of testing of parameters—for example, coming to the group late, coming and leaving, and disruptive behaviors, such as singing or shouting. Clients initially raised relatively safe subjects, and the staff involved tried to act very quickly on suggestions regarding the ward milieu. For example, there was concern expressed about the pay phone being just outside the ward rather than on the ward. The phone company was contacted and the phone was moved.

Gradually, the focus shifted from "What can the staff do?" to "What can we be doing together?" This paralleled the entry into the identification subphase of the working phase of the relationship. During this period, clients organized several activities and cooperative ventures, such as a "coffee club." The coffee club involved pooling money, purchasing jars of coffee and related items, and organizing coffee times. This was cheaper than other coffee sources and had no direct staff input.

Clients identified that one aspect of their life that was very institutional was the way each day was similar to the next. They contrasted this with a "normal" situation where the weekend is a time for rest. Continental breakfasts were organized for weekends so that clients could sleep in and have a less institutionalized lifestyle (i.e., weekends off). Staff arranged for communal supplies to be sent rather than individual meal trays, but the clients organized the activity and tidied up after themselves. The shift of activities from staff to clients was indicative of the exploitation phase of the relationship.

At regularly arranged periods, sessions of this ward community group were completed. Clients used this opportunity to review progress and also to evaluate directly the usefulness of the activity and make recommendations for future groups. Examples of recommendations were more groups per session and having clients participate in keeping minutes. The minutes were then read at the end of the group and beginning of the next group. This process and the end of each session reflected the resolution phase.

The phases of the relationship are useful for understanding group process. The staff participating in these groups would also use other aspects of Peplau's theory. They would attend to the anxiety level of the group and the language used. They would be aware of communication, both verbal and nonverbal, and of pattern integrations occurring on the personal and system levels. Changing from a common ward pattern of "helper-helpless" to a more collaborative style has been a difficult and ongoing process.

Peplau's theory has also been used to organize clinical programs. An example is the Community Mental Health Promotion Program of the Hamilton-Wentworth Department of Health Services (public health) in Hamilton, Ontario, Canada. This public health program offers case management services and counseling to individuals with a chronic mental illness who require service in their home. Staff found principles of Peplau's theory to be consistent with case management principles. This public health program is described in more detail in Forchuk et al. (1989).

The Relationship Form, outlining the phases of the relationship, is a part of the clinical record of the public health program. Similarly, a form based on Peplau's stages of learning is found on the chart. Only problems or issues agreed to by the client appear on the nursing care plan. The nurses use Peplau's theory as a guide to their practice. The program objectives (e.g., that clients will progress in therapeutic relationships) are drawn from the theory.

A formal evaluation consistent with Peplau's theory was used to evaluate the effectiveness of the overall public health program. Over a 2-year period, clients in the program were able to reduce hospitalization, develop therapeutic relationships, decrease social isolation, increase skills in activities of daily living, and increase their current stage of learning (Forchuk & Voorberg, 1991).

The Menninger Hospital in Topeka, Kansas has adopted Peplau's theory as a basis for nursing care. The theory has been used despite a great variety in clientele, focus, and length of stay on various inpatient units.

The clinical examples given (except for the Menninger example) are drawn from my clinical experience and therefore reflect a psychiatric-mental health focus. This is not to suggest that this clinical specialty is the only appropriate venue for applying Peplau's theory. The importance of nurse-client relationships and related concepts transcends clinical specialty areas.

The nurse working in an emergency department who uses Peplau's theory will recognize that relationships there are frequently in the orientation phase and that clients are generally experiencing high levels of anxiety. This anxiety will affect the current learning phase. The nurse will therefore give clear parameters and often use very short, simple sentences.

The nurse who uses Peplau's theory while working in a geriatric unit will be aware of the importance of establishing and maintaining a therapeutic relationship. That nurse may also find it particularly important to attend to language patterns as evidence of cognitive processes. The nurse observes pattern integrations, particularly family patterns, and attempts to promote ongoing healthy patterns.

The public health nurse using Peplau's theory may find the concept of stages of learning particularly useful in health teaching situations. The nurse is aware of the interrelationship between anxiety and learning. The nurse will at times work with clients who experience high levels of anxiety. Examples could be an inexperienced mother on a well-baby visit or a person receiving a disturbing diagnosis. The nurse adjusts the level of content appropriately and attends to the anxiety rather than focusing only on prepared content.

The nurse manager guided by Peplau's theory would be aware of the importance of the nurse-client relationships. Such a nurse manager will plan the organization of services so that consistent nurse-client assignment takes place. Every client will have a specific nurse assigned every shift and every effort will be made to maintain continuity of nurse-client assignments. When a client needs to undergo an anxiety-producing situation—for example, chemotherapy or an unpleasant diagnostic test—the nurse manager arranges for the regularly assigned nurse to accompany the client. The nurse manager is aware of the importance of the fit between the nurse and client and would not promote the old adage "a nurse is a nurse is a nurse." The nurse manager would also find the concept of pattern integrations particularly useful in examining patterns of care and interaction from a broader systems perspective.

The nurse educator using Peplau's theory would be aware of how his or her relationship with students parallels the stages of therapeutic relationships. This is well described in Buchanan (1993). The nurse educator would also be aware of current stages of learning and how these could be affected by anxiety levels. Communication, both verbal and nonverbal, would be viewed as an essential vehicle for the learning process. The nurse educator would realize that capacities become competencies through practice. He or she would therefore plan activities that encourage the practice of problem solving and other skills.

Peplau's theory is most commonly used in psychiatric mental health nursing. However, these examples illustrate that the clinical utility of the theory extends beyond this nursing specialty.

Research

Research based on Peplau's theory should consider both nurse and client factors. Ideally, such research should address the interpersonal factors and not just the intrapersonal factors of each participant in the relationship. Study of Peplau's theory can be done through quantitative and qualitative research designs. In this section, some of the past research involving Peplau's theory is reviewed. Also, my own program of research focusing on the orientation phase of the nurse-client relationship is described.

Peplau initially used a method similar to grounded theory in the development of her theory. In her 1952 book, she advocated the use of process recordings or "nursing process forms" to study the nurse-client relationship (Peplau, 1952a, p. 308). Process recordings generally use a column format to record verbal and nonverbal communication of the nurse and client as well as nurse interpretations.

Early studies based on Peplau's work tended to use such process recordings. These were frequently published as case studies. Manaser and Werner (1964) published a collection of instruments that could be used in analyzing process recordings in a manner consistent with Peplau's framework.

Several examples of single case studies can be found in Burd and Marshall (1971) and Hays and Larson (1963). Examples of extensive case studies using process recordings are Hays and Myers (1964), who analyzed 106 hours of nurse-client interactions with respect to the levels of learning described by Peplau (1971b), and Lemmer (1988), who analyzed a series of 17 nurse-client interactions. A disadvantage of this approach is that it has usually been limited to the study of a single nurse-client dyad at a time, and generally no comparisons between dyads have been made. An exception is Thompson (1986), who compared two women receiving short-term individual therapy based on Peplau's theory.

Lego (1980) reviewed nursing literature published on the nurse-client relationship from 1946 to 1976. The majority of these publications involved single case studies and "of 166 clinical papers, 78 were written by students and faculty colleagues of Peplau" (p. 81).

A number of nurse researchers have explored aspects of Peplau's theory through qualitative research methods. Morrison and Shealy (1992) have studied roles and role actions of the psychiatric nurse in the nurse-client relationship. This qualitative study included 30 registered nurses in 62 audiotaped interactions with children, adolescents, or adults who were psychiatric inpatients. Content analysis was conducted with respect to the roles undertaken by the nurses. The results were consistent with Peplau's (1964) contention that the counselor role was the primary role of the psychiatric nurse. There was a great deal of overlap among other common roles identified by Peplau, particularly leader and surrogate and resource person and teacher. A secondary role of friend was identified. This role was one that was discouraged by Peplau (1952a). The context of the caregiving situation and client acuity were seen as influences in the roles assumed by the nurses.

Buchanan (in progress) is studying nurse-client relationships from the perspective of a group of nurses who have completed a certificate program in mental health nursing. The nursing program includes teaching Peplau's theory. This grounded theory study involves interviewing the nurses no sooner than 1 year following their completion of the program. Peplau's theory is used as a guiding framework for the development of collaborative helping relationships as part of the structural component of the clinical experience of the certificate program. Buchanan is particularly interested in the practicalities of attempting to use a specific theory in the work setting.

Initial analysis is consistent with Peplau's (1952a) conceptualization of the phases of the nurse-client relationship. The practicalities of the work situation appear to influence the specific roles undertaken by the nurse. A discrepancy with Peplau's theory is that nurses tend to use self-disclosure more readily than the theory would recommend. This is very similar to the Morrison and Shealy (1992) finding regarding nurses' assuming a friend role with their clients.

Choiniere (1991) used a qualitative design to explore the development of trust between nurses and community mental health clients.

Grounded theory was used to explore six clients' perceptions of nurse behaviors that facilitated the development of trust. This study found that trust was slow to evolve and took as long as 3 years to develop. The development of trust occurred through interlocking, overlapping phases (caring presence, interactive caring, and mutual caring) that were synchronous with the phases of the nurse-client relationship described by Peplau (1952a).

Choiniere (1991) described trust as a learned end product of the exploitation subphase. Clients described a process that paralleled Peplau's stages of learning. Participants referred to *observed* patterns of the nurse that would be consistent with a trustworthy person. These patterns were then *described*—for example, as genuine concern and support. Participants *analyzed* the nurses' behaviors while *formulating* the belief that the nurses were trustworthy. This perception would be *validated* with the nurses, *tested, integrated,* and *used.*

The participants described the trust developed in the nurse-client relationship as having an effect beyond the dyad. Choiniere (1991) describes how clients stated that if their nurse believed them to be worthwhile persons, then perhaps they were. For example, one client stated that if her nurse could accept her as a worthwhile human being, then she could accept herself (p. 105).

The Relationship Form was developed by Forchuk and others (1986) to measure the phases of the nurse-client relationship as described by Peplau. It is a 7-point scale measuring the four phases of the relationship and three intermediate points. Forchuk and Brown (1989) have reported on the initial reliability and validity of the instrument. Peplau reviewed the Relationship Form for content validity. A panel of three independent clinical nurse specialists (CNSs), who functioned from an extensive theory-based practice, also reviewed the instrument. Interrater reliability was established by having an additional CNS act as a blind rater by reviewing clinical records and comparing the phase to that determined on the form by the clinician in the nurse-client relationship. Agreement within 1 point of the 7-point scale was 91%, but crude diagonal agreement was only 41%. A problem noted was that, in cases where disagreement existed, the CNS consistently rated the relationship 1 point higher than the clinician did.

To counterbalance the clinicians' hesitancy to note a change in the relationship until it has persisted for several encounters, a secondary confirmation was used in later studies by Forchuk and colleagues

(Forchuk, 1992a; Forchuk et al., in progress). For example, the assigned nurse would validate the current phase with a blind (to other measures) clinical nurse specialist who practices from Peplau's framework (Forchuk, 1992a).

Forchuk and colleagues (Forchuk, 1992a, 1992b; Forchuk et al., in progress) have conducted several studies examining the orientation phase of the nurse-client relationship. This phase has been given particular focus because progress through this initial phase has been related to psychotherapy and rehabilitation outcomes (Gehrs, 1991; Kirtner & Cartwright, 1958; Saltzman, Leutgert, Roth, Creaser, & Howard, 1976).

Forchuk (1992b) reported on a study examining client demographic factors and their relation to the duration of the orientation phase. The 73 subjects were community clients of a mental health program. All clients had been diagnosed as having a chronic mental illness. This study was interesting in what was found *not* to be related to the duration of the orientation phase. Psychiatric diagnosis, age of client, gender of client, age of first psychiatric hospitalization, age of first psychiatric contact, and type of service received (long-term case management or problem-specific counseling) were all unrelated to the time in the orientation phase.

The only demographic factors that were related to the orientation phase were the number and length of psychiatric hospitalizations. Those clients who took 11 or more months in orientation also tended to take much longer for each psychiatric hospitalization (average 70.3 months' stay over 5.7 hospitalizations) when compared to the group who completed orientation in 2 or fewer months (averaged 10.9 months' stay over 4.1 admissions). A suggestion made in this study is that it is possible that information that would facilitate movement through the orientation phase would also facilitate shorter hospital admissions.

Forchuk (1992b) also examined situations where the client returned to the orientation phase after completing this phase. Through a record review, 30 cases where this occurred were identified. The context of the return to the orientation phase is revealing. In 17 of the cases, the return to the orientation phase accompanied a change in staff. It is interesting to note that some of these staff changes were very brief— for example, for vacation coverage. Where staff changes occurred it seemed important that the client be informed well ahead of time. In cases where clients had only 2 weeks' notice of a staff permanently leaving the agency, the clients took longer to work through the orientation phase with the new nurse than with the initial nurse, whereas when the clients knew months in advance (with an obviously impending maternity leave), all clients were able to enter the working phase with the new nurse within 2 months.

The other 13 cases of clients' returning to the orientation phase accompanied a worsening of symptoms such as paranoia or depression. All of these clients returned to the working phase within 2 months, even if their symptoms persisted. Those clients with lengthier psychiatric hospitalizations appeared to be more likely to return to the orientation phase.

Forchuk (1992a) tested Peplau's theory regarding influences during the orientation phase. This investigation used a prospective design to examine the orientation phase of the nurse-client relationship. The sample consisted of 124 newly formed nurse-client dyads. Client subjects were individuals with a chronic mental illness.

The following variables predicted by Peplau's theory to be related to development of the therapeutic nurse-client relationship were examined: (a) nurses' preconceptions of their clients, (b) clients' preconceptions of their nurses, (c) other interpersonal relationships of clients, (d) other interpersonal relationships of nurses, and (e) anxiety of clients, and (f) anxiety of nurses. Variables were measured for both nurses and clients at 0, 3, and 6 months into their relationship.

Instruments used were the Relationship Form (Forchuk & Brown, 1989) to measure the duration of the orientation phase, the Working Alliance Inventory (Horvath & Greenberg, 1986) to measure the quality of the relationship, selected semantic differential scales (Osgood, Suci & Tannenbaum, 1957) to measure preconceptions, Personal Resource Questionnaire (Brandt & Weinert, 1981; Weinert, 1987) to measure other interpersonal relationships, and the Beck Anxiety Scale (Beck, Epstein, Brown, & Steer, 1988).

The preconceptions of both nurses and clients were most predictive of the developing relationship. Preconceptions of both nurses and clients were related to the duration of the orientation phase and development of the therapeutic alliance. There was support for the importance of clients' other interpersonal relationships but not nurses' other interpersonal relationships. Anxiety was not found to be significantly related to the development of the therapeutic relationship. A regression analysis including both nurse and client variables identified in the hypotheses was also completed. The explanatory power resulting from including both nurse and client variables was .38 ($R = .62$). This is considerably greater than client factors alone ($R^2 = .17$, $R = .42$) or the nurse factors alone ($R^2 = .14$, $R = .37$) as predictors of weeks in orientation.

This study therefore supported some tenets of Peplau's theory but not others. The finding that the combination of both nurse and client variables was most significant is supportive of an interpersonal approach. Many nursing theories focus on the client as the unit of attention, although the importance of the contribution of the nurse and larger social systems may be acknowledged. Peplau's theory recognizes that the nurse must use awareness of self and self-reflection as vigilantly as assessment of the client situation. This was reflected through the significance of the nurses' preconceptions.

A qualitative study examining the orientation phase of the relationship is currently being conducted (Forchuk et al., in progress). This naturalistic qualitative design will employ an interpersonal method drawing on the works of Peplau (1952a) and ethnonursing (Leininger, 1985a, 1987, 1990). This study also involves clients with a chronic mental illness.

Nurses and clients are being interviewed during the orientation phase to explore their thoughts and feelings regarding the emerging relationship. Each interview is conducted by a clinical nurse specialist who is also one of the principal investigators. The interviews are unstructured and employ broad, open-ended questions related to the evolving nurse-client relationship. No predetermined questions are used. The Relationship Form (Forchuk & Brown, 1989) is used to determine whether or not the dyad is still in orientation. Participants are encouraged to talk about issues related to the nurse-client relationship. These interviews are being audiotaped.

Nurse-client interactions are being videotaped during the orientation phase. Videotapes have been found particularly useful in identifying nonverbal issues. All audiotapes and videotapes are transcribed verbatim using Leininger's software program for qualitative data (Leininger, Templin, & Thompson, in progress).

The qualitative study involves the assistance of two well-known nursing theorists. Because the investigators have been primarily involved in work related to Peplau's theory (Forchuk, 1990, 1991a, 1991b, 1991c, 1992a, 1992b; Forchuk & Brown, 1989; Forchuk et al., 1989; Forchuk & Voorberg, 1991, Martin & Forchuk, 1989; Martin, Forchuk, Santopinto, & Butcher, 1992), it might be questionable how unbiased identification of themes might be. However, this investigation uses validation with the study participants and a different theorist, namely, Madeleine Leininger (1985b, 1988). Using a different theorist avoids what Smith (1990) refers to as an "ideological circle," which can develop when the research method is based on a specific theory and the researchers are already committed to that theory. After the themes have been identified, a comparison will be made to the concepts and themes within Peplau's theory. Peplau has agreed to assist with this phase of the analysis. The investigators could not find an example of another nursing study employing two nurse theorists in any similar manner.

The primary aim of the qualitative investigation (Forchuk et al., in progress) is to identify clients' and nurses' perceptions of important influences in the nurse-client relationship during the orientation phase. A secondary purpose is to determine how the clients' and nurses' perspectives regarding the orientation phase of the therapeutic relationship relate to the theoretical framework proposed by Peplau (1952a). It is anticipated that the findings will assist nurses and clients in the establishment of therapeutic relationships.

The earlier quantitative study by Forchuk (1992a) and the ongoing qualitative study (Forchuk et al., in progress) will complement each other from both theoretical and methodological perspectives. The next step in the research program phase will involve a meta-analysis of these two different studies. Future plans also include work with different clinical populations.

The examples of research using Peplau's theory reflect direct application to practice despite a broad diversity of methods used. Both qualitative and quantitative methods can be used in exploring issues from the perspective of Peplau's theory.

A key feature of such research is the inclusion of nurses and clients and the interpersonal focus.

Summary

Peplau's interpersonal theory of nursing identified the therapeutic nurse-client relationship as the crux of nursing. Her theory has been used extensively in nursing practice, particularly in mental health and psychiatric nursing. Peplau's theory allowed nursing to move away from "doing to" to "doing with" clients.

Glossary

Adaptation
A process employed to cope with the inevitable dilemmas of living. Synonyms include *adjust, fit,* and *conform* (Peplau, 1989a, p. 286).

Anxiety
An energy triggered by a perceived threat to the person's security. The threat could be real or imagined, internal or external. Levels of anxiety range from mild anxiety to moderate anxiety to severe anxiety to panic. Anxiety is considered a universally experienced phenomenon (Peplau 1952a, 1971a, 1973a, 1989a).

Behavior
Includes thoughts, actions, feelings and patterns (Peplau, 1989b, p. 201).

Capacities
Potential abilities that have not yet been developed.

Client
The recipient of nursing services. The client could be an individual, couple, family, group, or community (Forchuk, 1991c; Peplau, 1952b, 1987a, 1988). Synonymous with *patient.*

Competencies
Skills or abilities that have evolved through the use and practice of capacities. Competencies evolving in the nurse-client relationship

include problem-solving and interpersonal competencies (Peplau, 1973b).

Communication
An interpersonal process to transmit information (ideas, feelings, attitudes) that includes verbal language and nonverbal communication (Peplau, 1952a, pp. 289-307).

Environment
Physiological, psychological, and social fluidity that may be illness-maintaining or health-promoting (Peplau, 1952a, 1973c, 1987b).

Exploitation subphase
The second subphase of the working phase of the nurse-client relationship. This phase exists when the client is able to make full use of the services of the nurse and plans are put into operation (Peplau, 1952a, 1973g).

Goal of nursing
Forward movement of the personality (health) (Peplau, 1952a).

Health
Forward movement of personality and other ongoing human processes in the direction of creative, constructive, personal, and community living (Peplau, 1952a).

Identification subphase
The first part of the working phase of the nurse-client relationship. The client identifies with the nurse and the nurse-client encounters and begins to identify problems to be worked on within the nurse-client relationship (Peplau, 1952a, 1973g).

Illness maintenance
Pattern integrations that encourage the continued use of behaviors associated with the person's illness (Peplau, 1973c).

Interpersonal
Phenomena that occur between persons.

Interpersonal paradigm
The view that the therapeutic nurse-client relationship is the crux of nursing. This paradigm includes theorists such as Peplau, Orlando, Mellows, and Travelbee (Forchuk, 1991a).

Interpersonal relationships

Any processes occurring between two or more persons. Peplau includes Sullivan's (1952) perspective in specifying that all but one of the persons involved may be illusory (Forchuk, 1991c; Peplau, 1952a).

Intrapersonal

Phenomena that occur within the individual.

Investigative counseling

"An interviewing process that helps a person investigate life experiences" (Peplau, 1989b, p. 205).

Language

Verbal communication to express thoughts or feelings through words, images, concepts, or symbols. Peplau (1973d) views thought and language as integral to each other.

Learning

Skill development generally acquired through an active interpersonal process. Stages of learning are to (a) observe, (b) describe, (c) analyze, (d) formulate, (e) validate, (f) test, (g) integrate, and (h) use (Peplau, 1971b).

Nonverbal communication

Any form of information exchange between two or more people that is not dependent on the use of language. These forms include empathic linkages, gestural or body messages, and patterns (Peplau, 1987a, pp. 203-204).

Nurse

The medium of the art of nursing. "The unique blend of ideals, values, integrity, and commitment to the well-being of others, expressed in a nurse's self-presentation and responses to clients, makes each nurse a one-of-a-kind artist in nursing practice" (Peplau, 1988, p. 10).

Nurse-client relationship

The specific interpersonal relationship that develops between a nurse and a client. The relationship develops through interlocking and overlapping phases. These are: the orientation phase, the working phase (subdivided into identification and exploitation), and the resolution phase (Peplau, 1952a, 1962, 1964, 1965).

Nursing
An educative instrument, a maturing force, that aims to promote health (Peplau, 1952a).

Orientation phase
The initial phase of the nurse-client relationship. The nurse and client work through preconceptions, establish and meet parameters, develop initial trust, and begin to understand each other's roles (Peplau, 1952a, 1973e).

Panic
Extreme anxiety.

Patient
See *Client*.

Pattern integrations
Occur when the patterns of one person or system interact with the patterns of another person or system. The pattern integrations include complementary, mutual, antagonistic, and alternating. Pattern integrations may occur at several levels including intrapersonal, interpersonal, and systems phenomena (Peplau 1973c, 1987a, 1988).

Patterns
A characteristic mode of behavior, a configuration of separate acts or variations that have a similar aim or intention (Peplau, 1987a, p. 204).

Person
An individual, developed through interpersonal relationships, that lives in an unstable environment (Forchuk, 1991c; Peplau, 1952a).

Phases of the nurse-client relationship
Orientation, working (subdivided into identification and exploitation) and resolution (Peplau, 1952a, 1962, 1964, 1965).

Preconceptions
The initial thoughts, feelings, and assumptions one person has about another (Peplau, 1952a, pp. 21-30, 123).

Relief behaviors
Behaviors used to diminish or cope with anxiety (Peplau, 1989a).

Resolution phase
The final phase of the nurse-client relationship. It exists when all plans have been implemented until the nurse and client mutually agree to terminate the relationship (Peplau, 1952a, 1973f).

Roles of the nurse
The interlocking functions a nurse may undertake to assist a client (Forchuk, 1991e). Peplau (1952a) has identified common roles of the nurse as stranger, technical expert, surrogate for another person such as a parent or authority figure, teacher, resource person, and counselor. She further states that specific roles are variable within each nurse-client situation and are limited only by the imagination and skill of the nurse (Peplau, 1952a, pp. 43-72).

Self system
A person's concept of self that "is a product of socialization, a function in humans that evolves and is revised along constructive or destructive lines during interpersonal relationships throughout life" (Peplau, 1989a, p. 299).

Self-understanding
The extent to which a person has insight into his or her interpersonal and intrapersonal functioning. The self-understanding of the nurse will determine the extent to which the nurse can come to understand the situation confronting the client, from the client's perspective (Forchuk, 1991c; Peplau, 1952a).

Theory
"A formulation of the meaning of observed phenomena in an order or form that enables the formulation to be used to explain similar phenomena . . . and to guide the professional in choosing interventions relevant to the phenomena observed" (Peplau, 1989d, p. 27).

Thinking
A process, mediated by language, by which experience is incorporated, stored, organized and recalled. Thinking is used to link experiences and for learning (Peplau, 1973d).

Working phase
The middle phase of the nurse-client relationship that comprises the identification and exploitation subphases. Problems are identified and worked through in this phase (Peplau, 1973g).

References

Beck, A. (1976). *Cognitive therapy and the emotional disorders*. Madison, CT: International Universities Press.

Beck, A., Epstein, N., Brown, G., & Steer, R. (1988). An inventory for measuring clinical anxiety: Psychometric properties. *Journal of Clinical and Consulting Psychology, 56*, 893-897.

Brandt, P. A., & Weinert, C. (1981). PRQ—A social support measure. *Nursing Research, 30*(5), 277-280.

Buchanan, J. (1993). The teacher-student relationship: The heart of nursing education. In M. Rather (Ed.), *Transforming RN education: Dialogue and debate* (pp. 304-323). New York: National League for Nursing.

Buchanan, J. (in progress). *A grounded theory study of the nurse-client relationship*. Unpublished manuscript, University of New Brunswick, St. John, New Brunswick, Canada.

Burd, S. F., & Marshall, M. A. (Eds.). (1971). *Some clinical approaches to psychiatric nursing*. London: Macmillan.

Choiniere, J. (1991). *Clients' perceptions of nurse behaviors that facilitate trust in nurse-client relationships*. Unpublished master's thesis, Saint Joseph College, West Hartford, CT.

Ellis, A. (1962). *Reason and emotion in psychotherapy*. Secaucus, NJ: Citadel Press.

Forchuk, C. (1989). *Peplau's framework: Concepts and their inter-relationships*. Unpublished manuscript, Hamilton Psychiatric Hospital, Hamilton, Ontario, Canada.

Forchuk, C. (1990). Peplau's interpersonal theory. In A. Baumann, N. Johnson, & D. Atai-Otaong (Eds.), *Decision making in psychiatric and psychosocial nursing* (pp. 22-23). Toronto: B. C. Decker.

Forchuk, C. (1991a). A comparison of the works of Peplau and Orlando. *Archives of Psychiatric Nursing, 5*(1), 38-45.

Forchuk, C. (1991b). Conceptualizing the environment of the individual with a chronic mental illness. *Issues in Mental Health Nursing, 12,* 159-170.

Forchuk, C. (1991c). Peplau's theory: Concepts and their relations. *Nursing Science Quarterly, 4*(2), 54-60.

Forchuk, C. (1992a). *The orientation phase of the nurse-client relationship: Testing Peplau's theory.* Unpublished doctoral dissertation, Wayne State University, Detroit, MI.

Forchuk, C. (1992b). The orientation phase: How long does it take? *Perspectives in Psychiatric Care, 28*(4), 7-10.

Forchuk, C., Beaton, S., Crawford, L., Ide, L., Voorberg, N., & Bethune, J. (1986, August). *A marriage between Peplau's theory and case management: Instrument development.* Paper presented at the Nursing Theories Congress, Ryerson College, Toronto, Ontario, Canada.

Forchuk, C., Beaton, S., Crawford, L., Ide, L., Voorberg, N., & Bethune, J. (1989). Incorporating Peplau's theory and case management. *Journal of Psychosocial Nursing, 27*(2), 35-38.

Forchuk, C., & Brown, B. (1989). Establishing a nurse-client relationship. *Journal of Psychosocial Nursing, 27*(2), 30-34.

Forchuk, C., & Voorberg, N. (1991). Evaluating a community mental health program. *Canadian Journal of Nursing Administration, 4*(6) 16-20.

Forchuk, C., Westwell, J., Martin, M. L., Bamber, W., Kosterewa-Tolman, D., & Hux, M. (in progress). *The orientation phase of the nurse-client relationship: Exploration with an interpersonal method.* Unpublished manuscript, Hamilton Psychiatric Hospital, Hamilton, Ontario, Canada.

Gehrs, M. (1991). *The relationship between the working alliance and rehabilitation outcomes of clients with schizophrenia.* Unpublished master's thesis, University of Toronto, Ontario, Canada.

Gregg, D. (1954). The psychiatric nurse's role. *American Journal of Nursing, 54*(7), 848-851.

Hays, J., & Larson, K. (1963). *Interacting with patients.* New York: Macmillan.

Hays, J., & Myers, J. (1964). Learning in the nurse-patient relationship. *Perspectives in Psychiatric Care, 2,* 20.

Hirschmann, M. J. (1989). Psychiatric and mental health nurses' beliefs about therapeutic paradox. *Journal of Child Psychiatric Nursing, 2,*(1), 7-13.

Horvath, A. O., & Greenberg, L. (1986). The development of the Working Alliance Inventory. In L. Greenberg & W. Pinsof (Eds.), *Psychotherapeutic process handbook: A research handbook* (pp. 529-544). New York: Guilford.

Kirtner, W. L., & Cartwright, D. S. (1958). Success and failure in client-centered therapy as a function of initial in-therapy behavior. *Journal of Consulting Psychology, 22*(5), 329-333.

Lego, S. (1980). The one-to-one nurse-patient relationship. *Perspectives in Psychiatric Care, 18,* 67-89.

Leininger, M. M. (1985a). Ethnography and ethnonursing: Models and modes of qualitative data analysis. In M. M. Leininger (Ed.), *Qualitative research methods in nursing* (pp. 33-72). Orlando, FL: Grune & Stratton.

Leininger, M. M. (1985b). Transcultural care diversity and universality: A theory of nursing. *Nursing and Health Care, 6*(4), 209-212.

Leininger, M. M. (1987). Importance and use of ethnomethods: Ethnography and ethnonursing methods. In M. Cahoon (Ed.), *Recent advances in nursing* (pp. 12-15). London: Churchill Livingstone of Edinburgh.

Leininger, M. M. (1988). Leininger's theory of nursing: Cultural care diversity and universality. *Nursing Science Quarterly, 1*(4), 152-160.

Leininger, M. M. (1990). Ethnomethods: The philosophic and epistemic bases to explicate transcultural nursing knowledge. *Journal of Transcultural Nursing, 1*(2), 40-51.

Leininger, M. M., Templin, F., & Thompson, F. (in progress). *Leininger, Templin and Thompson program for qualitative analysis.* Unpublished manuscript, Wayne State University, Detroit, MI.

Lemmer, B. (1988). Care plan for a man receiving domiciliary care, using Peplau's model of nursing. In B. Collister (Ed.), *Psychiatric nursing: Person to person* (pp. 25-37). London: Edward Arnold.

Manaser, J. C., & Werner, A. M. (1964). *Instruments for the study of nurse-patient interaction.* New York: Macmillan.

Martin, M. L., & Forchuk, C. (1989, September). *Peplau's theory: Application of theory-based practice.* Paper presented at the First National Clinical Nurse Specialists Conference, Hamilton, Ontario, Canada.

Martin, M. L., Forchuk, C., Santopinto, M., & Butcher, H. (1992). Alternative approaches to nursing practice: Application of Peplau, Rogers, and Parse. *Nursing Science Quarterly, 5*(8), 80-85.

Martin, M. L., & Kirkpatrick, H. (1987). *Nursing theories used by staff nurses.* Unpublished manuscript, Hamilton Psychiatric Hospital, Hamilton, Ontario, Canada.

Martin, M. L., & Kirkpatrick, H. (1989). *Nursing theories used by staff nurses: Two year re-evaluation.* Unpublished manuscript, Hamilton Psychiatric Hospital, Hamilton, Ontario, Canada.

May, R. (1950). *The meaning of anxiety.* New York: Ronald Press.

Mead, G. H. (1934). *Mind, self and society.* Chicago: University of Chicago Press.

Mereness, D. (1966). *Psychiatric nursing* (Vols. 1-2). Dubuque, IA: Brown.

Miller, N. E., & Dollard, J. (1941). *Social learning and imitation.* New Haven, CT: Yale University Press.

Morrison, E. G., & Shealy, A. H. (1992, September). *Work roles of the psychiatric staff nurse.* Paper presented at the 14th Southeastern Conference of Clinical Specialists in Psychiatric-Mental Health Nursing, Lexington, KY.

Osgood, C. E., Suci, G. J., & Tannenbaum, P. H. (1957). *Measurement of meaning.* Urbana: University of Illinois Press.

Peplau, H. E. (1952a). *Interpersonal relations in nursing.* New York: G. P. Putnam.

Peplau, H. E. (1952b). Psychiatric nurses family groups. *American Journal of Nursing, 52,* 1475-1477.

Peplau, H. E. (1962). Interpersonal techniques: The crux of psychiatric nursing. *American Journal of Nursing, 62,* 50-54.

Peplau, H. E. (1964). *Basic principals of patient counselling.* Philadelphia: Smith, Kline & French Laboratories.

Peplau, H. E. (1965). The heart of nursing: Interpersonal relations. *Canadian Nurse, 61,* 273.

Peplau, H. E. (1971a). Anxiety. In S. F. Burd & M. A. Marshall (Eds.), *Some clinical approaches to psychiatric nursing* (pp. 323-327). London: Macmillan.

Peplau, H. E. (1971b). Process and concept of learning. In S. F. Burd & M. A. Marshall (Eds.), *Some clinical approaches to psychiatric nursing* (pp. 333-336). London: Macmillan.

Peplau, H. E. (Speaker). (1973a). *Anxiety* [Audiotape]. San Antonio, TX: P. S. F. Productions.

Peplau, H. E. (Speaker). (1973b). *The concept of psychotherapy* [Audiotape]. San Antonio, TX: P. S. F. Productions.

Peplau, H. E. (Speaker). (1973c). *Illness maintaining systems* [Audiotape]. San Antonio, TX: P. S. F. Productions.

Peplau, H. E. (Speaker). (1973d). *Language and its relation to thought disorders* [Audiotape]. San Antonio, TX: P. S. F. Productions.

Peplau, H. E. (Speaker). (1973e). *The orientation phase* [Audiotape]. San Antonio, TX: P. S. F. Productions.

Peplau, H. E. (Speaker). (1973f). *The resolution phase* [Audiotape]. San Antonio, TX: P. S. F. Productions.

Peplau, H. E. (Speaker). (1973g). *The working phase* [Audiotape]. San Antonio, TX: P. S. F. Productions.

Peplau, H. E. (1987a). Interpersonal constructs for nursing practice. *Nurse Education Today, 7*(5), 201-208.

Peplau, H. E. (1987b). Nursing science: A historical perspective. In R. Parse (Ed.), *Nursing science: Major paradigms, theories, and critiques* (pp. 13-30). Toronto: W. B. Saunders.

Peplau, H. E. (1988). The art and science of nursing: Similarities, differences and relations. *Nursing Science Quarterly, 1*, 8-15.

Peplau, H. E. (1989a). Anxiety, self and hallucinations. In A. W. O'Toole & S. R. Welt (Eds.), *Interpersonal theory in nursing practice: Selected works of Hildegard E. Peplau* (pp. 270-326). New York: Springer.

Peplau, H. E. (1989b). Investigative counseling. In A. W. O'Toole & S. R. Welt (Eds.), *Interpersonal theory in nursing practice: Selected works of Hildegard E. Peplau* (pp. 205-229). New York: Springer.

Peplau, H. E. (1989c). Loneliness. In A. W. O'Toole & S. R. Welt (Eds.), *Interpersonal theory in nursing practice: Selected works of Hildegard E. Peplau* (pp. 255-269). New York: Springer.

Peplau, H. E. (1989d). Theory: The professional dimension. In A. W. O'Toole & S. R. Welt (Eds.), *Interpersonal theory in nursing practice: Selected works of Hildegard E. Peplau* (pp. 21-41). New York: Springer.

Peplau, H. E. (1989e). Therapeutic nurse-patient interaction. In A. W. O'Toole & S. R. Welt (Eds.), *Interpersonal theory in nursing practice: Selected works of Hildegard E. Peplau* (pp. 192-204). New York: Springer.

Saltzman, C., Leutgert, M., Roth, C., Creaser, J., & Howard, L. (1976). Formation of a therapeutic relationship: Experiences during the initial phase as predictors of treatment duration and outcome. *Journal of Consulting and Clinical Psychology, 44*, 546-555.

Sills, G. M. (1978). Hildegard E. Peplau: Leader, practitioner, academician, scholar and theorist. *Perspectives in Psychiatric Care, 16*(3), 122-128.

Smith, D. E. (1990). *Conceptual practices of power.* Toronto: University of Toronto Press.

Sullivan, H. S. (1952). *The interpersonal theory of psychiatry.* New York: Norton.

Thompson, L. (1986). Peplau's theory: An application to short-term individual therapy. *Journal of Psychosocial Nursing, 24*(8), 26-31.

Tudor, G. E. (1952). A sociopsychiatric nursing approach to intervention in a problem of mutual withdrawal on a mental hospital ward. *Psychiatry: Journal for the study of Interpersonal Processes, 15*(2).

Weinert, C. (1987). A social support measure: PRQ85. *Nursing Research, 36,* 273-277.

Bibliography

Beeber, L., Anderson, C. A., & Sills, G. M. (1990). Peplau's theory in practice. *Nursing Science Quarterly, 3*(1), 6-8.

Belcher, J., & Fish, L. (1980). Hildegard E. Peplau. In J. B. George (Ed.), *Nursing theories: The base for professional nursing practice* (pp. 43-60). Englewood Cliffs, NJ: Prentice Hall.

Blake, M. (1980). The Peplau developmental model for nursing practice. In J. P. Riehl & C. Roy (Eds.), *Conceptual models for nursing practice* (2nd ed., pp. 53-59) . New York: Appleton-Century-Crofts.

Buchanan, J. (1993). The teacher-student relationship: The heart of nursing education. In M. Rather (Ed.), *Transforming RN education: Dialogue and debate* (pp. 304-323). New York: National League for Nursing.

Burd, S. F., & Marshall, M. A. (Eds.). (1971). *Some clinical approaches to psychiatric nursing.* London: Macmillan.

Carey, E. T., Rasmussen, L., Searey, B., & Stark, N. L. (1986). Hildegard E. Peplau: Psychodynamic nursing. In A. Marriner (Ed.), *Nursing theorists and their work* (pp. 181-195). Toronto: C. V. Mosby.

Chinn, P. L., & Jacobs, M. K. (1983). *Theory and nursing: A systematic approach.* Toronto: C. V. Mosby.

Choiniere, J. (1991). *Clients' perceptions of nurse behaviors that facilitate trust in nurse-client relationships.* Unpublished master's thesis, Saint Joseph College, West Hartford, CT.

Field, W. E. (1978). *Psychotherapy of Hildegard Peplau.* New Braunfels, TX: P. S. F. Productions.

Field, W. E., & Ruelke, W. (1973). Hallucinations and how to deal with them. *American Journal of Nursing, 73*(4), 638-640.

Fitzpatrick, J., & Whall, A. (1983). *Conceptual models of nursing: Analysis and application.* Bowie, MD: Brady.

511

Fitzpatrick, J., Whall, A., Johnson, R., & Floyd, J. (1982). *Nursing models and their psychiatric mental health applications*. Bowie, MD: Brady.

Forchuk, C. (1990). Peplau's interpersonal theory. In A. Baumann, N. Johnson, & D. Atai-Otaong (Eds.), *Decision making in psychiatric and psychosocial nursing* (pp. 22-23). Toronto: Decker.

Forchuk, C. (1991). A comparison of the works of Peplau and Orlando. *Archives of Psychiatric Nursing, 5*(1), 38-45.

Forchuk, C. (1991). Conceptualizing the environment of the individual with a chronic mental illness. *Issues in Mental Health Nursing, 12,* 159-170.

Forchuk, C. (1991). Peplau's theory: Concepts and their relations. *Nursing Science Quarterly, 4*(2), 54-60.

Forchuk, C. (1992). *The orientation phase of the nurse-client relationship: Testing Peplau's theory*. Unpublished doctoral dissertation, Wayne State University, Detroit, MI.

Forchuk, C. (1992). The orientation phase: How long does it take? *Perspectives in Psychiatric Care, 28*(4), 7-10.

Forchuk, C., Beaton, S., Crawford, L., Ide, L., Voorberg, N., & Bethune, J. (1989). Incorporating Peplau's theory and case management. *Journal of Psychosocial Nursing, 27*(2), 35-38.

Forchuk, C., & Brown, B. (1989). Establishing a nurse-client relationship. *Journal of Psychosocial Nursing, 27*(2), 30-34.

Forchuk, C., & Voorberg, N. (1991). Evaluating a community mental health program. *Canadian Journal of Nursing Administration, 4*(6) 16-20.

Gehrs, M. (1991). *The relationship between the working alliance and rehabilitation outcomes of clients with schizophrenia*. Unpublished master's thesis, University of Toronto, Ontario, Canada.

Goering, P. N., & Stylianos, S. K. (1988). Exploring the helping relationship between schizophrenic client and rehabilitation therapist. *American Journal of Orthopsychiatry, 58*(2), 271-280.

Gregg, D. (1954). The psychiatric nurse's role. *American Journal of Nursing, 54*(7), 848-851. (Reprinted in D. Mereness, *Psychiatric nursing,* 1966, Vol. 1, pp. 178-185)

Gregg, D. (1978). Hildegard E. Peplau: Her contributions. *Perspectives in Psychiatric Care, 16*(3), 118-121.

Hays, J. (1966). Analysis of nurse-patient communication. *Nursing Outlook, 14*(9), 32-35.

Hays, J., & Larson, K. (1963). *Interacting with patients*. New York: Macmillan.

Hays, J., & Myers, J. (1964). Learning in the nurse-patient relationship. *Perspectives in Psychiatric Care, 2,* 20.

Hirschmann, M. J. (1989). Psychiatric and mental health nurses' beliefs about therapeutic paradox. *Journal of Child Psychiatric Nursing, 2*(1), 7-13.

Lego, S. (1980). The one-to-one nurse-patient relationship. *Perspectives in Psychiatric Care, 18,* 67-89.

Lemmer, B. (1988). Care plan for a man receiving domiciliary care, using Peplau's model of nursing. In B. Collister (Ed.), *Psychiatric nursing: Person to person.* London: Edward Arnold.

Manaser, J. C., & Werner, A. M. (1964). *Instruments for the study of nurse-patient interaction*. New York: Macmillan.

Martin, M. L., Forchuk, C., Santopinto, M., & Butcher, H. (1992). Alternative approaches to nursing practice: Application of Peplau, Rogers, and Parse. *Nursing Science Quarterly, 5*(8), 80-85.

O'Toole, A. W., & Welt, S. R. (Eds.). (1989). *Interpersonal theory in nursing practice: Selected works of Hildegard E. Peplau.* New York: Springer.

Parse, R. R. (1987). *Nursing science: Major paradigms, theories, and critiques.* Toronto: W. B. Saunders.

Peplau, H. E. (1952). *Interpersonal relations in nursing.* New York: G. P. Putnam.

Peplau, H. E. (1952). Psychiatric nurses family groups. *American Journal of Nursing, 52,* 1475-1477.

Peplau, H. E. (1960, May). Anxiety in the mother-infant relationship. *Nurses Weekly,* p. 134.

Peplau, H. E. (1960). Talking with patients. *American Journal of Nursing, 60,* 964+.

Peplau, H. E. (1962). Interpersonal techniques: The crux of psychiatric nursing. *American Journal of Nursing, 62,* 50-54.

Peplau, H. E. (1964). *Basic principals of patient counselling.* Philadelphia: Smith, Kline & French Laboratories.

Peplau, H. E. (1965). The heart of nursing: Interpersonal relations. *Canadian Nurse, 61,* 273.

Peplau, H. E. (1967). Interpersonal relations and the work of the industrial nurse. *American Association of Industrial Nurses Journal, 15*(11), 7-12.

Peplau, H. E. (1969). Professional closeness as a special kind of involvement with a patient, client, or family group. *Nursing Forum, 8*(4), 342-360.

Peplau, H. E. (1971). Anxiety. In S. F. Burd & M. A. Marshall (Eds.), *Some clinical approaches to psychiatric nursing* (pp. 323-327). London: Macmillan.

Peplau, H. E. (1971). Process and concept of learning. In S. F. Burd & M. A. Marshall (Eds.), *Some clinical approaches to psychiatric nursing* (pp. 333-336). London: Macmillan.

Peplau, H. E. (Speaker). (1973). *Anxiety* [Audiotape]. San Antonio, TX: P. S. F. Productions.

Peplau, H. E. (Speaker). (1973). *The concept of psychotherapy* [Audiotape]. San Antonio, TX: P. S. F. Productions.

Peplau, H. E. (Speaker). (1973). *Illness maintaining systems* [Audiotape]. San Antonio, TX: P. S. F. Productions.

Peplau, H. E. (Speaker). (1973). *Language and its relation to thought disorders* [Audiotape]. San Antonio, TX: P. S. F. Productions.

Peplau, H. E. (Speaker). (1973). *The orientation phase* [Audiotape]. San Antonio, TX: P. S. F. Productions.

Peplau, H. E. (Speaker). (1973). *The resolution phase* [Audiotape]. San Antonio, TX: P. S. F. Productions.

Peplau, H. E. (Speaker). (1973). *The working phase* [Audiotape]. San Antonio, TX: P. S. F. Productions.

Peplau, H. E. (1976). What future for nursing? *American Operating Room Nursing Journal, 24,* 217-235.

Peplau, H. E. (1977). The changing view of nursing. *International Nursing Review, 24*(2), 43-45.

Peplau, H. E. (1987). Interpersonal constructs for nursing practice. *Nurse Education Today, 7*(5), 201-208.

Peplau, H. E. (1987). Nursing science: A historical perspective. In R. Parse (Ed.), *Nursing science: Major paradigms, theories, and critiques* (pp. 13-30). Toronto: W. B. Saunders.

Peplau, H. E. (1988). The art and science of nursing: Similarities, differences and relations. *Nursing Science Quarterly, 1,* 8-15.

Peplau, H. E. (1989). Anxiety, self and hallucinations. In A. W. O'Toole & S. R. Welt (Eds.), *Interpersonal theory in nursing practice: Selected works of Hildegard E. Peplau* (pp. 270-326). New York: Springer.

Peplau, H. E. (1989). Investigative counseling. In A. W. O'Toole & S. R. Welt (Eds.), *Interpersonal theory in nursing practice: Selected works of Hildegard E. Peplau* (pp. 205-229). New York: Springer.

Peplau, H. E. (1989). Loneliness. In A. W. O'Toole & S. R. Welt (Eds.), *Interpersonal theory in nursing practice: Selected works of Hildegard E. Peplau* (pp. 255-269). New York: Springer.

Peplau, H. E. (1989). Theory: The professional dimension. In A. W. O'Toole & S. R. Welt (Eds.), *Interpersonal theory in nursing practice: Selected works of Hildegard E. Peplau* (pp. 21-41). New York: Springer.

Peplau, H. E. (1989). Therapeutic nurse-patient interaction. In A. W. O'Toole & S. R. Welt (Eds.), *Interpersonal theory in nursing practice: Selected works of Hildegard E. Peplau* (pp. 192-204). New York: Springer.

Rix, G. (1988). Care plan for an aggressive person, based on Peplau's model of nursing. In B. Collister (Ed.), *Psychiatric nursing: Person to person* (pp. 119-127). London: Edward Arnold.

Sills, G. M. (1978). Hildegard E. Peplau: Leader, practitioner, academician, scholar and theorist. *Perspectives in Psychiatric Care, 16*(3), 122-128.

Silva, M. C. (1986). Research testing nursing theory: State of the art. *Advances in Nursing Science, 9*(1), 1-11.

Smith, M. J. (1988). Perspectives on nursing science. *Nursing Science Quarterly, 1,* 80-85.

Sullivan, H. S. (1952). *The interpersonal theory of psychiatry.* New York: Norton.

Thompson, L. (1986). Peplau's theory: An application to short-term individual therapy. *Journal of Psychosocial Nursing, 24*(8), 26-31.

Tudor, G. E. (1952). A sociopsychiatric nursing approach to intervention in a problem of mutual withdrawal on a mental hospital ward. *Psychiatry: Journal for the study of Interpersonal Processes, 15*(2).

Walker, L. O., & Avant, K. C. (1988). *Strategies for theory construction in nursing* (2nd ed.). Norwalk, CT: Appleton & Lange.

Woolridge, P. J., Schmitt, M. H., Skipper, J. K., & Leonard, R. C. (1983). *Behavioral science and nursing theory.* Toronto: C. V. Mosby.

PART XI

Betty Neuman

The Neuman Systems Model

KAREN S. REED

Biographical Sketch of the Nurse Theorist:
Betty Neuman, PhD, RN

Born: 1924, on a farm in southeastern Ohio

Family: Two brothers; husband, Kree; child, Nancy

Educational background: RN, Peoples Hospital, Akron, Ohio, 1947, as part of the Cadet Nurse Corps; BSN, UCLA, 1957; MS in public health-mental health, UCLA, 1966; PhD in clinical psychology, Pacific Western University, 1985

Positions: 1967, assumed chairmanship of the program from which she had graduated, where she began a program of post-master's-degree work for psychiatric nurses in the area of community mental health clinical specialty—the first such program in the nation; 1978-1979, Curriculum Consultant, Ohio University, Athens, Ohio; 1979-1980, Continuing Education Director, Ohio University; 1981 to present, consultant, lecturer, author

Basic philosophy: Helping each other live

Foreword

It has been 20 years since Betty Neuman published the first and primary article on the Neuman systems model in nursing research. Entitled "A Model for Teaching Total Person Approach to Patient Problems," the article reveals Neuman's creativity and purpose for her work. Nursing students needed a unifying focus in which to place their practice. Twenty years later, nursing students more than ever need to develop a client-centered and holistic context for their learning and their practice.

The Neuman systems model

- Provides a worldview of nursing that embraces a systems approach
- Maintains the centrality of the client to plans of care
- Clearly establishes nursing as a unique practice that addresses the client system (individual, family, or community) in relationship with the environment

The Neuman systems model systematically describes what occurs in nursing, provides a holistic approach to care, and, when used in practice and research, generates new concepts and theories relevant for nursing. To have been a pioneer in the application of the Neuman model to curriculum development and client approach and to have had the privilege of her trust and mentorship is to have received the most precious of gifts. Eagerly, I look forward to future developments in the use of the Neuman systems model in education, practice, and research that will be undertaken by those undergraduate students who become tomorrow's generation of nurse researchers.

I would like to acknowledge the work and wisdom of Karen Reed for providing the undergraduate student with this section on the Neuman systems model and Betty Neuman, author and theorist, for her relentless energy and commitment to knowledge development as a "letting go" process.

ROSALIE MIRENDA
Professor, Nursing
Neumann College, Aston, Pennsylvania

Acknowledgments

I am deeply grateful for the support and assistance of Betty Neuman and Rosalie Mirenda during this project. Their encouragement and willingness to help made this assignment the ultimate learning experience.

I also thank Donna Neff for her help in preparing the manuscript.

58

Origin of the Theory

In 1970, Betty Neuman designed a "teaching tool" for use with graduate students. She developed and coordinated a course requested by UCLA graduate nursing students that would provide an overview of course content. Selected faculty presented the overview course, which formed the new programming for clinical specialized teaching in areas such as psychiatric and gerontologic nursing. The purpose of the course was to aid entering graduate students in making appropriate clinical nurse specialization program choices.

A 2-year student evaluation confirmed the value of the "tool" for both course unification and integration of faculty lecture content. It also provided a comprehensive perspective from which to view the entire client situation. Neuman and a colleague published the diagram entitled "A Total Person Approach to Patient Problems," course evaluation, and results in the spring 1972 issue of *Nursing Research.* To date, the diagram remains unchanged but now is known as the "Neuman systems model." Her early work made explicit to nursing the importance of taking a holistic view of clients through identification of the five client system variables and the importance of their interrelationship with the environment.

In the first nursing models text, *Conceptual Models for Nursing Practice* (Riehl & Roy, 1974), Riehl classified the original diagram or

Author's Note: The author gratefully acknowledges the extensive use of material provided by Dr. Neuman in the writing of this section.

"tool" for the overview course as a systems model for nursing and titled it the "Betty Neuman health-care systems model," and then added its earlier title, "A Total Person Approach to Patient Problems," when presenting it in their text. Neuman developed an assessment/intervention tool and other data to clarify further the intent and purpose as well as how to use her work for the Riehl and Roy publication.

Further refinement of the model by Neuman and others in nursing continues. In 1982, Neuman edited her first book, *The Neuman Systems Model: Application to Nursing Education and Practice.* In this volume, 50 authors joined Neuman in describing the use of the model in a variety of educational and clinical settings. A more recent edition (Neuman, 1989) expanded on the original work. Plans are in progress for the third edition of the book, which will illustrate the work's increased usage worldwide.

Refinement of model concepts has continued over the past 20 years. Neuman has incorporated an additional fifth dimension, or variable (spirituality), that was not in the original work. The concept environment was expanded to include the created environment. A nursing process format, an assessment intervention tool, and a prevention-as-intervention process available in the 1974 Riehl and Roy text have been refined and expanded as "tools" for the implementation of the model.

Work continues in the use and clarification of the model in clinical and educational settings. Research focusing on testing of the model has begun. More than 50 countries worldwide are using the model in both educational and practice settings. Thus it is one of the three most widely used nursing models in existence.

Neuman continues to expand and clarify the model. She sees her present role as both networker and facilitator of the model's use. As such, she spends a large amount of time helping others understand and implement the model in a variety of health settings. During fall 1988, as a means to safeguard the integrity and further development of the Neuman systems model, she organized the Neuman systems model Trustees Group, Inc., her purpose being to "preserve, protect, and perpetuate the integrity of the Model for the future of nursing" (Neuman, 1989, p. 467).

59

The Neuman Systems Model:
Assumptions and Concepts

Assumptions of the Model

As with many nursing frameworks, the base of Neuman's work is from theoretical foundations outside nursing. The foundations of Neuman's model are primarily Selye's stress theory, von Bertalanffy's general systems theory, Caplan's levels of prevention, Lewis's field theory, and De Chardin's philosophy of life. These perspectives support the idea that a holistic viewpoint of humans is crucial (Fawcett, 1984). The Neuman model is considered a systems model. In a systems model the main focus is on the interaction of the parts, or subsystems, within the system. A systems perspective allows the nurse to view not only the pieces of the puzzle (or subsystems) but also the effect of each piece on all the other pieces. This perspective also illuminates the impact of the system on other systems. This multilevel, multifaceted method of viewing clients is one of the hallmarks of any systems model and, in particular, the Neuman model.

Some basic beliefs about person, health, environment, and nursing are necessary to understand when using the Neuman model. These basic beliefs are called assumptions: They provide the "bottom line" when using a theoretical framework.

The following assumptions are found in the Neuman model (Neuman, 1989, pp. 77, 21, 22):

1. Though each individual client or group as a client system is unique, each system is a composite of common known factors or innate characteristics within a normal, given range of response contained within a basic structure.

2. Many known, unknown, and universal environmental stressors exist. Each differs in its potential for disturbing a client's usual stability level, or normal line of defense. The particular interrelationships of client variables—physiological, psychological, sociocultural, developmental, and spiritual—at any point in time can affect the degree to which a client is protected by the flexible line of defense against possible reaction to a single stressor or combination of stressors.

3. Each individual client/client system, over time, has evolved a normal range of response to the environment that is referred to as a normal line of defense, or usual wellness/stability state.

4. When the cushioning, accordionlike effect of the flexible line of defense is no longer capable of protecting the client/client system against an environmental stressor, the stressor breaks through the normal line of defense. The interrelationships of variables—physiological, psychological, sociocultural, developmental, and spiritual—determine the nature and degree of the system reaction or possible reaction to the stressor invasion.

5. The client, whether in a state of wellness or illness, is a dynamic composite of the interrelationships of variables—physiological, psychological, sociocultural, developmental, and spiritual. Wellness is on a continuum of available energy to support the system in its optimal state.

6. Implicit within each client system is a set of internal resistance factors, known as lines of resistance (resources), which function to stabilize and return the client to the usual wellness state (normal line of defense) or possibly to a higher level of stability following an environmental stressor reaction.

7. Primary prevention relates to general knowledge that is applied in client assessment and intervention in identification and reduction or mitigation of risk factors associated with environmental stressors to prevent possible stressor reaction.

8. Secondary prevention relates to symptomatology following a reaction to stressors, appropriate ranking of intervention priorities, and treatment to reduce their noxious effects.

9. Tertiary prevention relates to the adjustive processes taking place as reconstitution begins and maintenance factors move the client back in a circular manner toward primary prevention.
10. The client is in dynamic constant energy exchange with the environment.

Concepts of the Model

Concepts are abstract ideas that describe a collection of thoughts or behaviors that often are hard to pinpoint. Happiness, life, and self-esteem are examples of concepts. Neuman's model concentrates on explaining a person's reaction to stressors in the environment. Six major concepts are used to describe this phenomenon: client, variables, environment, stressors, wellness, and nursing intervention (see Figure 59.1).

Client System

A series of concentric circles surrounding a core, or basic structure, depicts the client system in the Neuman model. Each line of defense or resistance has certain distinct properties, but the main function is to protect the basic structure and help maintain the system in a stable state.

In Neuman's model the term *client* is a synonym for the nursing metaparadigm concept "person." The term *client* indicates a collaborative relationship between caregiver and care receiver and focuses on the wellness perspective of the model. Neuman defines *client* as "an unlimited entity with an active personality system, whose evolution follows principles, symbolism, and systemic organizations. . . . It is not always possible to see the potential expansions of this entity and the ramifications of its actions" (Neuman, 1989, p. 11).

In the Neuman model, the client can be defined as any system that interacts with the environment. Therefore, the client may be defined as an individual, family, group, or community. The definition used for client depends on the nurse's population of interest.

Because Neuman believes the client to be open, the relationship of the client to the environment is reciprocal. Therefore, the client both influences and is influenced by the environment. For example, if a nonsmoker works in an office surrounded by smokers, the individual

CLIENT   ENVIRONMENT
    basic structure   internal
    lines of resistance   external
    normal line of defense   created
    flexible line of defense

VARIABLES   STRESSORS
    physiological   intrapersonal
    psychological   interpersonal
    developmental   extrapersonal
    sociocultural
    spiritual

NURSING INTERVENTIONS   WELLNESS
    primary intervention   entropy
    secondary intervention   negentropy
    tertiary intervention
    reconstitution

Figure 59.1. Key concepts of the Neuman systems model.
SOURCE: Reprinted by permission of Betty Neuman.

will be influenced by the environment. He or she may have an increase in respiratory illnesses due to the inhalation of secondary smoke. However, if the nonsmoker circulates a petition to designate smoking and nonsmoking sections within the office environment, he or she is influencing the environment to decrease the stressors.

A circle surrounded by a series of concentric rings graphically represents the client (see Figure 59.2). The rings act as a protective structure for the inner circle, known as the basic structure. The basic structure includes the innate energy resources necessary for the survival of the client. These resources are conceptualized as the survival factors of the species, the genetic features, and strengths and weaknesses of the system parts. For example, if the client is defined as an individual person, then the basic structure would include the mechanisms for maintaining a normal temperature range, the genetic response patterns, and the strength or weakness of body organs (Neuman, 1989).

If a family is considered the client, then the basic structure includes resources for survival of the family unit. This includes the genetic pool

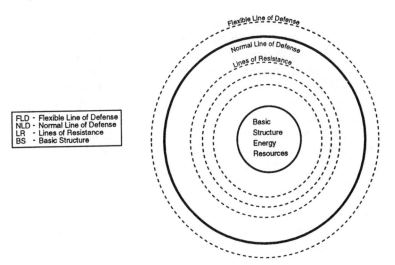

Figure 59.2. The client system.
SOURCE: Adapted from the Neuman systems model diagram by permission of Betty Neuman.

of the individuals within the family, financial resources to maintain the family, and the ethnic or cultural history that provides and maintains the family identity.

The concentric rings around the basic structure (Figure 59.3) form the basis of resource protection for the core of the system. The outer ring, known as the *flexible line of defense* (FLD), forms the outer boundary of the client. This boundary functions to protect the normal line of defense or the usual state of wellness of the client. The flexible line of defense is a buffer for the client and is the first line of defense in response to stressors from the environment. The client uses the flexible line of defense not only to keep the normal state of wellness from being compromised but also to improve the normal state of wellness. The flexible line of defense is accordionlike in nature, expanding or contracting, depending on the needs of the client. As the flexible line of defense expands, it provides more protection; as it contracts, it provides less protection. The ability of the flexible line of defense to function as a buffer relates directly to the type, amount, and strength of stressors within the environment in relationship to the response or reaction of the client. If the number and virility of environmental stressors increase, the buffer system is hard pressed to keep these stressors from impacting the normal functioning of the client. As with a bumper on a car, if the speed of the car increases (increased stressors) and the car comes into contact with a brick wall (increased stressor), the bumper will not be able to protect the car and passengers within the car from damage.

The *normal line of defense* (NLD) is the client's usual state of wellness. It becomes the baseline, or standard of functioning, for the client. The normal line of defense develops over time and is affected by not only internal factors that influence the ability to maintain wellness but also external factors. External factors influencing the baseline functioning of a client include environmental stressors of a chronic nature (such as pollution, altitude, etc.) to which the client has adapted. Internal factors influencing the baseline functioning include patterns of health behaviors, lifestyle, and cultural influences. If a stressor breaks through the flexible line of defense and comes in contact with the normal line of defense, a reaction will occur within the system. Typically, the client will exhibit symptoms of instability or illness, caused by the disruption of the normal stable state.

The *lines of resistance* (LR) are closest to the basic structure and function as a protective mechanism for the basic structure. The main purpose of the lines of resistance is to protect the basic structure's integrity. They become activated following a stressor invasion through the normal line of defense. If the lines of resistance are effective in their protection, the system is able to reconstitute and return to a steady state. When lines of resistance are ineffective, death of the system may occur.

Variables

In earlier writings, Neuman (1982) identified only four variables: physiological, sociocultural, psychological, developmental. She since has incorporated the spiritual variable into the model (Neuman, 1989). As she states, "The spiritual variable is viewed as an innate component of the basic structure, whether or not it is ever acknowledged or developed by the client or client system—it influences the system" (B. Neuman, personal communication, 1992).

According to Neuman, inherent within the client are five different variables that are similar to domains of function within the system:

(a) physiological, relating to body structure and function; (b) psychological, dealing with mental processes and relationships; (c) sociocultural, focusing on social and cultural influences; (d) developmental, including life developmental processes; and (e) spiritual, incorporating the belief influences, creative aspects, and essence of life.

These five variables may be at various levels of development. The variables pertaining to a child are not as developed as those of an adult. There is unlimited potential for interaction among the five variables. A term coined to describe the interaction has been "leaky margins" (C. Beynon, personal communication, 1991). For example, communication patterns used by the client (a psychological variable) often are influenced by the values of the society in which the client was raised (a sociocultural variable).

Environment

The environment is an important influencing concept of the Neuman model. It is defined as those forces surrounding man, both internal and external (Neuman, 1989). The internal and external environmental stress factors may have a positive or negative influence on the client. In the Neuman model, the three environmental typologies identified are *internal, external,* and *created.*

The *internal environment* (intrapersonal) "consists of all forces or interactive influences internal to or contained solely within the boundaries of the client" (Neuman, 1989, p. 31). The internal environment describes the result of relationships among the subsystems of the client. For the individual, this might be the interaction of one body subsystem with another. In a family as client, the interactions of subsystems would be those of the individual family members with one another.

The *external environment* consists of influences of an interpersonal, or extrapersonal, nature. These influences are outside the boundaries of the client. With an individual client, the external environment refers to the interaction of the client with another person such as a work colleague or a family member. With a family system as client, the external environment may include extended family or neighbors. Therefore, what may be an internal environment to one system may become an external environment to another. The crucial point is in defining the client system as one of interacting parts.

The *created environment,* a newer term to the Neuman systems model, is the client's attempt to create a safe setting for functioning (Neuman, 1990). An environment is created by the client if the client perceives a threat to the basic structure and function of the system. Neuman describes the created environment as largely made up of unconscious mechanisms that come into play as the system interprets the need. The client may use not only internal but also external cues to create a safe haven from which to operate.

An example of creating an environment is the process a person goes through when moving to a new location. The external environment is new and unfamiliar. It is a new city, new state, or new neighborhood. To decrease the feeling of discomfort or threat at the change in environment, one arranges furniture in the new house in a pattern similar to that in the previous home. Patterns of behavior also are kept, such as morning coffee and the newspaper or routines of exercise, all to ease into and feel less vulnerable in a new situation. This rearranging of the environment is not a conscious act to decrease stress. Rather, it is an unconscious attempt to reduce the disparity between the new and unfamiliar and the old and safe. The main goal of a created environment is to maintain system integrity, thereby allowing the system to function in a safe arena. When assessing the existence of a created environment it is important to consider what environment has been created, how it has been used, and how it will be used by the client to maintain optimal system functioning (Neuman, 1989).

Stressors

Stressors are a part of the environment. Neuman (1989) defines them as "tension producing stimuli with the potential for causing disequilibrium. . . . More than one stressor may be imposed upon the client at any given time" (p. 23). They may be present within or outside the client (see Figure 59.3). The typology of stressors includes the following:

1. *Intrapersonal stressors*—internal environmental interaction forces occurring within the boundary of the client, between client subsystems

Stressors
- Identified
- Classified as to knows
  or possibilities, i.e.
  - Loss
  - Pain
  - Sensory deprivation
  - Cultural change

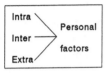

Stressors
- More than one stressor
  could occur
  simultaneously
- Same stressors could vary
  as to impact or reaction
- Normal defense line varies
  with age and development

Figure 59.3. Stressors within the environment.
SOURCE: Adapted from the Neuman systems model diagram by permission of Betty Neuman.

2. *Interpersonal stressors*—external environmental interaction forces occurring outside the boundary of the client but at proximal range
3. *Extrapersonal stressors*—external environmental interaction forces occurring outside the boundary of the client at distal range

The stressor's effect on the client is related to two factors: the strength of the stressor and the number of stressors impinging on the client at any given time. However, the stressor's effect also is related to the client's ability to protect against the stressor or change its effect on the system. Therefore, each client may have a different reaction to similar environmental stressors.

For example, an individual who makes a decision to return to school for an advanced degree may decide to continue working full-time. However, few students are able to manage the stress of being enrolled full-time in school while working full-time. The additional stress of class attendance, homework, and faculty expectations to the normal stress load typically decreases sleep time, disrupts patterns of eating and exercise, and reduces leisure time. Such activities help maintain the flexible line of defense. Therefore, the student has weakened the flexible line of defense and may find oneself more susceptible to infections and disease, thus becoming ill when he or she can least afford to.

Wellness

In the Neuman model, health status is reflected by the level of client *wellness*. Health and wellness are considered to be the same (Neuman, 1989). When system needs are fully met, a state of optimal wellness exists and the client is healthy. Conversely, unmet needs reduce the wellness state. Wellness is a condition where all subsystems are in balance and harmony with the whole of the client. Varying degrees of health exist, depending on the balance between met and unmet needs of the client. Thus health is on a continuum from wellness to illness. The wellness of the client is based on the actual or potential effect that environmental stressors have on the energy level of the system. For example, it requires less energy output to maintain a high degree of wellness for a client if the environment is not impaired by air and water pollution.

When more energy is produced than used, the client is moving toward *negentropy*, or a wellness state. When the system produces less energy than is required, movement of the client is toward *entropy*, or illness (Neuman, 1989). The greater the entropy state, the greater the imbalance between the needs of the system and the energy available. Energy conservation is critical to the goal of system stability.

Nursing Interventions

Nursing's goal is to keep the client stable. In systems terms, the maintenance of stability requires that interventions are directed toward counteracting movement toward entropy, or illness. Neuman (1989) describes nursing interventions by using the term *prevention*. There are three types of prevention: *primary*, *secondary*, and *tertiary*. The three levels of prevention are used to attain, maintain, and retain wellness by assisting system stability (see Figure 59.4).

Primary prevention is intervention aimed at protecting the normal line of defense by (a) increasing the flexible line of defense's ability to withstand environmental stressors and (b) decreasing risk factors.

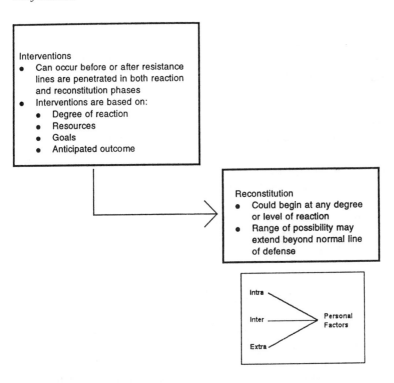

Figure 59.4. Levels of prevention and reconstitution.
SOURCE: Adapted from the Neuman systems model diagram by permission of Betty Neuman.

Nurses use *secondary prevention* interventions when the normal line of defense is disrupted, resulting in client symptoms. Secondary prevention is aimed at strengthening the system's lines of resistance and thus protecting the basic structure (see Figure 59.4). *Tertiary prevention* focuses on helping the client regain or return to a wellness state following treatment. The term *reconstitution* describes the process of returning to a wellness state: "Reconstitution may be viewed as feedback from the input and output of secondary intervention. The goal is to maintain an optimal wellness level by supporting existing strengths and conserving client energy" (Neuman, 1989, p. 37).

The Neuman model provides a framework from which to view the person as a system based on systems theory. The concepts—client system, variables, environment, stressors, wellness, and nursing interventions—are derived from a variety of systems-, stress-, and mental-health-related theories. The Neuman model is built on the assumption that the interaction of environment and client has both direct and indirect effects on the client's ability to maintain a state of wellness. The goal of nursing is to provide assistance for the client to best attain and maintain system stability as an optimal condition of wellness. When it becomes impossible for the client to conserve energy, the client is assisted in a peaceful and meaningful death.

In conclusion, the Neuman systems model comprises six major concepts that explain and examine the interaction of persons with the environment. The Neuman model provides a framework for describing the process that occurs as clients maintain, attain, or retain health during encounters with stressors. It is a multilevel, multidimensional systems model that allows for describing very complex situations (see Figure 59.5).

The Neuman Nursing Process

The nursing process as identified by Neuman includes all the common steps of the nursing process: assessment, planning, intervention, and evaluation. However, it was "designed specifically for nursing implementation of the Neuman systems model" (Neuman, 1989, p. 40) and contains three steps: nursing diagnosis, nursing goals, and nursing outcomes. The Neuman nursing process is used in conjunction with the "prevention as intervention" format, which is described later.

A nursing diagnosis is derived following assessment of the impact of stressors or potential stressors on the client system and the relative strength of the client system. The assessment process provides the evidence for a diagnostic statement that accurately describes the client's condition. Once the diagnosis is developed, it becomes the basis for nursing goals and outcomes. Nursing goals are developed to assist the client toward retaining a state of wellness. Nursing outcomes are determined by using primary, secondary, or tertiary interventions as necessary and evaluating the outcome goals once the intervention has taken place.

A unique aspect of the Neuman nursing process is the emphasis on client input. In the first step, the nurse verifies her or his perceptions with the client in terms of the meaning of the stressor and the

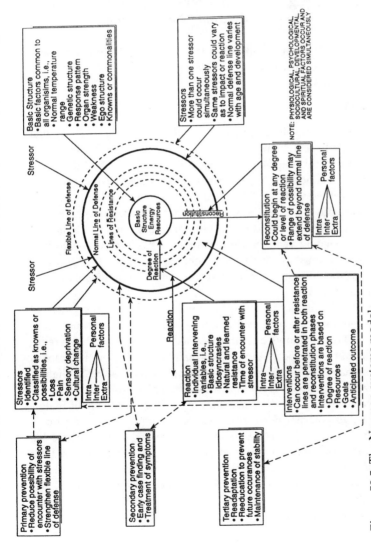

Figure 59.5. The Neuman systems model.
SOURCE: Reprinted by permission of Betty Neuman.
NOTE: Spiritual variable added.

535

strengths and weaknesses of the system. Client input also is important in terms of the nursing goals and evaluating outcome. Client negotiation is viewed as necessary in formulating the nursing intervention goals. Intervention outcomes also are verified with the client.

Using the Neuman Nursing Process
With an Individual Client System

The following is an example of the use of the Neuman nursing process with an individual.

Case Example

Mr. L is a 49-year-old divorced male with two children. He has come to the clinic to seek help for depression following the breakup of a long-term relationship. For the past 3 weeks he has had difficulty sleeping and concentrating. He obsessively thinks about the woman he was involved with. Mr. L finds himself crying and feeling as if his world has ended. He denies wanting to harm himself or others.

Mr. L has been divorced for 15 years. His marriage was a stormy one that lasted 12 years. Since that time he has been involved in a series of relationships. Only two were serious enough to think of marriage, including this most recent one. The last relationship was of 1½ years' duration.

Mr. L has a history of seven hospitalizations in his life. Three of these were for acute pancreatitis, and one was for treatment of acute gastritis. Mr. L acknowledges that he used to drink alcohol on a regular basis but for the past 8 months has maintained sobriety. He smokes approximately two packs of cigarettes per day. He appears slightly overweight and looks older than his stated age. His blood pressure is elevated at 180/90. There is a history of cardiac disease on his maternal side; his paternal side is negative for major physical illness but is positive for unipolar and bipolar depression. He eats most of his meals at fast-food restaurants and rarely cooks at home. He does little physical activity outside his job, which is fairly sedentary.

Mr. L has had custody of his children since they were ages 12 and 10. Both children have graduated from high school in the past 3 years and are gainfully employed. Mr. L himself did not finish high school but obtained a GED while in the army. He has been employed at the same factory since being discharged from the army.

Mr. L's family lives in the area. He is not particularly close to any of them and sees them infrequently. His relationship with his children is at present tenuous. His younger child, a son, is contemplating moving back home so he can go to school. Since Mr. L's last bout with alcohol, his daughter has refused to speak with him.

Mr. L does not have any hobbies or leisure activities that he pursues on a regular basis. He admits to being "crazy about cars" and has in the past bought several classic cars in order to restore them. However, he tends to lose interest in the middle of the project and often must pay others to complete the restorations. He spends most of his time working at the factory and seeing his friends in the bar. He acknowledges that this has been difficult for him lately because he is trying to maintain sobriety.

When asked to clarify why he has sought help, he states that he is tired of choosing the wrong kind of woman to have a relationship with and wants to learn how to make better choices. He cannot understand why his last girlfriend decided she needed to see other people and why their relationship wasn't enough to satisfy her.

The Neuman Nursing Process Applied

   I. Nursing Diagnosis
   A. Database
      1. Actual and potential stressors
         a. Actual: Mr. L has experienced the breakup of a long-term relationship, he recently quit drinking, and his relationship with his daughter is strained.
         b. Potential: Mr. L's adult child (son) is planning to move back into his home; there is a possibility of a relapse of alcoholic behavior. Mr. L has a potential for suicidal behavior.
      2. Structure assessment
         a. Basic structure (strengths and weaknesses): Mr. L is moderately obese and has a family history of alcoholism, cardiac disease, and depression. He has a history of alcohol use. Mr. L is financially stable at the present time. He has a history of difficulty maintaining close relationships with females.

    b. Lines of defense, resistance (strengths and weaknesses): Mr. L is a well-groomed, articulate 49-year-old male. He completed a GED while in the army. Mr. L has been gainfully employed at the same institution for 23 years. He has maintained sobriety for 8 months. There is no suicidal ideation present. Mr. L recognizes the need for help. He has experienced difficulty sleeping through the night and difficulty concentrating for the past 6 weeks. Mr. L has little insight into problems regarding romantic female relationships. He feels that others are responsible for most of his problems. Mr. L does no physical exercise on a regular basis. He eats out at restaurants and his diet is high in fat and sodium. Mr. L works the swing shift at the local factory, which limits his ability to establish a routine regarding sleep habits. Mr. L's leisure time is spent in bars. Since sobriety, he continues to go to the bars but drinks nonalcoholic beer. His relationship with his daughter is poor; his relationship with his son is good. Male friendships are limited to casual acquaintances. Mr. L has little interaction with other family members.

B. Variances From Wellness

    1. Synthesis of theory: The client has a weakened flexible line of defense as evidenced by lack of healthy routines established to help him cope with stressors. His past coping mechanisms have focused on the use of alcohol. Few psychological resources are used at present, as evidenced by the lack of social support and an unwillingness to look at the interpersonal dynamics of the situation. Mr. L prefers to blame others for his problems. There is a need for an external support system to stabilize the client system and begin reconstitution. Mr. L's structure is intact, but there are inherent weaknesses related to a familial history of alcoholism, cardiac illness, and depression.

    2. Hypothetical interventions: Provide psychoeducational readings on dependent behaviors, alcoholism, and medications. Monitor effects of antidepressant medications. Work with client to modify physical activity routines and dietary habits. Encourage Mr. L to develop hobbies and to increase interaction with others. Family counseling with son and daughter is recommended.

II. Nursing Goals
   A. Mr. L is willing to read materials on dependency and on medications. He refuses to discuss alcohol intake and states it is not a problem: "I've been sober for 8 months. I can control my drinking."
   B. Mr. L recognizes the need for changes in dietary habits and exercise routines. He sets a goal of walking twice a week for 45 minutes.
   C. Mr. L refuses to enter into family counseling with son and daughter. He states he doesn't need to be lectured by his daughter. He does agree to meet with the counselor after discharge to discuss his interpersonal problems with females.

III. Nursing Outcomes
   A. Readings are given to Mr. L on dependent personalities and on antidepressant medication.
   B. Dietary guidelines are given and discussed. A dietary plan for home is worked out.
   C. Information is given to the son and daughter regarding support groups for Adult Children of Alcoholics.

Intervention Format of the Neuman Model: Prevention as Intervention

One of the areas of the Neuman systems model that has received considerable attention and is in wide use is the prevention-as-intervention format of the model. Both Neuman (1989) and Fawcett (1989) believe this format is the beginning of an important theory to be derived from the Neuman model. However, concepts as yet have not been operationally defined or linked with specific propositions.

Neuman describes the prevention-as-intervention format as a typology. This means it is a way to view the links between environmental stressors, the reaction of the client to stressors, and the role of nursing in helping clients to retain, attain, or maintain wellness. The three levels described in the prevention-as-intervention format are primary, secondary, and tertiary.

In primary prevention, the goal is the retention of wellness. Wellness is retained by strengthening the flexible line of defense and reducing risk factors. Primary prevention interventions concentrate on decreasing the amount of stress in the environment or on increasing the client's ability to withstand stress. Increasing the ability to withstand stress, in Neuman model terms, is known as strengthening the flexible line of defense. Thus the goal of primary prevention intervention is to protect the client system's normal line of defense, or functioning at an optimal level.

Intervention may occur any time an actual or potential stressor is identified. Potential stressors are situations that have the potential for disrupting the client system. In potential stressful situations, the client system has not yet reacted to the stressor. For example, if the client system is identified as an expectant family, a potential stressor for the system would be the introduction of a new member into the system. Primary prevention activities for the parents might include attendance at prenatal classes to prepare for childbirth. In Neuman terms, this would be considered a measure to strengthen the family unit's flexible line of defense. Primary prevention also would include helping the parents look at ways to reduce the amount of stress in their environment by changing work schedules and increasing support systems.

Secondary prevention is used any time a reaction to a stressor occurs and the normal state of wellness is disrupted, resulting in overt symptoms being identified. In secondary prevention, the goal is to protect the client's basic functioning and facilitate a return to wellness. In Neuman terms, this means that because stressors have penetrated the normal line of defense, the internal lines of resistance must be strengthened to protect the basic structure. This strengthening is done by providing appropriate treatment, using client resources, and helping the client conserve energy to deal with the stressor effects.

To use the previous illustration, suppose the birth of the child was premature. Such an event would increase the strength of the original stressor, the addition of a family member. As such, the stressor has broken through the normal line of defense (state of wellness) for the family unit. This breakthrough is evidenced by the infant's hospitalization and the overt stress symptoms in the family. Symptoms seen within the family might include tension between parents, other siblings seeking increased attention from parents, financial strain on the family unit, physical exhaustion, and changes in work arrangements to be with the infant. Secondary prevention interventions would focus on the symptoms of system distress. These interventions would include actions such as providing opportunities for the family to witness the caregiving of the infant, teaching the parents about a premature infant, and helping the family mobilize adequate or needed support from outside resources.

Tertiary prevention is used to maintain wellness after treatment by supporting existing strengths and conserving client system energy. Tertiary prevention is closely linked to reconstitution. Reconstitution is defined as "the return and maintenance of system stability, following treatment of stressor reaction" (Neuman, 1989, p. 50). Because of stressor invasion the client system may or may not return to the previous level of wellness that was available before the stressor impact. Interventions at the tertiary level focus on helping the client system attain or maintain the best possible level of wellness following treatment and help the client conserve as much energy as possible.

Using the previous example, tertiary prevention would focus on helping the family incorporate a premature infant into the home following discharge from the hospital. This incorporation includes providing education and comfort to the family as well as monitoring the infant's physical and developmental progress. It also includes continuing to support parents as needed and determined by the parents in concert with the nurse.

60

Application to Practice and Research

In the past 20 years the use of the Neuman systems model to guide practice and research has grown exponentially. In the beginning the model was primarily used in academia, fulfilling Neuman's original idea that the model should be used as a teaching aid (Neuman, 1989). Initially, the model was used as a teaching method. Subsequently, it was used to organize the entire nursing curricula. The nursing program at Neumann College in Aston, Pennsylvania, was in the early 1970s the first college to do so. Since that time, numerous colleges and universities around the nation and the world have based both baccalaureate and graduate nursing programs on the model.

With students becoming cognizant and comfortable with the model during their educational experience, the next logical step was an increase in the application of the model in practice and research. In both editions of Neuman's book (1982, 1989), the vast majority of the material presented focuses on the application of the model in practice and research. Examples of application are not limited to these two volumes. A listing of material found in the literature that uses the Neuman systems model is included in the bibliography. Several of the sources included in the bibliography are discussed here in further detail as examples of how the Neuman model has been used in practice and research.

Practice

Individual Client Systems

The Neuman systems model has been used to describe individuals, families, and communities as client systems. With the individual as client system, the Neuman model has been used to support assessment and intervention models for a variety of age groups and clinical situations. The model has been used to develop a method of assessing nutritional status in both newborns (Torkington, 1988) and adult populations (Gavan, Hastings-Tolsma, & Troyan, 1988). Moore and Munro (1990) used the model to describe a method of assessing the mental health needs of older adults, and Herrick, Goodykoontz, Herrick, and Kackett (1991) developed a continuum of care for disturbed children: "The continuum provides a guide for nurses and other health care providers to achieve high quality care as economically as possible" (p. 41).

The Neuman model has been used in working with clients with multiple sclerosis (MS). Knight (1990) reports that the model is especially effective in describing the MS patient because the open system approach to viewing clients allows for the complex and often unpredictable situations found in MS clients. Brown (1988) used the model to examine risk-factor reduction in myocardial infarction patients, as well as to develop a plan of care.

Family Client Systems

Several authors have described the use of the Neuman model in assessment and planning of care for families in a variety of situations. Beckingham and Baumann (1990) presented an assessment and decision-making model for use with elderly families. Included is a schematic model of assessment that delineates the steps necessary for assessing elderly clients. With the same population, Delunas (1990) describes the process of assessing families who are at high risk for elder abuse. Using the model, an assessment system is iterated that focuses on intra-, inter-, and extrafamily stressors, giving nurses a means to assess the family as to their ability to care for an elder in the home without risk of abuse.

On the other end of the age spectrum, Wallingford (1989) describes the ability of the Neuman model to provide a framework for caring for families with a neurologically impaired child, including preparation for death. The stress of an impaired member, especially a child, can be devastating to a family. The article goes step by step to describe the impact of the chronic illness on the family system and specifies ways in which the nurse can help the family reconstitute.

The family and its interaction with the community also has been investigated. Authors such as Buchanan (1987) and Story and Ross (1986) describe the development of family assessment in community health nursing. One project that has been implemented is the system at the Middlesex-London Health Unit in London, Ontario, Canada. This health unit has implemented a family-based service model for the entire nursing division of the public health department (Drew, Craig, & Beynon, 1989).

Research

Use of the Neuman model as a conceptual framework for research has increased remarkably in the past 10 years. As examples, four studies are used here to illustrate the state of research with the Neuman model.

The Neuman model was used as a basis for an interview guide in a research study that examined the needs of cancer patients and their caregivers (Blank, Clark, Longman, & Atwood, 1989). The interview guides were developed to assess patient and caregiver stressors. Stressors were categorized as intra-, inter-, and extrapersonal. Blank et al. (1989) state, "The Neuman Framework is most appropriate for the purpose of addressing the home-care needs of cancer patients and their caregivers" (p. 81).

Leja (1989) investigated the effectiveness of guided imagery on depressed elderly clients following surgery using a quasi-experimental, nonequivalent control group design. The hypotheses for the study were that (a) older adults would have significantly lower depression scored 1 week following guided imagery teaching and (b) subjects who received guided imagery teaching would have significantly lower depression scores than subjects who received regular discharge teaching. Patients were asked to complete the Beck Depression Inventory prior to discharge. Following completion of the inventory, patients in the experimental group received guided imagery teaching; those in the control group received standard discharge teaching. Depression inventories were then mailed to the participants following discharge, with instructions to complete and return the material to the researcher.

Results of the study showed that patients who received guided imagery teaching did have lower scores of depression following discharge. This supported the first hypothesis. However, there was no difference between the experimental and control groups in post-discharge depression scores. Both groups were less depressed following discharge, no matter what type of intervention was used. Therefore, the author was not able to conclude that guided imagery was more effective than regular discharge teaching. The lack of support for the hypothesis may have been due to the small sample size ($n = 10$). However, the author identified discharge following surgical hospitalization as an additional stressor and the use of guided imagery as a primary prevention measure.

Ali and Khalil (1989) used the Neuman model to provide the theoretical rationale for studying the effect of psychoeducational preparation on patients' anxiety levels prior to cancer surgery. They hypothesized that the stress of a cancer diagnosis and the anticipation of surgery would increase the anxiety level of patients, thus weakening their flexible line of defense. The treatment, psychoeducational preparation, was to "raise the patients' line of defense and reduce their anxiety post operatively and before discharge" (Ali & Khalil, 1989, p. 238). The findings of the study supported their hypotheses and interventions.

Areas of congruence between personal and contextual factors and the assumptions of the Neuman model were explored by Hinds (1990). Quality-of-life issues were examined with a sample of lung cancer patients ($n = 87$). The seven factors studied accounted for 30% of the explained variance in reports of quality of life among the patients. Hinds described the fit of Neuman's assumptions with the client population. Lung cancer patients were described as systems whose "basic client structure is under attack and client survival is threatened" (p. 460).

Evidence of testing of the Neuman model can be found in the literature. Hoch (1987) compared the Roy's adaptation model and Neuman's model. She found no difference in the two approaches to patient care but did find a significant difference when comparing the groups who had nursing-theory-based care to those who did not. Quayhagen and Roth (1989) analyzed the fit of the Neuman model with available family assessment measurements. They identified 20 different scales, indexes, and inventories needed to measure the conceptual domains in the Neuman framework. Reed (1993) describes the process in developing a family assessment model to test placement of family concepts within the Neuman model.

In summary, the Neuman model is well represented in the nursing literature. The model is used in a wide variety of clinical settings with many different client populations. It has proven to be a most popular mechanism for structuring nursing care. Research supporting the model's concepts is at a beginning level of sophistication. Much work is needed in the area of concept development and measurement of constructs.

Glossary

Central core
The basic structure of survival factors "common to the species, such as variables contained within, innate or genetic factors, and strength and weakness of the system parts" (Neuman, 1989, p. 172).

Client/client system
An open system in interaction with the environment, composed of variables (physiological, psychological, sociocultural, developmental, and spiritual) that form the whole of the client. The client as a system is composed of a core or basic structure of survival factors and surrounding protective concentric rings. The client system may be an individual, group, family, or community (Neuman, 1989).

Created environment
Unconsciously developed by the client as a "symbolic expression of system wholeness." It is intrapersonal, interpersonal, and extrapersonal in nature. The created environment supersedes and encompasses both internal and external environments (Neuman, 1989, p. 70).

Client system stability
The best possible health state at any given point, where all variables are in balance or harmony with the whole of the client or client system.

Developmental variable
Developmental processes of client system.

Environment
All internal and external factors or influences surrounding the identified client or client system. The relationship between the client or client system and the environment is reciprocal. "Input, output and feedback between the client and environment is of a circular nature [such that] the client may influence or be influenced by environmental forces" (Neuman, 1989, p. 70).

External environment
All forces or interaction influences external to or existing outside the defined client or client system.

Extrapersonal factor
Forces occurring outside the client system.

Family
Primary system responsible for the transmission of social values, psychological growth, and spiritual strength of its members who reside within the system. These functions are transmitted through bonds developed by the interrelatedness and communication of individual members (Reed, 1989, p. 385).

Flexible line of defense
A "dynamic state of wellness; system's current, immediate state which is particularly susceptible to situational circumstances; e.g., amount of sleep, hormone level" (Neuman, 1982, p. 137). The flexible line of defense is the boundary between the client system and the environment.

Goal of nursing
To "facilitate for the client optimal wellness through either retention, attainment or maintenance of client system stability. . . . To assist the client in creating and shaping reality in a desired direction, related to retention, attainment and/or maintenance of optimal system wellness through purposeful interventions . . . directed at mitigation or reduction of stress factors and adverse conditions which affect or could affect optimal client functioning, at any given point of time." (Neuman, 1989, p. 72)

Health
Health "is reflected in the level of wellness. When system needs are met, a state of optimal wellness exists; conversely, unmet needs reduce the wellness state" (Neuman, 1989, p. 71).

Internal environment
All forces or interactive influences internal to or contained solely within the boundaries of the defined client or client system (Neuman, 1989).

Interpersonal factor
A force occurring among two or more client systems.

Intrapersonal factor
A force occurring within the individual.

Lines of resistance
Internal resistant forces that act to decrease the degree of reaction to stressors. They act as resources to help the client return to a stable health condition (B. Neuman, personal communication, 1992).

Normal line of defense
Adaptational state to stressors over time that is considered "normal" for the individual (Neuman, 1989).

Nursing diagnosis
"Acquisition of an appropriate date base that identifies, assesses, classifies, and evaluates the dynamic interactions among the physiological, psychological, sociocultural, developmental, and spiritual variables comprising the client system. This step of the nursing process takes into account the perceptions of both the client and the caregiver" (Fawcett, 1989, p. 177).

Nursing outcomes
Determined by nursing interventions using one or more of the three prevention modes (Neuman, 1989). Outcomes are the desired results of nursing interventions and are stated behaviorally in terms of the patient. They are derived from the nursing diagnoses and correlate with them. They are classified as short term and long term; they also may be classified as immediate, intermediate, and future. Outcomes will change as the patient/client's status and priorities change. The actual outcomes of the prescribed nursing interventions are evaluated in terms of their relation to the stated outcomes (Neuman, 1989).

Neuman nursing process
Designed to implement and facilitate the use of the Neuman systems model for nursing. The nursing process has been systemized into three categories: nursing diagnosis, nursing goals, and nursing outcomes.

Physiologic variable
Bodily structure and function of the client system.

Prevention as intervention
Modes for facilitating integrative processes necessary to retain/attain/maintain stability and integrity of the client or client system. Intervention modes are used within the structure of each of the preventions: primary, secondary, and tertiary (Neuman, 1989).

Primary prevention
Relates to general knowledge that is applied to individual patient assessment in an attempt to identify and allay the possible risk factors associated with environmental stressors. Decreases the possibility of encounter with stressors and strengthens the flexible line of defense in the system to protect the integrity of the normal line of defense.

Psychological variable
Mental processes and relationships of the client system.

Reconstitution
"Represents the return and maintenance of system stability, following treatment of stressor reaction, which may result in a higher or lower level of wellness than previously" (Neuman, 1989, p. 50).

Sociocultural variable
Social and cultural functions of the client system.

Spiritual variable
"Aspects of spirituality. A continuum from complete unawareness or denial to a consciously developed high level of spiritual understanding" (Neuman, 1989).

Stressor
"Any environmental stimulus, problem, or condition capable of causing instability of the system by penetration of the normal line of defense; this may be intra-, inter-, or extrapersonal in nature" (Neuman, 1982, p. 137).

Secondary prevention
Relates to symptomatology, appropriate ranking of intervention priorities, and treatment protocol. Treats system response following stressor penetration of normal line of defense.

Tertiary prevention
Relates to the adaptive process as reconstitution begins, and ultimately moves back in a circular manner toward primary prevention. Assists in repatterning for restoration of the functions that have been altered as a consequence of the response to stressor penetration of the normal line of defense.

Variances from wellness
Determined by comparing the normal health state with what is taking place at a given time period (Neuman, 1989).

References

Ali, N. S., & Khalil, H. Z. (1989). Effect of psychoeducational intervention on anxiety among Egyptian bladder cancer patients. *Cancer Nursing, 12,* 236-242.

Beckingham, A. C., & Baumann, A. (1990). The aging family in crisis: Assessment and decision-making models. *Journal of Advanced Nursing, 15,* 782-787.

Blank, J. J., Clark, L., Longman, A. J., & Atwood, J. R. (1989). Perceived home care needs of cancer patients and their caregivers. *Cancer Nursing, 12,* 78-84.

Brown, M. W. (1988). Neuman's systems model in risk factor reduction. *Cardiovascular Nursing, 24*(6), 43.

Buchanan, B. F. (1987). Human-environment interaction: A modification of the Neuman systems model for aggregates, families, and the community. *Public Health Nursing, 4,* 52-64.

Delunas, L. R. (1990). Prevention of elder abuse: Betty Neuman health care systems approach. *Clinical Nurse Specialist, 4,* 54-58.

Drew, L. L., Craig, D. M., & Beynon, C. E. (1989). The Neuman systems model for community health administration and practice: Provinces of Manitoba and Ontario, Canada. In B. Neuman (Ed.), *The Neuman systems model* (2nd ed., pp. 315-342). Norwalk, CT: Appleton & Lange.

Fawcett, J. (1984). *Analysis and evaluation of conceptual models of nursing.* Philadelphia: F. A. Davis.

Fawcett, J. (1989). *Analysis and evaluation of conceptual models of nursing* (2nd ed.). Philadelphia: F. A. Davis.

Gavan, C. A. S., Hastings-Tolsma, M. T., & Tryan, P. J. (1988). Explication of Neuman's model: A holistic systems approach to nutrition for health promotion in the life process. *Holistic Nursing Practice, 3*(1), 26-38.

Herrick, C. A., Goodykoontz, L., Herrick, R. H., & Kacket, B. (1991). Planning a continuum of care in child psychiatric nursing: A collaborative effort. *Journal of Child and Adolescent Psychiatric and Mental Health Nursing, 4,* 41-48.

552

Hinds, C. (1990). Personal and contextual factors predicting patients' reported quality of life: Exploring congruency with Betty Neuman's assumptions. *Journal of Advanced Nursing, 15,* 456-462.

Hoch, C. C. (1987). Assessing delivery of nursing care: Roy adaptation model and the Neuman health care systems model. Increasing life satisfaction in retired individuals. *Journal of Gerontological Nursing, 13*(1), 10-17.

Knight, J. B. (1990). The Betty Neuman systems model applied to practice: A client with multiple sclerosis. *Journal of Advanced Nursing, 15,* 447-455.

Leja, A. M. (1989). Using guided imagery to combat postsurgical depression. *Journal of Gerontological Nursing, 15*(4), 6-11.

Moore, S. L., & Munro, M. F. (1990). The Neuman systems model applied to mental health nursing of older adults. *Journal of Advanced Nursing, 15,* 293-299.

Neuman, B. (1982). *The Neuman systems model: Application to nursing education and practice.* New York: Appleton-Century-Crofts.

Neuman, B. (1989). *The Neuman systems model* (2nd ed.). Norwalk, CT: Appleton & Lange.

Neuman, B. M. (1990). Health as a continuum based on the Neuman systems model. *Nursing Science Quarterly, 3,* 129-135.

Quayhagen, M. P., & Roth, P. A. (1989). From models to measures in assessment of mature families. *Journal of Professional Nursing, 5,* 144-151.

Reed, K. S. (1989). Family theory related to the Neuman systems model. In B. Neuman (Ed.), *The Neuman systems model* (2nd ed., pp. 385-395). Norwalk, CT: Appleton & Lange.

Reed, K. S. (1993). Adapting the Neuman systems model for family nursing. *Nursing Science Quarterly, 6*(2), 93-97.

Riehl, J. P., & Roy, C. (1974). *Conceptual models for nursing practice.* New York: Appleton-Century-Crofts.

Story, E. L., & Ross, M. M. (1986). Family centered community health nursing and the Betty Neuman systems model. *Nursing Papers, Perspectives in Nursing, 18,* 77-88.

Torkington, S. (1988). Nourishing the infant. *Senior Nurse, 8*(2), 24-25.

Wallingford, P. (1989). The neurologically impaired and dying child: Applying the Neuman systems model. *Issues in Comprehensive Pediatric Nursing, 12,* 139-157.

Bibliography

References Related to Neuman's Work

Aggleton, P., & Chalmers, H. (1989). Neuman's systems model. *Nursing Times, 85*(51), 27-29.

Ali, N. S., & Khalil, H. Z. (1989). Effect of psychoeducational intervention on anxiety among Egyptian bladder cancer patients. *Cancer Nursing, 12,* 236-242.

Baerg, K. L. (1991). Using Neuman's model to analyze a clinical situation. *Rehabilitation Nursing, 16,* 38-39.

Barrett, M. (1991). A thesis is born. *Image: Journal of Nursing Scholarship, 23,* 261-262.

Bass, L. S. (1991). What do parents need when their infant is a patient in the NICU? *Journal of Neonatal Nursing, 10*(1), 25-38.

Beckingham, A. C., & Baumann, A. (1990). The aging family in crisis: Assessment and decision-making models. *Journal of Advanced Nursing, 15,* 782-787.

Berkey, K. M., & Hanson, S. M. H. (1991). *Family assessment and intervention.* St. Louis: C. V. Mosby.

Beyea, S., & Matzo, M. (1989). Assessing elders using the functional health pattern assessment model. *Nurse Educator, 14*(5), 32-37.

Biley, F. (1990). The Neuman model: An analysis. *Nursing* (London), 4(4), 25-28.

Biley, F. C. (1989). Stress in high dependency units. *Intensive Care Nursing, 5,* 134-141.

Blank, J. J., Clark, L., Longman, A. J., & Atwood, J. R. (1989). Perceived home care needs of cancer patients and their caregivers. *Cancer Nursing, 12,* 78-84.

Bonner, M., Sr. (Ed.). (1988). *Proceedings of the First International Nursing Symposium: Neuman systems model.* Aston, PA: Neumann College Nursing Program.

Bourbonnais, F. F., & Ross, M. M. (1985). The Neuman systems model in nursing education, course development and implementation. *Journal of Advanced Nursing, 10,* 117-123.

Bowdler, J. E., & Barrell, L. M. (1987). Health needs of homeless persons. *Public Health Nursing, 4,* 135-140.

Breckenridge, D. M., Cupit, M. C., & Raimond, J. N. (1982). Systematic nursing assessment tool for the CAPD client. *Nephrology Nurse, 24,* 26-27, 30-31.

Brown, M. W. (1988). Neuman's systems model in risk factor reduction. *Cardiovascular Nursing, 24*(6), 43.

Buchanan, B. F. (1987). Human-environment interaction: A modification of the Neuman systems model for aggregates, families, and the community. *Public Health Nursing, 4,* 52-64.

Burke, S. O., & Maloney, R. (1986). The women's value orientation questionnaire: An instrument revision study. *Nursing Papers, 18*(1), 32-44.

Burritt, J. E. (1988). The effects of perceived social support on the relationship between job stress and job satisfaction and job performance among registered nurses employed in acute care facilities. *Dissertation Abstracts International, 49,* 2123B.

Campbell, V. (1989). The Betty Neuman health care systems model: An analysis. In J. P. Riehl-Sisca (Ed.), *Conceptual models for nursing* (3rd ed., pp. 63-72). Norwalk, CT: Appleton & Lange.

Cantin, B., & Mitchell, M. (1989). Nurses' smoking behavior. *The Canadian Nurse, 85*(1), 20-21.

Capers, C. F. (1986). Some basic facts about models, nursing conceptualizations, and nursing theories. *Journal of Continuing Education in Nursing, 17,* 149-154.

Carroll, T. L. (1989). Role deprivation in baccalaureate nursing students pre and post curriculum revision. *Journal of Nursing Education, 28,* 134-139.

Clark, C. C., Cross, J. R., Deane, D. M., & Lowry, L. W. (1991). Spirituality: Integral to quality care. *Holistic Nursing Practice, 5,* 67-76.

Courchene, V. S., Patelski, E., & Martin, J. (1991). A study of the health of pediatric nurses administering Cyclosporine A. *Pediatric Nursing, 17,* 497-500.

Cross, J. R. (1990). Betty Neuman. In J. B. George (Ed.), *Nursing theories: The base for professional nursing practice* (3rd ed., pp. 259-278). Norwalk, CT: Appleton & Lange.

Dale, M. L., & Savala, S. M. (1990). A new approach to the senior practicum. *Nursing Connections, 3*(1), 45-51.

DeBrun, K. T. (1988). *An investigation of the relationships among standing, sitting, recumbent postures, judgement of time duration and preferred personal space in adult females.* Unpublished doctoral dissertation, New York University.

Decker, S. D., & Young, E. (1991). Self-perceived needs of primary caregivers of home-hospice clients. *Journal of Community Health Nursing, 8*(3), 147-151.

DeLoughery, G. W., Gibbie, K. M., & Neuman, B. M. (1974). Teaching organizational concepts to nurses in community mental health. *Journal of Nursing Education, 13,* 18-24.

Delunas, L. R. (1990). Prevention of elder abuse: Betty Neuman health care systems approach. *Clinical Nurse Specialist, 4,* 54-58.

Derstine, J. B. (1992). Theory-based advanced rehabilitation nursing: Is it a reality? *Holistic Nursing Practice, 6*(2), 1-6.

Drew, L. L., Craig, D. M., & Beynon, C. E. (1989). The Neuman systems model for community health administration and practice: Provinces of Manitoba and Ontario, Canada. In B. Neuman (Ed.), *The Neuman systems model* (2nd ed., pp. 315-342). Norwalk, CT: Appleton & Lange.

Edwards, P. A., & Kittler, A. W. (1991). Integrating rehabilitation content in nursing curricula. *Rehabilitation Nursing, 16*(2), 70-73.

Field, P. A. (1987). The impact of nursing theory on the clinical decision making process. *Nurse Educator, 13*, 563-571.

Flannery, J. (1991). FAMILY-RESCUE: A family assessment tool for use by neuroscience nursing in the acute care setting. *Journal of Neuroscience Nursing, 23*, 111-115.

Flannery, J. C. (1988). Validity and reliability of levels of cognitive functioning assessment scale for adults with closed head injuries. *Dissertation Abstracts International, 48*, 3248B.

Foote, A. W., Piazza, D., & Schultz, M. (1990). The Neuman systems model: Application to a patient with a cervical spinal cord injury. *Journal of Neuroscience Nursing, 22*, 302-306.

Forchuk, C. (1991). Reconceptualizing the environment of the individual with a chronic mental illness. *Issues in Mental Health Nursing, 12*, 159-170.

Freiberger, D., Bryant, J., & Marino, B. (1992). The effects of different central venous line dressing changes on bacterial growth in a pediatric oncology population. *Journal of Pediatric Oncology Nursing, 9*(1), 2-7.

Fulbrook, P. R. (1991). The application of the Neuman systems model to intensive care. *Intensive Care Nursing, 7*(1), 28-39.

Gavan, C. A. S., Hastings-Tolsma, M. T., & Tryan, P. J. (1988). Explication of Neuman's model: A holistic systems approach to nutrition for health promotion in the life process. *Holistic Nursing Practice, 3*(1), 26-38.

Gavigan, M., Kline-O'Sullivan, C., & Klumpp-Lybrand, B. (1990). The effect of regular turning on CABG patients. *Critical Care Quarterly, 12*(4), 69-76.

Gibson, D. E. (1988). *A Q-analysis of interpersonal trust in the nurse-client relationship.* Unpublished doctoral dissertation, University of Alabama at Birmingham.

Gries, M., & Gernsler, J. (1988). Patient perceptions of the mechanical ventilation experience. *Focus on Critical Care, 15*, 52-59.

Harbin, P. D. O. (1989). *The Q-analysis of the stressors of adult female nursing students enrolled in baccalaureate schools of nursing.* Unpublished doctoral dissertation, University of Alabama at Birmingham.

Heffline, M. S. (1991). A comparative study of pharmacological versus nursing interventions in the treatment of postanesthesia shivering. *Journal of Post Anesthesia Nursing, 6*, 311-320.

Herrick, C. A., & Goodykoontz, L. (1989). Neuman's systems model for nursing practice as a conceptual framework for a family assessment. *Journal of Child and Adolescent Psychiatric Mental Health Nursing, 2*, 61-67.

Herrick, C. A., Goodykoontz, L., Herrick, R. H., & Kackett, B. (1991). Planning a continuum of care in child psychiatric nursing: A collaborative effort. *Journal of Child and Adolescent Psychiatric and Mental Health Nursing, 4*, 41-48.

Hiltz, D. (1990). The Neuman systems model: An analysis of a clinical situation. *Rehabilitation Nursing, 15*, 330-332.

Hinds, C. (1990). Personal and contextual factors predicting patients' reported quality of life: Exploring congruency with Betty Neuman's assumptions. *Journal of Advanced Nursing, 15,* 456-462.

Hinton-Walker, P., & Raborn, M. (1989). Application of the Neuman model in nursing administration and practice. In B. Henry, C. Arndt, M. DiVincenti, & A. Marriner-Tomey (Eds.), *Dimensions of nursing administration* (pp. 711-723). Boston: Blackwell Scientific.

Hoch, C. C. (1987). Assessing delivery of nursing care: Roy adaptation model and the Neuman health care systems model. Increasing life satisfaction in retired individuals. *Journal of Gerontological Nursing, 13*(1), 10-17.

Hoeman, S. P., & Winters, D. M. (1990). Theory-based case management: High cervical spinal cord injury. *Home Healthcare Nurse, 8*(1), 25-33.

Huch, M. H. (1991). Perspectives on health. *Nursing Science Quarterly, 1*(1), 33-40.

Johnson, S. E. (1989). A picture is worth a thousand words: Helping students visualize a conceptual model. *Nurse Educator, 14*(3), 21-24.

Kaku, R. V. (1992). Severity of low back pain: A comparison between participants who did and did not receive counseling. *AAOHN Journal, 10*(2), 81-89.

Knight, J. B. (1990). The Betty Neuman systems model applied to practice: A client with multiple sclerosis. *Journal of Advanced Nursing, 15,* 447-455.

Laschinger, H. K., & Duff, V. (1991). Attitudes of practicing nurses towards theory-based nursing practice. *Canadian Journal of Nursing Administration, 1*(1), 6-10.

Leja, A. M. (1989). Using guided imagery to combat postsurgical depression. *Journal of Gerontological Nursing, 15*(4), 6-11.

Lindell, M., & Olsson, H. (1991). Can combined oral contraceptives be made more effective by means of a nursing care model? *Journal of Advanced Nursing, 16,* 475-479.

Loescher, L. J., Clark, L., Atwood, J. R., Leigh, S., & Lamb, G. (1990). The impact of the cancer experience on long-term survivors. *Oncology Nursing Forum, 17,* 223-229.

Louis, M. (1989). An intervention to reduce anxiety levels for nurses working with long-term care clients using Neuman's model. In J. P. Riehl-Sisca (Ed.), *Conceptual models for nursing practice* (3rd ed., pp. 95-103). Norwalk, CT: Appleton & Lange.

Lowry, L. W. (1988). Operationalizing the Neuman systems model: A course in concepts and process. *Nurse Educator, 13*(3), 19-22.

Lowry, L. W., & Jopp, M. C. (1989). An evaluation instrument for assessing an associate degree nursing curriculum based on the Neuman systems model. In J. P. Riehl-Sisca (Ed.), *Conceptual models for nursing practice* (3rd ed., pp. 73-85). Norwalk, CT: Appleton & Lange.

Maynihan, M. M. (1990). *Nursing theories in practice: Implementation of the Neuman systems model in an acute care nursing department* (NLN Publication No. 15-2350, pp. 263-273). New York: National League for Nursing.

McDaniel, G. M. S. (1989). *The effects of two methods of dangling on heart rate and blood pressure in post-operative abdominal hysterectomy patients.* Unpublished doctoral dissertation, University of Alabama at Birmingham.

Mirenda, R. (1986). The Neuman model in practice. *Senior Nurse, 5*(3), 26-27.

Mirenda, R. (1986). Neuman systems model. In P. Winstead-Fry (Ed.), *Case studies in nursing theory* (NLN Publication No.15-2152, pp. 127-166). New York: National League for Nursing.

Mischke-Berkey, K., Warner, P., & Hanson, S. (1989). Family health assessment and intervention. In P. J. Bomar (Ed.), *Nurses and family health promotion: Concepts, assessment and interventions* (pp. 115-154). Baltimore: Williams & Wilkins.

Moore, S. L., & Munro, M. F. (1990). The Neuman systems model applied to mental health nursing of older adults. *Journal of Advanced Nursing, 15,* 293-299.

Moynihan, M. M. (1990). Implementation of the Neuman systems model in an acute care nursing department. In M. E. Parker (Ed.), *Nursing theories in practice* (pp. 263-273). New York: National League for Nursing.

Mrkonich, D. E., Hessian, M., & Miller, M. W. (1989). A cooperative process in curriculum development using the Neuman health-care systems model. In J. P. Riehl-Sisca (Ed.), *Conceptual models for nursing practice* (3rd ed., pp. 87-94). Norwalk, CT: Appleton & Lange.

Neuman, B. (1982). *The Neuman systems model: Application to nursing education and practice.* New York: Appleton-Century-Crofts.

Neuman, B. (1989). The Neuman nursing process format: Family. In J. P. Riehl-Sisca (Ed.), *Conceptual models for nursing practice* (3rd ed., pp. 49-62). Norwalk, CT: Appleton & Lange.

Neuman, B. (1989). *The Neuman systems model* (2nd ed.). Norwalk, CT: Appleton & Lange.

Neuman, B. (1990). The Neuman systems model: A theory for practice. In M. E. Parker (Ed.), *Nursing theories in practice* (pp. 241-261). New York: National League for Nursing.

Neuman, B., & Wyatt, M. (1981, January 20). Prospects for change: Some evaluation reflections from one articulated baccalaureate program. *Journal of Nursing Education,* pp. 40-46.

Neuman, B., & Young, J. (1972). A model for teaching total person approach to patient problems. *Nursing Research, 21,* 264-269.

Neuman, B. M. (1990). Health as a continuum based on the Neuman systems model. *Nursing Science Quarterly, 3,* 129-135.

Norman, S. E. (1991). The relationship between hardiness and sleep disturbances in HIV-infected men. *Dissertation Abstracts International, 51,* 4780B.

Norris, E. W. (1989). *Physiologic response to exercise in clients with mitral valve prolapse syndrome.* Unpublished doctoral dissertation, University of Alabama at Birmingham.

Parker, M. E. (Ed.). (1991). *Nursing theories in practice.* New York: National League for Nursing.

Peoples, L. T. (1991). *The relationship between selected client, provider, and agency variables and the utilization of home care services.* Unpublished doctoral dissertation, University of Alabama at Birmingham.

Piazza, D., Foote, A., Wright, P., & Holcombe, J. (1992). Neuman systems model used as a guide for the nursing care of an 8-year-old child with leukemia. *Journal of Pediatric Nursing, 9*(1), 17-24.

Pierce, J. D., & Hutton, E. (1992). Applying the new concepts of the Neuman systems model. *Nursing Forum, 27*(1), 15-18.

Quayhagen, M. P., & Roth, P. A. (1989). From models to measures in assessment of mature families. *Journal of Professional Nursing, 5,* 144-151.

Reed, K. S. (1989). Family theory related to the Neuman systems model. In B. Neuman (Ed.), *The Neuman systems model* (2nd ed., pp. 385-395). Norwalk, CT: Appleton & Lange.

Reed, K. S. (1993). Adapting the Neuman systems model for family nursing. *Nursing Science Quarterly, 6*(2), 93-97.

Riehl-Sisca, J. P. (1989). *Conceptual models for nursing practice* (3rd ed.). Norwalk, CT: Appleton & Lange.

Ross, M. M., Bourbonnais, F. F., & Carroll, G. (1987). Curricular design and the Betty Neuman systems model: A new approach to learning. *International Nursing Review, 34*(3/273), 75-79.

Ross, M. M., & Helmer, H. (1988). A comparative analysis of Neuman's model using the individual and family as the units of care. *Public Health Nursing, 5,* 30-36.

Rowe, M. L. (1989). *The relationship of commitment and social support to the life satisfaction of caregivers to patients with Alzheimer's disease.* Unpublished doctoral dissertation, University of Texas at Austin.

Schlosser, S. P. (1986). The effect of anticipatory guidance on mood state in primparas experiencing unplanned cesarean delivery (metropolitan area, Southeast). *Dissertation Abstracts International, 46,* 2627B.

Simmons, L., & Borgdon, C. (1991). The clinical nurse specialist in HIV care. *Kansas Nurse, 66*(1), 6-7.

Sipple, J. E. A. (1989). *A model for curriculum change based on retrospective analysis.* Unpublished doctoral dissertation, University of South Carolina, Columbia.

Sirles, A. T., Brown, K., & Hilver, J. C. (1991). Effects of back school education and exercise in back injured municipal workers. *AAOHN Journal, 39*(1), 7-12.

Smith, M. C. (1989). Neuman's model in practice. *Nursing Science Quarterly, 2,* 24-25.

Speck, B. J. (1990). The effect of guided imagery upon first semester nursing students performing their first injections. *Journal of Nursing Education, 29,* 346-350.

Story, E. L., & DuGas, B. W. (1988). A teaching strategy to facilitate conceptual model implementation in practice. *Journal of Continuing Education in Nursing, 19,* 244-247.

Story, E. L., & Ross, M. M. (1986). Family centered community health nursing and the Betty Neuman systems model. *Nursing Papers: Perspectives in Nursing, 18,* 77-88.

Terhaar, M. F. (1989). The influence of physiologic stability, behavioral stability and family stability on the preterm infant's length of stay in the neonatal intensive care unit. *Dissertation Abstracts International, 50,* 1328B.

Torkington, S. (1988). Nourishing the infant. *Senior Nurse, 8*(2), 24-25.

Vaughn, M., Cheatwood, S., Sirles, A. T., & Brown, K. C. (1989). The effect of progressive muscle relaxation on stress among clerical workers. *American Association of Occupational Health Nurses Journal, 37,* 302-306.

Vincent, J. L. M. (1988). A Q analysis of the stressors of fathers with an infant in an intensive care unit. *Dissertation Abstracts International, 49,* 3111B.

Wallingford, P. (1989). The neurologically impaired and dying child: Applying the Neuman systems model. *Issues in Comprehensive Pediatric Nursing, 12,* 139-157.

Webb, C. A. (1988). *Q cross-sectional study of hope, physical status, cognitions and meaning and purpose of pre- and post-retirement adults.* Unpublished doctoral dissertation, University of Pittsburgh.

Weinberger, S. L. (1991). Analysis of clinical situation using the Neuman systems model. *Rehabilitation Nursing, 16,* 278, 280-281.

Whatley, J. H. (1988). *Effects of health locus of control and social network on risk-taking in adolescents.* Unpublished doctoral dissertation, University of Alabama at Birmingham.

Wheeler, K. (1989). Self-psychology's contributions to understanding stress and implications for nursing. *Journal of Advanced Medical Surgical Nursing, 1*(4), 1-10.

Wiens, A. G. (1985). Rehabilitation assessment—A nursing perspective: The Neuman nursing model. *Rehabilitation Nursing, 10*(2), 25-27.

Williamson, J. W. (1989). *The influence of self-selected monotonous sounds on the night sleep pattern of postoperative open heart surgery patients.* Unpublished doctoral dissertation, University of Alabama at Birmingham.

PART XII

Ida Jean Orlando

A Nursing Process Theory

NORMA JEAN SCHMIEDING

Biographical Sketch of the Nurse Theorist: Ida Jean Orlando, BS, MA, RN

Born: August 12, 1926
Diploma: New York Medical College, Lower Fifth Avenue
    Hospital, School of Nursing, New York
BS: St. John's University, Brooklyn, NY
MA: Teachers College, Columbia University, New York
Previous Positions: Associate Professor of Nursing and
    Director of the Graduate Program in Mental Health
    Psychiatric Nursing, Yale School of Nursing, New
    Haven, CT; Clinical Nursing Consultant, McLean
    Hospital, Belmont, MA, and Director, Research Project:
    Two Systems of Nursing in a Psychiatric Hospital;
    Assistant Director of Nursing for Education and
    Research, Metropolitan State Hospital, Waltham, MA;
    National and international consultant and speaker

Foreword

A major value of nursing theory is its utility in helping nurses distinguish actions that form the core of professional nursing practice from actions that are the responsibility of other health-care providers. At the time that Orlando's theory was evolving, much of nursing care practice involved assisting physicians so more effective medical care could be provided to patients. Nursing science was in the embryonic phase and practices were based on medically derived principles or on anecdotal data. Comparatively few nurses questioned this approach and many perceived their professional obligations to patients as secondary to their medical assistant responsibilities.

Orlando had the wisdom to question the prevailing mode of thinking about nursing practice. She recognized that nursing could not be a profession unless it had a distinct function or goal. Without the articulation of that goal, she knew that nurses would continue to function as paraprofessionals to medicine and would never develop a science of nursing. Orlando's inductive studies revealed that outcomes improved when the nurse was *patient* centered. Her data enabled her to define the nurse's professional responsibility and to delineate the process for fulfilling that obligation. This section provides an excellent description and analysis of that important work.

The author, Norma Jean Schmieding, is eminently qualified to present this theory. As a young nurse, Schmieding found herself questioning many aspects of the nurse's role. She wondered about all of the activities that consumed nurses' time without benefiting patients and knew the value of nursing to patients was being diluted by these routines. She recognized that tasks rather than patients often preoccupied nurses and yet was not sure how to change all of this. Then she encountered Ida Jean Orlando, who was teaching deliberative nursing process at McLean Hospital in Massachusetts. Her response was relief. Her concerns about nursing practice and her belief in the salience of the discipline to patients were validated.

Schmieding used the process she learned from Orlando in her own practice. Later, upon assuming the role of director of nursing, she used the theory to guide practice within the nursing service she administered. This helped other nurses identify their professional role, and the quality of nursing care improved greatly. While a doctoral student and recently, Schmieding has authored numerous articles based on the theory. In fact, Orlando's work was the focus of her doctoral dissertation.

This section provides the reader with an understanding of Orlando's work from the perspective of an individual who has practiced, studied, and taught it. The theory has laid a foundation for nursing practice and nursing science. Schmieding has presented it with skill and precision.

Lois A. Haggerty, PhD, RN
Associate Professor
Boston College School of Nursing

Preface

Nursing, as a noble profession, occurs through a process that involves the nurse and the individual in need of the nurse's help. When a nurse and a patient first meet, neither has much information about the other. Nurses never know in advance what reaction they will have toward the patient nor the patient's reaction toward them. Nonetheless, what transpires in this contact has implications for the patient's welfare as well as the nurse's fulfillment of her or his professional responsibility and work satisfaction. Because the majority of practice occurs in face-to-face contact, nurses need skills to discover the meaning of the situation.

Each nursing theory provides a different view of nursing that is intended to help the nurse to nurse. The focus may be the patient, the nurse, or the nurse-patient process. Orlando's theory focuses on the nurse-patient process and helps the nurse understand what happens, how it happens, and its relationship to the process of helping the patient. The patient is an active participant in this process.

This section is not a critique of Orlando's theory but, rather, a distillation of the theory's major components. The sections on propositions, research, and clinical application are intended to convey the relevance of Orlando's theory to practice as well as to pose areas for further research. The literature references provide sources for those who wish to explore further the theory and related works.

To understand a theory one must study it and experiment with its application to practice. Only in this way can nurses select a theory most helpful to their practice. I hope students will find Orlando's theory useful. The beauty of Orlando's theory is that it does not preclude the use of other theories and concepts, including nursing theories. Rather, they are resources from which the nurse can draw to help the patient.

For years I have studied and used Orlando's theory in practice, teaching, research, and administration and can attest to its usefulness. Each time I delve into Orlando's theory I am amazed by its clarity and the simplicity with which she describes the theory. I hope the readers of this section will find the theory as compelling as I have.

61

Origin of the Theory

Orlando formulated her nursing process theory in the late 1950s while principal investigator of the Yale School of Nursing Project. This project, funded by a National Institute of Mental Health Grant, was entitled "Integration of Mental Health Principles in the Basic Nursing Curriculum." The grant's purpose was to identify factors inhibiting and enhancing the integration of mental health concepts in the nursing curriculum. To establish these factors, principles guiding effective nursing practice had to be identified. Orlando's book *The Dynamic Nurse-Patient Relationship*,[1,2] published in 1961, was an outcome of this project and has been highly acclaimed for its influence on nursing education and practice. According to Orlando (1961), the book's content was to contribute to concerns about (a) the nurse-patient relationship, (b) the nurse's professional role and identity, and (c) knowledge development distinct to nursing. Orlando's theory radically shifted the nurse's focus from the medical diagnosis and automatic activities, decided upon without patient participation, to the patient's immediate experience and whether the patient was helped by the nurse's action. Orlando was, and remains, one of a few nurse theorists who explicitly include active patient participation as integral to their theory. Orlando's formulations are integrated into much of current education and practice literature, often unintentionally, without recognition of the source. Orlando's theory has become a part of many nurses' thinking and practice.

Following her initial work at Yale, Orlando further refined her theory through a National Institute of Mental Health Public Health Service research grant while she was a clinical nurse consultant at McLean Hospital in Belmont, Massachusetts. In this grant Orlando assessed the relevance of her previous formulations, trained and evaluated nurses in the use of these formulations, and tested the validity of her formulations. Her second book, *The Discipline and Teaching of Nursing Process*, published in 1972, contained the study's research results and the extended formulations of her theory, which included a definition of the entire nursing practice system.

It is important to place in a historical context the critical nursing issues at the time of a theory's development. In the 1950s, nursing was struggling to define its work and to move nursing education into the mainstream of higher education and away from apprentice models of learning. In nursing schools there was a move to incorporate new knowledge, such as psychiatric principles, into nursing curricula and to move away from the medical model as the basis of nursing education.

These issues are reflected in Orlando's (1961) thinking. For example, she writes that principles and concepts from other fields enable nurses to explain their observations of patients and the activities that are carried out in relation to these observations. However, she cautions that these principles are derived from the study of particular aspects of the behaving human organism and not from nursing practice. Orlando (1961) recognizes the importance of making this distinction because general principles, which explain behavior or promote health, remain valid even when the immediate and individual nature of the nursing situation is not considered. Nurses, however, have to deal with specific situations to which general knowledge cannot be arbitrarily applied. Nonetheless, Orlando (1961) acknowledges that theories and practices from other fields may be used by nurses as needed; therefore, the broader the nurse's knowledge, the greater the resources on which the nurse may draw when necessary to help the patient. This belief supports incorporating a liberal arts foundation into basic nursing education. Thus Orlando recognizes the importance of using knowledge developed in other fields while at the same time emphasizing the distinctiveness of the discipline of professional nursing.

Orlando (1972) maintains that nursing problems were associated with the absence of a distinct function of professional nursing, which, in turn, left nurses without a clear concept of what outcome should be achieved with patients. Because professional authority is derived from a distinct professional function, she believed this lack of specificity of function had interfered with the development of a framework to evaluate professional nurses' activities. It also had interfered with the study of the nursing process and the development of the content needed to achieve the outcome of a distinct function (Orlando, 1972).

A practice discipline needs theories to guide the practitioners' actions. Theories unique to nursing are derived from the observation of nursing phenomena. Many nursing theories have been developed from borrowed theories adopted or adapted to nursing. Orlando was one of the earliest nurse theorists and one of the first to develop a nursing theory inductively from the empirical study of nurses' practice.

The development of scientific knowledge, according to Kuhn, must take into account how that science is actually practiced (cited in Schmieding, 1983). The origin of Orlando's theory emanates from her systematic observations of nursing practice. She was the first nurse to use a participant observer field methodology approach to theory development. This qualitative methodology more recently has become an accepted approach for knowledge development in nursing.

For years Orlando was preoccupied with the thought that she did not know what a nurse should produce when professionally trained. Her principal investigator position at Yale provided her with a clinical setting to observe the interactions between nurses and patients directly. For 3 years Orlando recorded "only what I heard the person say and what I saw in the sequence in which it took place" (Pelletier, 1976, p. 18).[3] She then examined the content of these 2,000 nurse-patient records and only was able to categorize them into two mutually exclusive sets that she labeled "good nursing" and "bad nursing." Recommendations from psychiatrists and sociologists for a different approach to the data's categorization failed to establish mutually exclusive categories. Orlando then presented a random selection of these records to nurses with dissimilar characteristics and backgrounds. Strikingly, all these nurses agreed with Orlando's categorization of what was judged good and bad nursing. Orlando exclaimed,

And then the light dawned. I decided that if the anecdotal account was the only material available to base the judgment on, then what made good or bad nursing happen had to be contained in the anecdotal record from which all those uniform judgments were made. Stated another way: specific items and/or conditions producing the good or bad outcomes had to be contained in the records which were so judged and could therefore be commonly identified. (Pelletier, 1976, p. 22)

Deliberative formulations were found in the outcomes judged good nursing, whereas in bad nursing the outcomes contained automatic nursing formulations:

In the records judged as good the nurse's focus was on the immediate verbal and nonverbal behavior of the patient from the beginning through the end of the contact; whereas in those judged as bad the nurse's focus was on prescribed activity or something that had nothing to do with the patient's behavior. (Pelletier, 1976, p. 23)

In contacts where good nursing occurred the nurse found out, from the patient's viewpoint, what was happening to the patient and identified the patient's distress. The nurse also determined why the patient was distressed and recognized that the patient was unable to relieve the distress without the nurse's help. This observation led Orlando to "the inescapable conclusion that the function of professional nursing is to find out and meet the patient's immediate needs for HELP" (Pelletier, 1976, p. 24). These findings led Orlando to conclude that the outcome of the professional nurse's work is found in the immediate behavior of the patient and that a professional service had not transpired until the patient's immediate behavior was improved from the patient's point of view.

Orlando does not acknowledge any previous work as the source of her theoretical thinking. Some scholars believe she was influenced by and influenced other nurse theorists. Andrews (1989), Leonard and Crane (1990), and Meleis (1991) note the similarities of her work to that of Peplau (1952) in terms of Orlando's focus on interpersonal relationships and the commonality of their definition of nursing. Peplau and Orlando have similarities in that they both view nursing as a dynamic process that includes the patient as an integral part of the problem-solving process and their theories each evolved from their direct work with patients. Despite these similarities, Peplau's thinking was greatly influenced by Harry Stack Sullivan, whereas Orlando's thinking and her theory's content appear to have been more significantly influenced by people with whom she was associated at Teachers College, Columbia University.

During the time while Orlando was enrolled at Teachers College in the master's program for mental health consultation, its dean, Louise McManus, was involved nationally in defining nursing. She wrote about the nature of professional nursing and stressed the uniqueness of each situation and that automatic fixed habits of response were insufficient or inadequate as the basis of nursing practice (McManus, 1948). The uniqueness of each situation and the inadequacy of nursing actions based on automatic fixed responses can be seen in Orlando's formulations. Ruth Gilbert (1940, 1951),[4] who wrote *The Public Health Nurse and Her Patient*, was Orlando's teacher for public health nursing. Gilbert focused attention on the dynamics of behavior and on establishing the nurse-patient relationship. In stressing the benefits of mental hygiene for nursing practice, Gilbert (1940) notes that it provides "a deliberate, observant, objective way of working, a habit of stopping to question and to think through what the behavior of the patient may mean in relation to a situation, and how the nurse herself relates to that situation" (p. 1). Some similarities between Gilbert's work and Orlando's can be noted in that both place emphasis on the deliberativeness of the nurse's action and on understanding the dynamics and meaning of a patient's behavior.

L. Thomas Hopkins, another person at Columbia whose work may have influenced Orlando, taught educational courses in which Orlando was enrolled. Orlando specifically identifies him as attracting her attention through his conception of the learning process (I. Orlando, personal communication, October 25, 1985). The core of Hopkins's (1941, 1954) work centers around the influence of past experiences on the meaning of the present situation and on the importance of perceptions in determining behavior. He stressed that behavior emanates from and is validated in experience. The origin of his work can be traced to Kilpatrick (1925, 1941), who in turn acknowledges John Dewey as having the most formative influence on his work. The similarity to Dewey's (1933, 1938) ideas can be seen in the writings of the three people just cited as well as in Orlando's theory.

Regardless of the origin of Orlando's theory, the centrality of the patient is ever present in her theoretical thinking. She believes that the " 'core of practice' 'should' be what it has been and continues to be—the inability of the individual(s) 'to nurse' the self and the self alone cannot identify or get the needed help" (Pelletier, 1980, p. 8). According to Orlando, professional nursing is required when the cause of the inability to care for the self is not known or clearly understood by the person or the nurse before the nurse's investigation of the situation is conducted (Pelletier, 1980).

Orlando's emphasis on obtaining the patient's perspective and involvement in determining the nurse's activity as well as for evaluating the results of the activity is of central importance to her nursing process theory. Orlando's theory was a major force in shifting the nurse's focus away from assisting the physician to finding out and meeting the patient's immediate needs.

Notes

1. Republished by the National League for Nursing in 1990. Quotes from Orlando (1961) are used by permission from the National League for Nursing. Quotes from Orlando (1972) are used by permission from Ida J. Orlando (Pelletier).

2. When Orlando developed her theory the term *patient* was used; therefore throughout this book *patient* rather than *client* is used. In addition, masculine pronouns were used for patients and feminine for nurses; this is noted in some direct quotes.

3. Pelletier is Orlando's married name.

4. Ruth Gilbert recommended Orlando for her position at Yale University School of Nursing.

62

Assumptions of the Theory

Each nursing theory contains assumptions that are explicit or implied. Assumptions are premises accepted by the theorist as given and true, self-evident, and unquestioned (Barnum, 1990). They "are the taken-for-granted statements of the theory. . . . They may or may not represent the shared beliefs of the discipline" (Meleis, 1991, p. 13). Assumptions are important because "they describe that state of being out of which the nursing theory grows. Underlying assumptions are the starting points of the . . . [theorist's] reasoning" (Barnum, 1990, p. 20). In evaluating a theory's assumptions a nurse should consider whether they reflect the real world of nursing and whether the theory is logically consistent with its assumptions. According to Marriner-Tomey (1989), to accept as true the theory about the phenomenon, one must accept the assumptions as true.

Orlando developed her theory in the late 1950s before the nursing profession began to study theory development systematically. Therefore, Orlando, like most of the early nurse theorists, did not explicitly identify the theory's concepts, assumptions, and propositions systematically. Nonetheless, her theory contains assumptions about the nursing profession, nurses, patients, and the nature of nurse-patient interaction. The following implied assumptions are presented along with Orlando's thoughts related to them.

Assumptions About Nursing

Assumption 1

Nursing is a distinct profession separate from other disciplines. Orlando (1987) asserts that nurses are independent professionals by virtue of their license to practice nursing. Her view that doctor's orders are for the patient, not the nurse, conveys the thrust of her conviction of this assumption (Pelletier, 1967). She believes that nursing's failure to articulate a function distinct from medicine, and other professions, has kept nursing on a dependent path. As a result, health administrators, medical authorities, and health policies continue to push nursing down a dependent path that has served nonnursing interests (Orlando, 1985, 1987). Only a radical independent path would cause health care policymakers to consider fully the importance of professional nursing services (Orlando & Dugan, 1989). This distinction would help nurses, as a collective body, to develop the independent organization and delivery of services within the competitive health care system (Orlando & Dugan, 1989). A distinct professional function provides the independent authority and autonomy needed to achieve this distinctiveness.

Assumption 2

Professional nursing has a distinct function and product (outcome). Nursing's failure to identify a distinct function has thwarted the development of a theoretical framework upon which to base professional nursing practice and the training of professional nurses (Orlando, 1972). It also has undermined the profession's ability to build a coherent knowledge base (Orlando & Dugan, 1989). The distinct function should characterize every activity of every nurse while practicing nursing; therefore, it must be identifiable in each nurse-patient contact (Pelletier, 1976). The function justifies nursing's work as a profession and remains constant regardless of the patient's age, diagnosis, medical care status, or whether cared for at home or in an institution or agency (Orlando, 1972). The focus of professional nursing is the patient's immediate experience. Orlando (1987) believes nursing might lose its intrinsic character and go down the dependent path if nursing does not collectively clearly articulate its unique function.

Orlando thinks the lack of a distinct function has inhibited nursing's demonstration of the product (outcome) of that function through practice and research, as well as interfered in the development of the content required to achieve the product of the distinct function (Pelletier, 1976). A distinct product would clarify what form the result would take after the nurse fulfills the function. This distinct product is something the patient cannot produce alone or get from anyone else who is not trained to practice professional nursing (Pelletier, 1976). Implicit in this assumption is that effective practice can be empirically identified.

Assumption 3

There is a difference between lay and professional nursing. Orlando (1983) thinks the nursing profession should provide the public with the distinction between lay and professional nursing. According to Orlando (1961), any person nurses another when she or he carries the burden of responsibility for those things that the person cannot do alone. Orlando and Dugan (1989) write that lay nursing is a transmitted social behavior found in all cultures and includes encouragement, nurturance, nourishment, protection, and curative care. This assistance can be provided to the self or to another by almost anybody. The activity is routine, repetitive, or custodial in nature. When these efforts fail, people suffer distress and are helpless because they are unaware of and unable to identify the cause of the distress: "In contrast to 'lay' nursing, professional nursing is required when the 'causes' of the individual's inability 'to nurse' the self (or another as with family members) are NOT known or clearly understood by the individual(s) or the nurse. That is, not known *before* the nurse's professional investigation is conducted" (Pelletier, 1980, pp. 4-5).

A professional nurse identifies both the cause of the distress and the individual help required to relieve the distress and designs the activity to meet the need for help. The effect of the activity, the alleviation of distress, is noted in the patient's verbal and nonverbal behavior (Orlando & Dugan, 1989). The distinction between lay and professional nursing would clarify nursing's societal responsibility.

Assumption 4

Nursing is aligned with medicine. In Orlando's early work, the nurse's access to the patient was through medicine. Although she states that traditionally nursing has been aligned with medicine, Orlando consistently emphasizes the difference in the two professions' responsibility to the patient. Physicians place patients under the nurse's care when patients cannot meet their own needs for help or because they need help in following the prescribed treatment or diagnostic plan (Orlando, 1961). Medicine is responsible for the prevention and treatment of disease, whereas nursing is responsible for offering help to patients for their physical and mental comfort while they are under medical treatment or supervision (Orlando, 1961). In her later writings, Orlando clearly states that nursing is practiced wherever a person is in need of its service. This service is provided to people both sick and well, with or without a diagnosed disease, and takes place within or outside institutions (Orlando, 1972, 1987).

Assumptions About Patients

Assumption 1

Patients' needs for help are unique. Because patients are unique the help a nurse provides must be specifically geared to each patient's immediate needs for help (Orlando, 1961). Orlando developed specific guidelines for nurses to use to uncover the meaning of a patient's unique experience.

Assumption 2

Patients have an initial inability to communicate their needs for help. According to Orlando (1961), nurses must realize that patients cannot clearly state the nature and meaning of their distress or need without the nurse's help or without having a previously established helpful relationship (Orlando, 1961). Without this recognition patients' distress will not be identified. Consequently, this delay may seriously threaten the patient's condition or exacerbate his or her discomfort

(Orlando, 1961). Considering patients' initial inability to communicate clearly, nurses should assume that patients' behavior is evidence of distress or an unmet need for help.

Assumption 3

When patients cannot meet their own needs they become distressed (Orlando, 1961). When patients become distressed they are dependent on the nurse for help. If patients are able to meet their own needs and follow prescribed activities unaided, they do not require the nurse's help. Therefore, nurses must be able to validate whether or not patients require their help at a given time (Orlando, 1961).

Assumption 4

The patient's behavior is meaningful. Although the behavior has a specific meaning to the patient this meaning is not self-evident. On the surface a patient's problem may look simple and the nurse may think she or he can apply some knowledge from another field to solve the problem. However, what becomes apparent from Orlando's (1961) theory is that the meaning of the patient's behavior is rarely what it appears; thus arbitrary solutions are seldom helpful. Consequently, the nurse, after observing a patient's behavior, realizes that she or he does not understand the meaning without further exploration with the patient (Orlando, 1961).

Assumption 5

Patients are able and willing to communicate verbally (and nonverbally when unable to communicate verbally). Implicit in the theory is that it is most useful with patients who are able and willing to communicate verbally. Although it can be used with babies and comatose or unconscious patients, it does rely heavily on verbal communications. If patients are unable to speak or are unconscious, nurses could enlist family or significant others to participate on the patient's behalf or rely on their own observations of nonverbal vocal behavior and/or nonverbal physiological manifestations in carrying out a deliberative nursing process (Schmieding, 1986).

Assumptions About Nurses

Assumption 1

The nurse's reaction to each patient is unique. According to Orlando (1961, 1972), each nurse's immediate reaction is based on how the nurse experiences her or his participation in the nurse-patient situation. The nurse never knows in advance what her or his reaction to the patient will be. Orlando notes that in each situation the nurse has to find out more about her or his own reaction and action in order to understand its particular meaning to the patient (Orlando, 1961).

Assumption 2

Nurses are responsible for helping patients avoid or alleviate distress. Because they are responsible to alleviate patients' distress or to help patients avoid distress nurses must focus on eliminating things that interfere with the patient's mental and physical comfort. Conversely, nurses should not add to the patient's distress (Orlando, 1961).

Assumption 3

The nurse's mind is the major tool for helping patients. Similar to Burr, Hill, Nye, and Reiss (1979), Orlando regards the nurse's mind as the chief vehicle for converting mental processes, perceived from an immediate situation, into action. What occurs in the mind is in large part a function of what occurs in the interaction. The nurse's mind, therefore, is the intervening variable between the nurse's unique perception and its conversion into action. Orlando (1961) notes that what a nurse automatically perceives or thinks is not as important as what the nurse does. What the nurse says or does is an outcome of the nurse's reaction in the situation. Thus the nurse's behavior is influenced by the meaning the nurse attaches to the thought she or he has in mind. Therefore, the nurse's mind, and its content, is the nurse's major tool. Orlando describes how the nurse should use her or his reaction in an exploratory way to find the meaning of the patient's behavior (Orlando, 1961). Orlando assumes that nurses are logical thinkers who can convert the content of their minds into actions that ultimately will benefit the patient.

Assumption 4

The nurse's use of automatic responses prevents the responsibility of nursing from being fulfilled. When a nurse acts without deliberations with the patient, the action often is not helpful because the nurse does not consider the patient's perception. Automatic personal responses are based on assumptions and are rarely reliable for decision making or action. Because the nurse's automatic response does not include the patient, communications between patient and nurse become unclear or stop (Orlando, 1961). The patient's distress or sense of helplessness continues because the nurse's action is based on reasons other than the patient's immediate need for help (Orlando, 1961).

Assumption 5

A nurse's practice is improved through self-reflection. The nurse's words and actions are the exclusive mode through which the patient is served. Therefore, the focus of improvement is on what nurses say and do and how these practices influence the process of care. As nurses comprehend how their practice helped or did not help the patient, this understanding comprises the material out of which nurses develop and improve their knowledge and skill in practice (Orlando, 1961). Self-reflection, as a method to improve a practitioner's practice, is supported by action science as developed by Argyris and Shön (1978).

Assumptions About the Nurse-Patient Situation

Assumption 1

The nurse-patient situation is a dynamic whole. Because the patient and the nurse are people, they interact and a process occurs between them. In this process, what the nurse says and does affects the patient and what the patient says and does affects the nurse (Orlando, 1961). This process is unique for each situation. Orlando (1961) notes that when the nurse expresses her or his perceptions or thoughts as questions or wonderings it enables the patient to express the meaning the patient has of the nurse's expression. When nurses explore the meaning of the patient's behavior, the patient is more willing to express her or his concerns. Once patients have been helped and trust the nurse, their communications are more spontaneous and explicit (Orlando, 1961).

Assumption 2

The phenomenon of the nurse-patient encounter represents a major source of nursing knowledge. The nurse's perception of a patient's behavior, and her or his subsequent thoughts and feelings, are objective and subjective data acquired through the nurse's direct experience with the patient. Although they require investigation, these data represent the knowledge base out of which the patient's plan of care will be developed.

Accepting these assumptions is prerequisite to the theory's acceptance. These assumptions are the foundation for the formulations of the interrelated concepts that constitute Orlando's theory.

63

Major Dimensions of the Theory

Theories allow a systematic way to look at the world in order to describe, explain, predict, and control it (Torres, 1990). Theories are invented to help people solve problems. In nursing, theories help the nurse make decisions and take actions in practice situations. A theory is an intellectual tool that directs one's focus of investigation or exploration of specific phenomena. It is like a map that picks out the most important parts of the phenomena (Barnum, 1990). Because it emphasizes certain aspects of a phenomenon it restricts the boundaries of inquiry (Dewey, 1938), thus ferreting out irrelevant data and making the processing of the remaining complex data more manageable. Therefore, when nurses are caring for patients, theories help nurses select and organize direct patient observations and indirect patient data from records and reports to use in deciding their approach to a patient's care. Theories give nurses a sense of purpose and direction for their actions, and without their use patient outcomes are achieved on a hit-or-miss basis. When selecting a theory a nurse should assess its effectiveness in solving practice problems; the theory also should be easy to use.

Concepts are the building blocks of a theory; thus a theory contains a set of interrelated concepts. Concepts are mental images or ideas that come to mind when one observes the phenomenon of interest. They help one impose intellectual organization upon observations (Harré, 1989). They are ideas that one carries around in one's mind.

For a theory to be useful to nursing practice it should contain a sufficient number of concepts for the nurse to use to comprehend complex phenomena. However, if a theory has too many concepts it is difficult to grasp the phenomenon. A theory's concepts are abstract; therefore they are inferred or indirectly observed. In nursing, the more abstract a concept, the more difficult it is to grasp its meaning and thus the more difficult to infer it empirically through patient observations.

An elaboration of the five major concepts of Orlando's theory illuminates their logical relationship and describes the nursing practice that results from the systematic use of the theory's concepts. Although the concepts are interrelated, they are discussed separately here. Other secondary nursing concepts related to the theory's major concepts are integrated throughout the discussion.

Professional Nursing Function

Orlando (1961) believed that inadequate patient care was caused by the profession's lack of a clearly articulated nursing function. According to Orlando, professional authority is derived from the profession's distinct function; therefore, without this distinctiveness nursing practice cannot be autonomous because it lacks authority. Orlando (1961) thinks the lack of a distinct function has interfered with the development of a framework to evaluate the influence of the nurse's actions on patient outcomes.

Orlando formulated her concept of the nursing function by analyzing the outcomes of nurse-patient contacts in problematic situations. The context within which this concept evolved relates to Orlando's view of nursing, which focuses on the patient's immediate needs for help in the immediate experience. She states,

Nursing . . . is responsive to individuals who suffer or anticipate a sense of helplessness; it is focused on the process of care in an immediate experience; it is concerned with providing direct assistance to individuals in whatever setting they are found for the purpose of avoiding, relieving, diminishing or curing the individual's sense of helplessness. (Orlando, 1972, p. 12)

According to Orlando (1961), helplessness, need, or stress originate from the patient's physical limitations, adverse reactions to the setting, and experiences that prevent the patient from communicating her or his needs. When a patient is ill or in some state of difficulty she or he often is unable to meet her or his own needs: *"Need is situationally defined as a requirement of the patient which, if supplied, relieves or diminishes his immediate distress or improves his immediate sense of adequacy or well-being"* (Orlando, 1961, p. 5). Therefore "learning how to understand what is happening between herself and the patient is the central core of the nurse's practice and comprises the basic framework for the help she gives to patients" (Orlando, 1961, p. 4).

The function of professional nursing is the principal organizing concept of Orlando's theory, which means it is the fundamental concept around which the theory's other concepts revolve. She envisions the nursing function as "finding out and meeting the patient's immediate needs for help" (Orlando, 1972, p. 20). The patient's "immediate needs for help" should not be confused with basic human needs. Basic needs are shared by all people, whereas the need for help is highly individualized and varied (Orlando, 1987). Orlando's conception of need is specific to *the help* a person requires in an immediate situation. The distinct function clarifies the nurse's role and guides inquiry by directing the nurse's focus to the patient's immediate experience. Thus the patient's experience is the focal point of the nurse's investigation. According to Orlando (1972), the "distinct professional function is constant regardless of the patient's age, diagnosis or treatment, whether housed at home or in an institution or agency" (p. 20).

Orlando (1972) notes that at the onset of nurse-patient contact it is not known to the nurse whether the patient is in need of help. However, information is available through exploration with the patient for achieving a correct understanding of the patient's behavior and determining whether the patient is in need of help. If the patient is in need and the need for help is met by the nurse, the professional function has been fulfilled. Orlando (1972) describes the results in the following way: "The product of meeting the patient's immediate need for help is . . . 'improvement' in the immediate verbal and nonverbal behavior of the patient. This observable change allows the nurse to believe or disbelieve that her activity relieved, prevented or diminished the patient's sense of helplessness" (p. 21). In Orlando's theory, both the aim and the end result of nursing are improvement in the patient's behavior.

Repetitious use of the concept—finding out and meeting the patient's immediate need for help—guides the nurse's investigation and makes the nurse sensitive to specific stimuli in nurse-patient situations. Finding out and meeting the patient's immediate needs for help becomes an acquired way of thinking; thus in each situation the nurse's underlying thought is "Does the patient have an immediate need for help or not?" The nurse then explores her or his observations with the patient to confirm or refute an immediate need for help (Schmieding, 1987). Because it directs the nurse's focus to the patient this concept provides specific boundaries to the nurse's practice, thereby increasing intellectual efficiency and decreasing confusion. The nurse also can use the concept of function to decide whether an activity or task is nonnursing. The question to be answered is "Does the activity help the nurse find out and meet the patient's immediate need for help?"

The concept of the nursing function, as articulated by Orlando, clearly establishes the nurse's accountability to the patient and provides an evaluative framework. Orlando (1972) stresses that evaluation must take place each time a nurse acts. Orlando (1972) considers that it is the nurse's direct responsibility to meet the patient's immediate need, either personally or by calling in the services of others. With the emphasis that Orlando places on the patient's immediate experience, it is logical that the patient's behavior is another major concept of her theory.

The Patient's Presenting Behavior

Orlando's theory focuses exclusively on understanding the complexities of problematic situations. Nursing practice is made up of frequent nurse-patient contacts in which patients may make remarks such as "Can I have something for pain?"; "I can't get out of bed!"; "My baby is not getting enough to eat."; "How long have you been a nurse?"; or "Please pull down my blind." In these contacts it is not clear whether or not patients are experiencing distress or are in need of help. The nurse is responsible, and should be professionally prepared, to help patients communicate their need for help and to see that their immediate need is met. Because this identification of need is the foundation of the nurse-patient relationship, nurses must develop skills in exploring with patients the meaning of their verbal and nonverbal behavior (Orlando, 1961).

The discovery and meeting of patients' immediate needs for help are not straightforward. Patients often are unable to express the nature of their distress without the nurse's help. Orlando (1961) believes the reasons why patients may not clearly communicate distress could be related to not knowing in a real sense how the nurse might help and experiencing ambivalence about their dependency needs. Whatever the cause, the nurse must assume that the patient's behavior may indicate an unmet need for help unless the nurse has contrary evidence (Orlando, 1961). Therefore the nurse should view patients' behavior as not immediately understandable but as a means to understanding. From her observations of practice Orlando (1961) formulated the following concept to guide the nurse's observation: *"The presenting behavior of the patient, regardless of the form in which it appears, may represent a plea for help"* (p. 40).

Patients' behavior can be manifested in the following forms: (a) verbal, such as asking a question, making a demand or request, or making a statement to the nurse; (b) nonverbal vocal, such as coughing, moaning, crying, and wheezing; and (c) nonverbal, such as tears in the eyes, skin color, pacing, reddened face, clenched fist, or physiological manifestations such as blood pressure and pulse (Orlando, 1961). Whatever the behavior, it causes the nurse to take notice. However, the initial behavior is unreliable for interpreting the meaning of patients' behavior because the behavior may *not* indicate that patients are distressed or the true nature of the distress. In other words, the behavior may not mean what it appears to mean. Therefore the nurse must be able to find out the meaning of the behavior and then determine the patient's immediate need for help.

Because the patient's behavior may be a cue or signal to the nurse, the patient's presenting behavior always should be explored. Orlando specifies that both the patient and the nurse participate in this exploratory communication process to identify the problem as well as the solution. She writes,

> First, *the nurse must take the initiative in helping the patient express the specific meaning of his behavior in order to ascertain his distress.* Second, *she must help the patient explore the distress in order to ascertain the help*

he requires for his [immediate] need [for help] to be met. (Orlando, 1961, p. 26)

Because the patient's behavior stimulates the nurse's perceptions it becomes the starting point of the nurse's investigation. According to Orlando, the nurse's perception of the patient's presenting behavior forms the basis of the nurse's thoughts and feelings. This perception is discussed in the next section.

Immediate Reaction

The nurse's direct observation of the patient's presenting behavior is the basis of the nurse's perceptions, thoughts, and feelings, which occur in an automatic, almost instantaneous sequence (Orlando, 1972). This observation represents the first data and the only resource the nurse can use in understanding the meaning of the patient's behavior. The nurse's reaction, stimulated by the patient's behavior, comes from the nurse's past experiences and knowledge, which combine with the nurse's understanding of the immediate situation to produce the nurse's unique reaction.

According to Orlando (1961), a nursing situation is composed of the patient's behavior, the nurse's reaction, and the nurse's action. The interaction of these is called the nursing process. To describe the process more specifically, Orlando (1972) identified four distinct items in any person's action process and described the sequence of their occurrence. She notes,

These separate items reside within an individual and at any given moment occur in the following automatic, sometimes instantaneous, sequence: (1) The person perceives with any one of his five sense organs an object or objects; (2) The perceptions stimulate automatic thought; (3) Each thought stimulates an automatic feeling; and (4) Then the person acts. (Orlando, 1972, p. 25)

The first three items are defined as the person's immediate reaction and cannot be observed; only the action, which is what the person says and conveys nonverbally, can be observed.

Orlando (1961) views the immediate reaction as unique to each situation and notes that in a nursing situation what a nurse perceives, thinks, and feels about the patient's behavior reflects the nurse's individuality. She explains that the nurse's automatic thoughts about the perception reflect the nurse's meaning or interpretation attached to the perception. From the patient's viewpoint, the nurse's meanings may or may not be correct. However, regardless of the extent of their accuracy, the perceptions that provoke the nurse's thoughts are communications from the patient and as such are "raw" data for the nurse to use in her or his investigation of the patient's behavior. Orlando (1961) notes that if the nurse was preoccupied with the application of principles this preoccupation would condition the nurse's first thoughts.

Orlando views the nurse's appropriate use of the immediate reaction as critical to understanding the meaning of the patient's behavior. Orlando formulated a deliberative nursing process to help the nurse use her or his immediate reactions.

Deliberative Nursing Process

Orlando's (1961) deliberative nursing process[1] formulations reflect her view of the nurse-patient situation as a dynamic whole; the patient's behavior affects the nurse and the nurse's behavior (action) affects the patient. In developing her theory, Orlando carefully analyzed nurse-patient contacts to determine what nurse action resulted in a positive patient outcome as well as what contributed to negative outcomes. Nurse actions with positive results were called a deliberative nursing process, whereas nurse actions that produced negative patient outcomes were called automatic personal responses.

According to Orlando (1972), the use of a deliberative nursing action requires that a shared communication process occur between the nurse and the patient in order to determine: (a) the meaning of the patient's behavior, (b) the help required by the patient, and (c) whether the patient was helped by the nurse's action.

To comprehend this approach, it is necessary to explain Orlando's (1972) conception of a person's action process. In a person-to-person contact each person experiences an immediate reaction that contains the person's perception about the observed behavior of another person, the thought about the perception, and a feeling associated with the thought. These items remain a secret from the other person unless the first individual openly discloses them. Only the first individual's

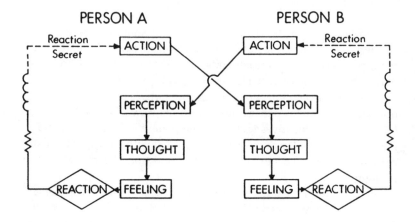

Figure 63.1. The action process in a person-to-person contact functioning in secret. The perceptions, thoughts, and feelings in each individual are not directly available to the perception of the other individual through the observable action.
SOURCE: Orlando (1972, p. 26). Reprinted by permission.

action is available to the other person (see Figures 63.1 and 63.2 to visualize these processes). In other words, if a nurse makes a statement to the patient and does not share what perception, thought, or feeling formed the basis of the action, the patient remains unaware of them. This sequential process, whether disclosed or not, continues throughout the entire contact.

Although the separation of perceptions, thoughts, and feelings is extremely difficult, this process helps nurses see how one aspect of their reaction affects the other aspects (Orlando, 1961). Orlando developed guidelines (1972) that specify how a person should use the content of her or his immediate reaction in a deliberative way, through open disclosure, to achieve a helpful patient outcome. The guidelines include the following: (a) in a situation a person verbally states to the other person any or all the items in her or his immediate reaction, (b) the stated item must be expressed as self-designated, and (c) the person asks the other person to verify or correct the item verbally expressed. In a nurse-patient contact, Orlando's deliberative nursing process can be described as follows: Whatever the nurse perceives about the patient with any one of the five sense organs and thinks and feels about this perception must, at least in part, be verbally expressed

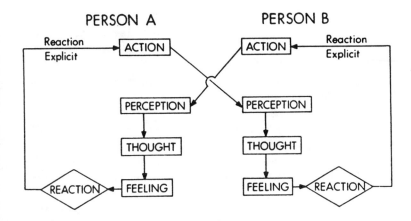

Figure 63.2. The action process in a person-to-person contact
functioning in open disclosure. The perceptions, thoughts, and feelings
of each individual are directly available to the perception of the other
individual through the observable action.
SOURCE: Orlando (1972, p. 26). Reprinted by permission.

as self-designated to the patient and then asked about. Only the
person involved in the person-to-person contact can verify ownership of the items. An example would be "I noticed your face got red
as you talked about your doctor (a visual perception stated as self-
designated). I thought you might be angry with him (thought about
the perception stated as self-designated). Could that be or not (requests verification or correction)?" The nurse continues this process
until she or he observes and verifies, with the patient, improvement
in the patient's verbal and nonverbal behavior.

The nurse who uses this type of action is more likely to find out
and meet the patient's immediate needs for help because when the
nurse expresses her or his immediate reaction the patient also is more
likely to do so (Orlando, 1972). The nurse's expression of his or her
reaction minimizes the opportunity for the nurse to make assumptions and increases the chance to correct or verify the nurse's private
interpretations of the patient's action. Both people have a better
understanding of how the other experienced the immediate situation
(Orlando, 1972). "Failure to impose the entire discipline on the nurse's
own process at least some of the time with any one person may result
in misinterpretation of actions on both sides" (Pelletier, 1968, p. 4).

Orlando (1961) provided helpful guidelines for the nurse to use in expressing her or his immediate reactions in a deliberate, exploratory way. To explore the observed behavior, she wrote, *"Any observation [perception] shared and explored with the patient is immediately useful in ascertaining and meeting his need or finding out that he is not in need at that time"* (pp. 35-36). An example is "I notice tears in your eyes. Could that be or not?" Because the patient is more likely to agree with the correctness of the nurse's perception, its use is more efficient than first exploring thoughts (Orlando, 1961). Efficiency is important because the longer that patients are frustrated in getting help, the more distressful their presenting behavior and the more obscure its meaning (Orlando, 1961).

The nurse's automatic thoughts about perceptions also can be used to explore the patient's behavior. Because the nurse's thoughts about her or his perception are likely to be inadequate, incorrect, or only partially correct, the nurse should explore their validity. In describing the nurse's use of the immediate thoughts, Orlando (1961) wrote, *"The nurse does not assume that any aspect of her reaction* [here meaning thought] *to the patient is correct, helpful or appropriate until she checks the validity of it in exploration with the patient"* (p. 56). Therefore the nurse should use her or his thoughts deliberatively, namely, through exploration for their relevance to the present situation. In understanding the nature of thoughts, Orlando (1961) cautions that a nurse is more likely to assume that her or his thoughts about a perception are correct if they are not tentatively formulated as questions or wonderings. When the nurse states her or his thoughts as a tentative possibility the patient is more likely to respond with her or his own negative reaction. For example, "I saw you close your eyes when I started to change your colostomy bag. I thought you might be frightened about having to learn how to do this yourself. Could that be or not?"

After the thought about the perception the nurse experiences a feeling, which may be positive or negative. Regardless of whether the feeling is negative or positive it can be as useful as perceptions and thoughts, provided the patient has an opportunity to respond to it (Orlando, 1961). When the nurse explores her or his feeling, Orlando (1972) proposes that the nurse also state the perception that provoked the thought rather than stating only the feeling. For example, if the nurse was angry because the patient kept asking for a bedpan and the nurse thought the patient did not need it, the nurse would state, "I get angry when you keep asking for the bedpan because I don't think you need it. Am I right or not?" If the nurse does not resolve her or his feelings with the patient, these same feelings may occur again when in contact with the patient. In addition, if these feelings are not expressed and explored, they may show in the nurse's nonverbal behavior (Orlando, 1961).

Determining the meaning of the patient's behavior and identifying the patient's immediate need for help do not end the nurse's responsibility to the patient. Therefore, in each situation the nurse initiates an exploratory process to ascertain how the patient is affected by what she or he says or does (Orlando, 1961). Orlando stresses that it is not the nurse's activity that is evaluated but rather its effects upon the patient. Only through this evaluative process can a nurse become aware of how and whether her or his action helped the patient.

Unlike the current usage of the term *nursing process*, Orlando's deliberative nursing process is *not* a linear process of assessing, diagnosing, planning, implementing, and evaluating, with each step following the other in unvaried sequence. Rather, the deliberative nursing process is a "muddy," serial, back-and-forth process because it has elements of continuous reflection as the nurse attempts to understand the patient's meaning of the behavior and what help the patient needs from the nurse in order to be helped. These responses are stimulated by the nurse's unfolding awareness of the particulars of the individual situation (Orlando, 1961). Orlando thinks the use of the deliberative nursing process helps the nurse fulfill the nursing function because the nurse finds out and meets the patient's immediate needs for help. However, when a nurse uses an automatic personal response the patient's distress is not relieved because communication between them becomes unclear (Orlando, 1961).

Automatic Personal Responses

Orlando (1961) asserts that people's automatic reactions and actions, inherent in a nursing situation, are likely to cause unclear communication, which creates a situational conflict. Therefore, understanding the nature of automatic responses is necessary to recognize the problems associated with their use. This understanding helps the nurse to avoid the pitfall of having a "ready" answer or solution to the problem at hand. Orlando (1961) characterizes automatic personal responses as being decided upon without the patient's perception of the situation and for reasons other than the patient's immediate need for help.

Orlando (1961) observed that automatic responses contribute to inadequate communications because items of a person's immediate reaction are withheld from the other person. Thus the first person makes assumptions about the situation that are never verified or corrected. For the nurse these assumptions form an unreliable basis for decision making and action because the patient does not participate in the process. Orlando (1972) specifies why automatic responses, which are contrary to the nurse's use of a deliberative process of action, are not helpful:

1. When a nurse withholds his or her immediate reaction, the patient cannot verify or correct it. This withholding allows the patient to make assumptions about the nurse's verbal and nonverbal behavior.
2. If the nurse's response is not stated as self-designated, the patient is allowed to make assumptions about the origin of what is heard (the use of "we" does not clearly provide the origin).
3. If the nurse's response is not in the form of a question, the other person may not feel free to correct or verify what was heard. As a result neither person in the contact knows the immediate reaction of the other; therefore, each is left with an unverified understanding of the other's action (Orlando, 1972).

Figure 63.1 reinforces this description.

Orlando (1961) stresses that actions based on the nurse's conclusion, arrived at without deliberation with the patient, often are not helpful. Thus an action carried out automatically, without the patient's participation, could be correct but ineffective in helping the patient (Orlando, 1961).

The nurse's experience of the immediate situation is not sufficient to understand a patient's presenting behavior. Rather, in each nurse-patient experience a deliberative process of inquiry is needed to prevent the use of automatic responses and activities.

Orlando's deliberative nursing process is an integral part of her formulations, thus making it a practical theory to use. The simplicity of this deliberative approach, however, disguises the complexity of its use. As with any skill the use of the deliberative nursing process must be developed through practice. Self-reflection through the analysis of one's action process helps the nurse recognize when she or he does not act in a deliberative manner.

Improvement

The last major concept in Orlando's theory is improvement in the patient's behavior. If the nurse's activity meets the patient's immediate needs for help, the patient's behavior improves from what it had been; if the patient's behavior does not change, the nursing function has not been met:

> In both situations the results are available immediately after the activity is performed. . . . The product of meeting the patient's immediate need for help is . . . "improvement" in the verbal and nonverbal behavior of the patient. This observable change allows the nurse to believe or disbelieve that her activity relieved, prevented or diminished the patient's sense of helplessness. (Orlando, 1972, p. 21)

When the patient's behavior has improved the situation loses its problematic character; the equilibrium changes to a unified whole. The nurse uses this concept of improvement to evaluate whether her or his activity has produced a change in the patient's condition (the product of professional nursing). Namely, did the nurse help the patient communicate clearly and did this process help direct how the patient's need for help would be met? Orlando (1961) believes improvement is relative to what condition existed when the nurse and patient started the process, the length of their relationship, what they were able to accomplish, and whether the patient notes an increased sense of well-being. She asserts that the nurse's "own individuality and that of the patient require that she go through this each time she is called upon to render service to those who need her" (Orlando, 1961, p. 91).

Orlando (1961) states that she did not deal with long-range nursing goals. She believes the process of helping a patient occurs in the immediate situation and the outcome for the patient depends on the help provided in that immediate experience.

The nature of the concepts in this nursing process theory demonstrates that Orlando envisions nursing as a creative process that begins and ends in the patient's immediate experience. Her formulations of a person's action process and her prescriptions on how to use the elements of the nurse's immediate reaction make it a practical nursing practice theory.

Note

1. *Deliberative nursing process* was renamed *nursing process discipline* in 1972. Deliberative nursing process is used in this section to provide consistency.

64

The Theory's Propositions and Implied Research

"Propositions are statements of relationships between concepts in the theoretical system" (Kim, 1983, p. 11). "Until one has propositional statements about the relationship between the concepts one does not have a usable theory" (Burr et al., 1979, p. 52). Propositions state the theory's concepts in an associational or causal way that indicates that the relationship can be measured. Thus propositions provide a means for developing hypotheses so the theory can be tested through research. Without research, the theory's influence on nursing practice can only be assumed. It is only through research that these assumptions can be confirmed or refuted. It is through research that a theory can be further developed or refined.

Orlando did not formulate explicit propositions of her theory; however, propositional statements can be derived from her concepts. Following each proposition, research implied by the proposition is suggested.

> Proposition 1: There is a relationship between the *patient's presenting behavior* and the presence of patient distress *(an immediate need for help)*.

When patients have an unmet need for help they become distressed (Orlando, 1961). This distress is manifested through their behavior.

Behaviors can be conveyed to the nurse through verbal and nonverbal communications.

A research study could be undertaken to categorize the following types of verbal communication to the nurse: questions, complaints, and requests. Nurses trained in the use of Orlando's deliberative nursing process would explore the meaning to the patient of the verbal communications and categorize results into types of distress or no distress. Although the patient's distress is unique, knowledge about the type of behavior that is most often used by patients to communicate certain types of distress, and their associated need for help, would be a helpful resource to nurses for exploration of similar situations in the future. Also, these findings would be useful for developing further research, and for educational purposes.

> Proposition 2: There is a relationship between a nurse's use of
> Orlando's *distinct nursing function* and the nurse's ability to rec-
> ognize the need for inquiry *(deliberative nursing process)* into the
> meaning of the *patient's presenting behavior.*

Dewey (1938) and Kuhn (1970) both believe that the use of an organizing principle (such as Orlando's function of nursing) allows a person to recognize a situation as problematic. Early recognition of a patient's immediate need for help is important because the longer the patient experiences distress, the greater the distress becomes and the more obscure the patient's behavior (Orlando, 1961). The more obscure the behavior, the more difficult it is for the nurse to find out what the patient is distressed about. According to Orlando (1961) the treatment and prevention of a disease proceeds best when patients are not distressed.

Research could be designed to examine differences in nurse responses in patient encounters between nurses who use "finding out and meeting the patient's immediate need for help" and nurses who use a different theory and/or no nursing theory. Implied in this research is the relationship between the nurse's immediate reaction to a patient's verbal request and the use of all or part of the immediate reaction in the nurse's response.

> Proposition 3: The more competent the nurse is in labeling her or his
> perceptions, thoughts, and feelings *(immediate reaction)*, the more

apt she or he is to find out *(deliberative nursing process)* the nature of the patient's distress.

According to Orlando (1961), although it is difficult to separate the items of the immediate reaction, it is important to do so because it helps the nurse understand how the items influence each other. If the nurse does not understand the basis of her or his process of action it is difficult for the nurse to use the immediate reaction effectively in exploration of the patient's behavior. Orlando (1961) believes the exploration of any part of the nurse's reaction is immediately helpful in determining the patient's need for help.

A research study that includes the education of nurses in the use of Orlando's theory could be designed to compare nurses' identification of patient distress and associated need for help between nurses who can accurately separate their immediate reaction with nurses unable to do so. A secondary research component in this study could be to identify types of patient behavior that are more likely associated with the nurse's ability or inability to accurately separate the items of her or his immediate reaction.

Proposition 4: If the nurse explores her or his *immediate reaction* with the patient the patient's distress is lessened *(improvement)*.

The major aim of Orlando's (1961) theory is to bring about improvement in the patient's verbal and nonverbal behavior, thus improving the nursing care of patients. If the patient's immediate needs for help are not found out and met, the patient's condition remains the same or worsens. A patient's condition might be seriously threatened if the distress is not relieved. After the nurse's action, the nurse is able to determine immediately whether the distress was relieved by observing changes in the patient's verbal and nonverbal behavior. Research that compares patient outcomes when nurses explore and when they do not explore the patient's presenting behavior could be used to test the theory.

In addition to research on the effects of improvement in the patient's immediate behavior, other indicators reflecting improvement might be studied. For example, experimental research could compare randomly assigned patients who have deliberative nursing care with those who have automatic nursing care by measuring patient levels of anxiety, depression, or helplessness after each shift. This study would measure the immediate influence of nursing on patients. A variety of standardized instruments are available to measure these concepts. Patient distress also could be operationalized as increased dependence, which could be measured with standardized instruments.

> Proposition 5: The nurse's use of the *deliberative nursing process* will be less costly than the nurse's use of *automatic personal responses* (a secondary concept of the theory).

Because automatic actions are based on conclusions arrived at independently of the patient they most often are not helpful, as they do not consider the patient's perception of the situation. Because the nurse arbitrarily applies a solution to what she or he thinks the patient's problem is, that solution often is ineffective and therefore costly in terms of the nurse's time, materials, and drugs. It also may prolong the patient's hospitalization or use of ambulatory services. Recently, reducing health care costs has been a major national goal. Therefore the nurse's use of a deliberative nursing process might be both effective and efficient.

One research question would be "Are nurses who use a deliberative nursing process approach to explore the patient's behavior more likely to reduce costs than those who use automatic personal actions?" The study could measure such costs as length of stay or health care visits, use of analgesics and hypnotics, and nursing contact hours.

> Proposition 6: Patients experiencing repeated *improvement* as the result of *deliberative nursing* will have positive cumulative effects.

Orlando (1961) often refers to the cumulative effects of repeated patient improvement as the result of deliberative nursing. She notes that although improvement is always relative to the patient's condition at the start of the nurse-patient contact, these repeated improvements may positively contribute to the patient's improved self-care. At another time she notes that improvement is related to the length of the nurse-patient contact and to what they accomplish in each contact. Even though the changes might be small they may have cumulative value (Orlando, 1961).

Research could be designed to measure the degree of self-care competence in colostomy care on discharge in two groups of patients, one receiving deliberative nursing and the other nondeliberative nursing care. A research question for obstetrical nursing is "Do primiparous women feel more confident about self- and newborn care at discharge when they have received deliberative nursing care versus nondeliberative nursing care?" Also, a researcher could compare patients' sense of self-care confidence immediately prior to discharge in cohorts of patients receiving deliberative and nondeliberative care.

Orlando's propositions provide a way to study systematically the elements of her theory. These proposed research studies would provide information to further assess the theory's internal validity as well as to determine how the nurse's use of the theory influences the outcome of the patient's condition.

65

Research of the Theory

Whereas the understanding of a professional discipline is gained through its theories, to a great extent, knowledge of that discipline is gained through research (Walker, 1992). One way to expand nursing knowledge is through research of its theories. According to Barnum (1990), for a nursing theory to be relevant it must meet three criteria: (a) It addresses essential nursing issues, (b) it contributes to knowledge development in nursing, and (c) it has research potential. Research tests a theory's description or explanation as well as providing a body of related knowledge (Barnum, 1990).

In nursing, research of a theory serves to develop and refine theory and to improve practice. As new knowledge is implemented into practice it stimulates further research. The theory-research-practice process continues in a circular fashion and results in improvement and/or refinement of practice.

Because nursing is a practice discipline it has an obligation to society to generate new knowledge continually so nursing care can be based on validated research. Tradition, habit, or intuition are insufficient as the basis of practice (Torres, 1990). The use of theories in practice, and the research of them, provides the means for a profession to progress; it also helps fulfill the profession's obligation to society.

Research of Orlando's theory began at Yale University shortly after the theory's development. These studies are hallmarks in clinical nursing research. Some investigators used elements of Orlando's theory without acknowledgment; some of these are included in the bibliography. In this section, clinical research is briefly summarized, according to major focus areas, followed by a section on the theory's use in education and administration.

Studies on Patient's Presenting Behavior

In a study to determine whether patients clearly and adequately expressed their need for help, Elder (1963) found that initially patients did not adequately communicate their need and that the patient's behavior was unreliable for assessing the patient's degree of discomfort. Research on postpartum patients' perceptions of needs by Faulkner (1963) revealed that the patient's expression of one need for help may have several associated needs. She also found that patients rarely summon nurses for emotional needs. Gowan and Morris (1964) found that 81% of postoperative patients had other needs that were unexpressed because "the nurse was perceived as too busy," "hated to bother nurse," or thought the "nurse would disapprove."

Fischelis (1963) conducted a study to determine whether nurses who labeled patients explored the patient's behavior and whether the labels led to beneficial activities. She found that nurses who labeled patients had not explored the meaning of the patient's behavior. Interviews with patients revealed that none of the nurses' explanations of the patient's behavior were correct and that the nurses' activities had not benefited the patient.

Studies on the
Effectiveness of Deliberative Nursing

Four studies were designed to examine whether deliberative nursing relieved specific patient distress. In an experimental study of patients experiencing sleeplessness, Gillis (1976) found that patients in the experimental group used fewer sleep medications than those in the control group. Three studies have indicated that deliberative nursing reduced distress from pain (Barron, 1966; Bochnak, Rhymes, & Leonard, 1962, also reported in Bochnak, 1963; Tarasuk [Bochnak],

Rhymes, & Leonard, 1965). The major findings of these studies were that patients receiving deliberative nursing used fewer pain medications and experienced greater speed and degree of pain relief than did those patients receiving other forms of nursing.

Cameron (1962, 1963) found that nurses using questions to clarify and interpret were more effective in removing barriers that interfered with patient comfort or capability than questions seeking factual information. In a study of patient-initiated interactions, Dye (1963a, 1963b) found that patient distress was more often relieved by deliberative nursing. The results also indicated that most nursing actions were nondeliberative and that adverse reactions to the setting were the major cause of patient distress.

Studies documenting the positive effects of deliberative nursing actions on specific patient physiological outcomes are found in the upcoming studies.

In two pilot studies of patients admitted to an emergency room and to a psychiatric hospital, Anderson, Mertz, and Leonard (1965; also reported in Mertz, 1963) found a statistically significant difference in patient vital signs between patients receiving deliberative and nondeliberative nursing.

In an exploratory study of patients scheduled for gynecological elective surgery, Elms's (1964) results revealed that pulse rate showed a significant decrease as the result of deliberative nursing and more of these patients indicated that their distress was relieved by the nurse's approach. In a larger study using the same design and type of patient, a difference did not exist in pulse rate but more patients in the experimental group cited nursing as a factor in distress relief than did those in the control group (Elms & Leonard, 1966).

The use of a deliberative nursing process with gynecological patients was studied by Dumas and her colleagues. In three experimental studies, one of which was a pilot, Dumas and Leonard (1963; also reported in Dumas, 1963) found the incidence of postoperative vomiting to be significantly less in patients whose nurse used deliberative nursing. Patients whose distress was not relieved preoperatively tended to vomit more postoperatively. However, contradictory results were found in a subsequent study on the same unit but with a different nurse providing care (Dumas, Anderson, & Leonard, 1965). In another experimental study, Dumas and Johnson [Anderson] (1972) measured the effects of a deliberative nursing process on seven variables associated with postoperative recovery. The stress level of patients who received deliberative nursing preoperatively was significantly lower than that of patients who did not. However, little difference was found between the two groups on the other indicators of recovery. Type of surgery was thought to be a significant confounding variable. Studying the incidence of vomiting in general postoperative patients, Rhymes (1964) found that the difference between patients who did not vomit or need catherization was related to deliberative nursing care.

In a study of patients in labor, Tryon (1962; also reported in Tryon & Leonard, 1964) found that patients who participated in the preoperative plans had more effective enema results than those who did not participate. This finding lends some support to Orlando's theory that automatic activities, even though prescribed, often are not effective if the patient's reaction to the activity has not been considered. In a second study, Tryon (1966) postulated that a deliberative nursing approach to routine "support" measures would increase patient participation; the results were inconclusive.

The next two studies tested the influence of deliberative nursing on physiological measurements other than vital signs. Using electively hospitalized medical patients, Pride (1968) tested the causal connection between experimental nursing, friendly unfocused nursing, and "no approach" on patient stress, as measured by urine potassium and the IPAT Anxiety Scale, a physiochemical index of patient welfare. Pride found that urine potassium was lower in patients receiving experimental nursing than for patients receiving other forms of nursing. However, there was no relationship between patient's level of anxiety and type of nursing. Clausen [Cameron] (1983) found breast-feeding mothers who received deliberative nursing care exhibited higher level functioning of the milk ejection reflex than those who did not.

Research related to the care of children was the focus of the next two studies. Wolfer and Visintainer (1975) found that children who received deliberative nursing care prior to minor surgery had less upset behavior, were more cooperative, and had fewer postsurgery adjustment problems than children who did not. When comparing parents' knowledge of illness, care prescribed, and compliance with treatment, Thibaudeau and Reidy (1977) found that mothers who had received deliberative nursing, as compared with those who had not, had significantly more knowledge of illness and complications and complied more fully with the prescribed treatment.

Characteristics of Nurses
Who Use Deliberative Nursing

With adult cancer patients Ponte (1988) correlated primary nurses' use of empathy skill and their use of Orlando's deliberative process. A positive relationship was found between empathy skills and nurses' use of a deliberative nursing process. Surprisingly, these primary nurses scored low both on use of empathy skills and deliberative nursing process.

Education and Administration Research

In addition to the previously mentioned research by Orlando (1972), investigators have used Orlando's theory in nursing education and administration. Haggerty (1987) applied Orlando's theory to the analysis of student nurses' responses to videotapes of patients with differing distress behaviors and found that deliberative responses were not associated with type of educational program, but were related to the type of patient distress.

Schmieding (1988) adapted Orlando's theory to the study of nurse administrators' actions and found that in the majority administrators did not view situations posed to them by their staff as problematic, their feelings in the situation were overwhelmingly negative, and they would act without further investigation. Subsequent research by Schmieding revealed that (a) nurses preferred that their supervisor use exploratory actions with them, but the majority thought their supervisor would use nonexploratory actions (1990b); (b) head nurses seldom involved staff nurses in the problem-solving process (1990a); and (c) a relationship was found between the head nurse's response to a staff nurse and the staff nurse's response to patients (1992).

Conclusion

These research findings lend some support to the validity of Orlando's theory but further research, with stronger controls on threats to internal validity and larger, randomly assigned samples, should be developed. The use of Orlando's theory could provide a means for increasing the influence of nursing on positive patient outcomes.

66

Application to Practice

"One of the most important tests of a theory is its applicability in practice" (Barnum, 1990, p. 19). Orlando's theory is characterized as a practice theory that provides a framework to guide nurses' actions. A theory's language can influence its use. If the language is too abstract or esoteric nurses will have difficulty clearly understanding it and applying it to their practice. Orlando uses language nurses can readily understand and use in everyday practice.

According to Barnum (1990), "The function of theory is to guide practice and to direct the mind-set of nurses. If it fails to do that, it is useless" (p. 69). The ultimate criterion of a practice theory is whether the patient is helped through its use. Some criteria for selecting a practice theory are the following:

- Does it provide conceptual direction to the nurse about how to use it to help the patient?
- Can the nurse verify through empirical observations of the patient that the theory's use influenced the outcome?
- Can it be incorporated into the nurse's mind-set and become an integral part of the nurse's practice?

Orlando's theory focuses the nurse's mind-set to the patient's immediate experience and emphasizes that only the patient can verify what he or she is experiencing. Orlando's theory is a process rather than a content theory, which becomes integrated into the nurse's total practice. Thus a nurse does not have to stop and think "Should I apply Orlando's theory in this case?" Rather, it is a theory that nurses consistently use with all patients, and its concept of improvement enables nurses to verify their results immediately by observing changes in the patient's behavior.

The four cases in this section are brief examples of situations where nurses used Orlando's deliberative process. The first three have been previously published (Schmieding, 1986). The fourth is presented in a nursing process record form, designed by Orlando (1972), which depicts the nurse's action process. The examples are representative of situations where nurses feel frustrated, label patients, react against patients, or feel a concern for patients.

A 78-year-old man with compromised circulation caused by Raynaud's disease had recent skin grafts to his foot that were not healing as rapidly as expected. When his primary nurse was about to change his foot dressing she noticed that the patient had eaten only bites of his lunch (presenting behavior). The nurse's first two nursing actions were automatic personal responses that failed to help the patient express his distress. She said, "Didn't you like the food?" The patient replied, "It was OK." The nurse responded, "Then why didn't you eat it?" The patient responded, "I didn't feel hungry." The nurse was feeling frustrated and stopped to clarify what she was thinking and feeling. She then said, "I feel frustrated. The reason I asked why you didn't eat more was that I'm concerned that your skin graft won't properly heal if you do not eat enough protein. Can you understand my frustration?" The gentleman abruptly looked up at the nurse and said, "Gee, I didn't think anyone around here cared for an old man like me [the patient's distress]. Bring back the food and I'll try to eat more." Within a short time the patient had eaten all the food on the tray and thereafter continued to eat the food brought to him. His wound began to steadily heal and he was discharged within 1 week.

Referring to patients by behavioral terms or diagnostic labels can adversely influence the patient's care because the nurse bases her or his action on assumptions about the patient's label rather than on the patient's immediate behavior. The following case conveys how basing action on patient labels might interfere with individualized care.

A 62-year-old woman, diagnosed as schizophrenic, was admitted to a gynecology unit for uterine bleeding. The head nurse expressed concerns to her supervisor about caring for "schizophrenics" because nurses on the unit did not know how to talk to this type of patient. The supervisor assured the head nurse that, as with other patients, the nurse's exploration of her or his immediate reaction with the patient was most effective in determining what help this patient needed. Shortly after the conversation, the head nurse heard the patient yelling, "Don't take my blood, don't take my blood!" (presenting behavior). When the head nurse entered the room three people were assuring the patient that they were not trying to hurt her but that they needed to test her blood to find out what was causing her illness (automatic actions based on their assumption that the patient thought they wanted to hurt her). The head nurse stepped to the patient's side and said, "I'd like to know why you are saying, 'Don't take my blood' " (exploring the head nurse's perception). The patient looked up, hesitated a moment, and then, pointing at the lab technician, resident, and staff nurse, said, "You, you, and you, get out." Then, pointing to the head nurse, she said, "You sit down and stay." The patient revealed to the head nurse that she was afraid the test would require too much blood and only make her weaker than she already was (the distress). After being assured that the test required only a little blood the patient consented to have the blood drawn.

Another incident occurred with the above patient when low census on two units required that the patients on both units be placed in one. Nurses on one unit told the head nurse it would be too upsetting to move the schizophrenic patient and therefore the patients from the other unit should be transferred to accommodate this patient even though there were more patients on the other unit. The head nurse agreed with this plan only if the nurse first validated this assumption with the patient. The nurse explained the problem to the patient and explored the assumption by stating, "The nurses and I think it would be too upsetting to you to move. Would it be?" The patient replied, "That's the problem! Get the wheelchair, honey, I'm ready to move." These two situations convey that Orlando's theory is useful both in clinical nursing and for making administrative decisions.

Nurses are human and thus at times have negative personal reactions toward patients that interfere with their ability to help those patients. Often, these reactions are based on assumptions about the patient's behavior on which the nurse has placed a value judgment. If these thoughts are withheld, the patient is left to make her or his interpretation about the nurse's verbal and nonverbal behavior. In the following situation, several nurses had negative reactions to the patient; one nurse expressed and explored her feeling to the patient and found out that her interpretation of the patient's behavior was incorrect.

A 39-year-old diabetic patient who was 4 months pregnant was admitted with vomiting. She spoke only when spoken to and remained in bed even though she could be up (presenting behavior). She said she had vomited, but the nurses had not observed it. During reports, nurses speculated, "I don't think she really is vomiting" and "I don't think she really wants this baby." These remarks were passed from shift to shift and eventually these speculations were passed on as facts even though no one had confirmed them with the patient. One nurse was shocked to learn that the patient did not want her baby. Although apprehensive, the nurse decided to express her feeling to the patient. She stated, "I'm shocked because I hear you don't want this baby. Is that true?" Immediately the patient's eyes began to well over with tears and she sobbed, "That's not true. I want the baby, it's just that I'm afraid I'll die in labor [the patient's distress]. Fifteen years ago when my other child was born I wasn't diabetic." The nurse was stunned by the patient's remark and asked, "Does your doctor or anyone know of this?" The patient replied, "No, I thought if I told people they would think I was a hysterical woman." The patient then agreed to discuss this with both her doctor and her family. Nurses on the unit, when hearing about this, became sympathetic toward the patient. It must be emphasized that the misunderstanding might not have happened if the first nurse who had a negative reaction would have explored her or his assumption with the patient.

The fourth situation involves a 67-year-old man with terminal carcinoma of the lung. His condition was steadily deteriorating as evidenced by increased cyanosis and dyspnea. Radiation treatment was being done only for palliative purposes. While the patient was being transferred to the stretcher for treatment his dyspnea and cyanosis increased, whereupon he was returned to bed and his oxygen was increased. The nurse was concerned about how she could help this patient. The nurse's action processes are recorded in the nursing process record shown in Table 66.1. It dramatically shows how a nurse can help relieve distress in a dying patient.

TABLE 66.1 Nursing Process Record

Perception of or About the Patient	Thought and/or Feeling About the Perception	Said and/or Did to, With, or for the Patient
Patient staring into space. One arm over forehead. Tightly holding my hand.	I thought he was frightened. I felt concern for him.	"I think you're feeling frightened; is that so?"
"Yes." Then he sighed. Tightly holding my hand.	I thought it might help him to talk about his fears.	"I think it would be helpful if you talked about your fears. Could you?"
"I'm thinking about being sick." Removes arm from forehead.	I don't think I know what this means to him.	"Could you tell me more about what that means to you?"
"I'm scared because I know I'm not going to get better." Continues to hold my hand, but less tightly.	I thought he was right and that I needed to let him talk more about it. I felt sad.	"I think you're right. Can you talk more about it?"
"Well, I've asked God to speed it up."	My thought was that he made God part of his life.	"It sounds like God is part of your life. Do you feel that way?"
"Yes, he is always there." Less dyspnic and less cyanotic. Releases hand and folds both arms over chest.	I wonder if he wants to talk more about this or if he wants to rest.	"I'm wondering if there is anything else you'd like to say."
"No, I'd just like to rest for a while." He closed his eyes and was asleep in 5 minutes.		

SOURCE: Orlando (1972).

67

Conclusion

Orlando's theory remains one of the most effective practice theories. It is appealing because it clearly describes what nurses perceive as "good nursing." Nurses participated in the theory's development by allowing their practice to be observed. They validated Orlando's categorization of nursing situations into "good" and "bad" nursing. Nurses know what good nursing is, and Orlando's theory provides the means to help nurses achieve this excellence in practice.

Glossary

Automatic activities
Automatic activities are those decided upon by the nurse for reasons other than the patient's immediate need (Orlando, 1961).

Automatic personal response
An automatic personal response is defined as the withholding of the items of a person's immediate reaction from the other person (Orlando, 1972).

Deliberative nursing process (renamed "nursing process discipline" in 1972)
The requirements of the deliberative nursing process (nursing process discipline) are (a) what the nurse says verbally or conveys nonverbally to the individual must match any or all of the items of her or his immediate reaction, (b) the nurse must clearly express it as self-designated, and (c) the nurse must ask correction or verification from that other person (Orlando, 1972).

Distress
Patients become distressed when they cannot, without help, cope with their needs (Orlando, 1961).

Evaluation of nurse activity
Because a nurse's activity is professional only when the nurse deliberately achieves the purpose of helping the patient, the activity is

not the criterion by which it may be evaluated. The relevance and significance of an activity are determined by whether it helps the patient communicate his or her needs and how the need for help is being met (Orlando, 1961).

Immediate reaction
A person's perception through one of the five sense organs, the automatic thought stimulated by the perception, and the feeling the person experiences following the thought.

Improvement (also see Product)
The patient's immediate improvement is relative to what it was when the process started, and is concerned with increases in the patient's sense of well-being or a change for the better in his or her condition (Orlando, 1961).

Need
"Need is situationally defined as a requirement of the patient which, if supplied, relieves or diminishes his immediate distress or improves his immediate sense of adequacy or well-being" (Orlando, 1961, p. 5).

Nurse's practice
"Learning how to understand what is happening between herself and the patient is the central core of the nurse's practice and comprises the basic framework for the help she gives to patients" (Orlando, 1961, p. 4).

Nursing
"Nursing . . . is responsive to individuals who suffer or anticipate a sense of helplessness; it is focused on the process of care in an immediate experience; it is concerned with providing direct assistance to individuals in whatever setting they are found for the purpose of avoiding, relieving, diminishing or curing the individual's sense of helplessness" (Orlando, 1972, p. 12).

Nursing process
The elements of nursing process are the patient's behavior, the nurse's reaction, and the nursing action (Orlando, 1961).

Nursing process discipline (see Deliberative nursing process")

Nursing situation
Three basic elements make up a nursing situation: (a) the patient's behavior, (b) the nurse's reaction, and (c) the nursing actions designed for the patient's benefit (Orlando, 1961).

Nursing's purpose
"The purpose of nursing is to supply the help a patient requires for his needs to be met" (Orlando, 1961, p. 8).

Presenting behavior
"The presenting behavior of the patient, regardless of the form in which it appears, may represent a plea for help" (Orlando, 1961, p. 40).

Product
"The product of meeting the patient's immediate need for help is . . . 'improvement' in the immediate verbal and nonverbal behavior of the patient" (Orlando, 1972, p. 21).

"The product of professional nursing must be formulated in terms of what professional nursing aims to accomplish, that is, the individual's restoration or improvement in the capacity to care for the self" (Orlando & Dugan, 1989, p. 79).

Professional function of nursing
"The function of professional nursing is . . . conceptualized as finding out and meeting the patient's immediate needs for help" (Orlando, 1972, p. 20).

Situational conflict
At the start of any nurse-patient contact, an almost inevitable conflict occurs between an automatic activity and the patient's immediate need, which may be described as a *situational conflict* (Orlando, 1961).

References

Anderson, B. J., Mertz, H., & Leonard, R. C. (1965). Two experimental tests of a patient-centered admission process. *Nursing Research, 14*(2), 151-157.

Andrews, C. M. (1989). Ida Orlando's model of nursing practice. In J. J. Fitzpatrick & A. L. Whall (Eds.), *Conceptual models of nursing analysis and application* (2nd ed., chap. 6). Norwalk, CT: Appleton & Lange.

Argyris, C., & Schön, D. (1978). *Organizational learning: A theory of action perspective.* Reading, MA: Addison-Wesley.

Barnum, B. J. S. (1990). *Nursing theory analysis, application, evaluation* (3rd ed.). Glenview, IL: Scott, Foresman/Little, Brown Education.

Barron, M. A. (1966). The effects varied nursing approaches have on patients' complaints of pain. *Nursing Research, 15*(1), 90-91.

Bochnak, M. A. (1963). The effect of an automatic and deliberative process of nursing activity on the relief of patients' pain: A clinical experiment. *Nursing Research, 12*(3), 191-192.

Bochnak, M. A., Rhymes, J. P., & Leonard, R. C. (1962). The comparison of two types of nursing activity on the relief of pain. In *Innovations in nurse-patient relationships: Automatic or reasoned nurse action* (Clinical Paper No. 6). New York: American Nurses' Association.

Burr, W. R., Hill, R., Nye, F. I., & Reiss, I. L. (Eds.). (1979). *Contemporary theories about the family.* New York: Free Press.

Cameron, J. (1962). The patient needs to be understood. In *Innovations in nurse-patient relationships: Automatic or reasoned nurse action* (Clinical Paper No. 19). New York: American Nurses' Association.

Cameron, J. (1963). An exploratory study of the verbal responses of the nurse-patient interactions. *Nursing Research, 12*(3), 192.

Clausen [Cameron], J. C. (1983). Clinical nursing research on the science and art of breastfeeding using a deliberative nursing care approach. *Western Journal of Nursing Research, 5*(3), 29.

Dewey, J. (1933). *How we think: A restatement of the relation of reflective thinking to the educative process.* Boston: D. C. Heath.

Dewey, J. (1938). *Logic: The theory of inquiry.* New York: Holt, Rinehart & Winston.

Dumas, R. G. (1963). Psychological preparation for surgery. *American Journal of Nursing, 63*(8), 52-55.

Dumas, R. G., Anderson, B. J., & Leonard, R. C. (1965). The importance of the expressive function in preoperative preparation. In J. K. Skipper, Jr., & R. C. Leonard (Eds.), *Social interaction and patient care* (pp. 16-29). Philadelphia: J. B. Lippincott.

Dumas, R. G., & Johnson [Anderson], B. A. (1972). Research in nursing practice: A review of five clinical experiments. *International Journal of Nursing Studies, 9,* 137-149.

Dumas, R. G., & Leonard, R. C. (1963). The effect of nursing on the incidence of postoperative vomiting. *Nursing Research, 12*(1), 12-15.

Dye, M. C. (1963a). Clarifying patients' communication. *American Journal of Nursing, 63*(8), 56-59.

Dye, M. C. (1963b). A descriptive study of conditions conducive to an effective process of nursing activity. *Nursing Research, 12*(3), 194.

Elder, R. G. (1963). What is the patient saying? *Nursing Forum, 2*(1), 25-37.

Elms, R. R. (1964). Effects of varied nursing approaches during hospital admission: An exploratory study. *Nursing Research, 13*(3), 266-268.

Elms, R. R., & Leonard, R. C. (1966). Effects of nursing approaches during admission. *Nursing Research, 15*(1), 39-48.

Faulkner, S. A. (1963). A descriptive study of needs communicated to the nurse by some mothers on a postpartum service. *Nursing Research, 4*(12), 260.

Fischelis, M. C. (1963). An exploratory study of labels nurses attach to patient behavior and their effect on nursing activities. *Nursing Research, 12*(3), 195.

Gilbert, R. (1940). *The public health nurse and her patient.* New York: Commonwealth Fund.

Gilbert, R. (1951). *The public health nurse and her patient* (2nd ed.). Cambridge, MA: Harvard University Press.

Gillis, Sister L. (1976). Sleeplessness: Can you help? *The Canadian Nurse, 72*(7), 32-34.

Gowan, N. I., & Morris, M. (1964). Nurses' responses to expressed patient needs. *Nursing Research, 13*(1), 68-71.

Haggerty, L. A. (1987). An analysis of senior nursing students' immediate responses to distressed patients. *Journal of Advanced Nursing, 12,* 451-461.

Harré, R. (1989). *The philosophies of science* (2nd ed.). Oxford and New York: Oxford University Press.

Hopkins, L. T. (1941). *Interaction: The democratic process.* Boston: D. C. Heath.

Hopkins, L. T. (1954). *The emerging self in school and home.* New York: Harper & Brothers.

Kilpatrick, W. H. (1925). *Foundations of method: Informal talks in teaching.* New York: Macmillan.

Kilpatrick, W. H. (1941). *Selfhood and civilization: A study of the self-other process.* New York: Teachers College Press.

Kim, H. S. (1983). *The nature of theoretical thinking in nursing.* Norwalk, CT: Appleton-Century-Crofts.

Kuhn, T. S. (1970). *The structure of scientific revolutions* (2nd ed.). Chicago: University of Chicago Press.

Leonard, M. K., & Crane, M. D. (1990). Ida Jean Orlando. In J. B. George (Ed.), *Nursing theories: The base for professional nursing practice* (3rd ed., chap. 10). Norwalk, CT: Appleton & Lange.

Marriner-Tomey, A. (Ed.). (1989). *Nursing theorists and their work* (2nd ed., chap. 19). St. Louis, MO: C. V. Mosby.

McManus, R. L. (1948). *The effect of experience on nursing achievement*. New York: Teachers College Press.

Meleis, A. I. (1991). *Theoretical nursing development and progress* (2nd ed.). Philadelphia: J. B. Lippincott.

Mertz, H. (1963). A study of the process of the nurse's activity as it affects the blood pressure readings and pulse rate of patients admitted to the emergency room. *Nursing Research, 12*(3), 197-198.

Orlando, I. J. (1961). *The dynamic nurse-patient relationship, function, process and principles*. New York: G. P. Putnam.

Orlando, I. J. (1972). *The discipline and teaching of nursing process: An evaluative study*. New York: G. P. Putnam.

Orlando [Pelletier], I. J. (1983, October). *Comments on ANA's social policy statement of 1980*. Paper presented at Southeastern Massachusetts University College of Nursing Honor Society, South Dartmouth.

Orlando, I. J. (1985, October). *Nursing in the 21st century: Alternate paths*. Paper presented at Oakland University School of Nursing, Rochester, MI.

Orlando, I. J. (1987). Nursing in the 21st century: Alternate paths. *Journal of Advanced Nursing, 12*, 405-412.

Orlando, I. J., & Dugan, A. B. (1989). Independent and dependent paths: The fundamental issue for the nursing profession. *Nursing and Health Care, 10*(2), 77-80.

Pelletier, I. J. (1976, August). *The fundamental issue in professional nursing*. Paper presented at University of Tulsa College of Nursing, Tulsa.

Pelletier, I. O. (1967). The patient's predicament and nursing function. *Psychiatric Opinion, 4*, 25-29.

Pelletier, I. O. (1968, May 3). *Nursing process and the problem of evaluating its effectiveness*. Unpublished presentation at the Academic Conference, McLean Hospital, Belmont, MA.

Pelletier, I. O. (1980). *Commentary on ANA draft report, The nature and scope of nursing practice characteristics of specialization: A social policy statement*. Unpublished manuscript.

Peplau, H. E. (1952). *Interpersonal relations in nursing: A conceptual frame of reference for psychodynamic nursing*. New York: G. P. Putnam.

Ponte, P. R. (1988). *The relationship among empathy and the use of Orlando's deliberative process by the primary nurse and the distress of the adult cancer patient*. Doctoral dissertation, Boston University, Boston.

Pride, L. F. (1968). An adrenal stress index as a criterion measure of nursing. *Nursing Research, 17*(4), 292-303.

Rhymes, J. (1964). A description of nurse-patient interaction in effective nursing activity. *Nursing Research, 13*(4), 365.

Schmieding, N. J. (1983). The analysis of Orlando's nursing theory based on Kuhn's theory of science. In P. Chinn (Ed.), *Advances in nursing theory development* (pp. 63-87). Rockville, MD: Aspen Systems.

Schmieding, N. J. (1986). Orlando's theory. In P. Winstead-Fry (Ed.), *Case studies in nursing theory* (pp. 1-36). New York: National League for Nursing.

Schmieding, N. J. (1987). Problematic situations in nursing: Analysis of Orlando's theory based on Dewey's theory of inquiry. *Journal of Advanced Nursing, 12*(4), 431-440.

Schmieding, N. J. (1988). Action process of nurse administrators to problematic situations based on Orlando's theory. *Journal of Advanced Nursing, 13*(1), 99-107.

Schmieding, N. J. (1990a). Do head nurses include staff nurses in problem solving? *Nursing Management, 21*(3), 58-60.

Schmieding, N. J. (1990b). A model for assessing nurse administrator's actions. *Western Journal of Nursing Research, 12*(3), 293-306.

Schmieding, N. J. (1992). Relationship between head nurse responses to staff nurses and staff nurse response to patients. *Western Journal of Nursing Research, 13*(6), 746-760.

Tarasuk [Bochnak], M. B., Rhymes, J., & Leonard, R. C. (1965). An experimental test of the importance of communication skills for effective nursing. In J. K. Skipper, Jr., & R. C. Leonard (Eds.), *Social interaction and patient care* (pp. 110-120). Philadelphia: J. B. Lippincott.

Thibaudeau, M., & Reidy, M. M. (1977). Nursing makes a difference: A comparative study of the health behavior of mothers in three primary care agencies. *International Journal of Nursing, 14,* 97-107.

Torres, G. (1990). The place of concepts and theories within nursing. In J. B. George (Ed.), *Nursing theories: The base for professional nursing practice* (3rd ed., chap. 1). Norwalk, CT: Appleton & Lange.

Tryon, P. A. (1962). The effect of patient participation in decision making on the outcome of a nursing procedure. In *Nursing and the patients' motivation* (Clinical Paper No. 19). New York: American Nurses' Association.

Tryon, P. A. (1966). Use of comfort measures as support during labor. *Nursing Research, 15*(2), 109-118.

Tryon, P. A., & Leonard, R. C. (1964). The effect of patients' participation on the outcome of a nursing procedure. *Nursing Forum, 3*(2), 79-89.

Walker, L. O. (1992). Theory, practice, and research in perspective. In L. H. Nicoll (Ed.), *Perspectives on nursing theory* (2nd ed., chap. 5). New York: J. B. Lippincott.

Wolfer, J., & Visintainer, M. A. (1975). Pediatric surgical patients' and parents' stress response and adjustment as a function of psychological preparation and stress point nursing care. *Nursing Research, 24*(4), 244-255.

Bibliography

References Related to Orlando's Work

Allen, M., Frasure-Smith, N., & Gottlieb, L. (1982). What makes a "good" nurse? *The Canadian Nurse, 78,* 42-45.

Bottorff, J. L., & D'Cruz, J. V. (1984). Towards inclusive notions of "patient" and "nurse." *Journal of Advanced Nursing, 9,* 549-553.

Chapman, J. S. (1969). *Effects of different nursing approaches upon psychological and physiological responses of patients.* Cleveland, OH: Case Western Reserve University, Frances Payne Bolton School of Nursing.

Dracup, K. A., & Breu, C. S. (1978). Using nursing research findings to meet the needs of grieving spouses. *Nursing Research, 27*(4), 212-216.

Eisler, J., Wolfer, J. A., & Diers, D. (1972). Relationship between need for social approval and postoperative recovery and welfare. *Nursing Research, 21*(5), 520-525.

Farrell, G. A. (1991). How accurately do nurses perceive patients' needs? A comparison of general and psychiatric settings. *Journal of Advanced Nursing, 16,* 1062-1070.

Forchuk, C. (1991). A comparison of the works of Peplau and Orlando. *Archives of Psychiatric Nursing, 5,* 38-45.

Haggerty, L. A. (1985). A theoretical model for developing students' communication skills. *Journal of Nursing Education, 24*(7), 296-298.

Hampe, S. O. (1975). Needs of grieving spouses in a hospital setting. *Nursing Research, 24*(2), 113.

Harrison, C. (1966). Deliberative nursing process versus automatic nurse action. *Nursing Clinics of North America, 1*(3), 387-397.

Kokuyama, T., & Schmieding, N. J. (in press). Responses staff nurses prefer compared with their perception of head nurse responses. *Japanese Journal of Nursing Administration.*

Kumata, M., & Goto, H. (1984). What I learned from Orlando—Individuality and determination in actual interaction with a patient. *Gekkan Nursing, 4*(4), 129-133.

Lego, S. (1975). The one-to-one nurse-patient relationship. In *Psychiatric nursing 1946 to 1974: A report on the state of the art—Completed by Florence L. Huey* (pp. 1-61). New York: American Journal of Nursing Company.

Mahaffy, P. P. (1965). The effects of hospitalization on children admitted for tonsillectomy and adenoidectomy. *Nursing Research, 14*(1), 12-19.

Marriner-Tomey, A., Mills, D. I., & Sauter, M. K. (1989). Ida Jean Orlando (Pelletier) nursing process theory. In A. Marriner-Tomey (Ed.), *Nursing theorists and their work* (2nd ed., chap. 19). St. Louis: C. V. Mosby.

Nelson, B. (1978). A practical application of nursing theory. *Nursing Clinics of North America, 13*(1), 157-169.

New England Board of Higher Education. (1977). *Mental health continuing education for associate degree nursing faculties: Project report* (NIH Training Grant No. 715 MH13182). Wellesley, MA: Author.

Peitchinis, J. A. (1972). Therapeutic effectiveness of counseling by nursing personnel. *Nursing Research, 21*(2), 138-148.

Perry, J. (1985). Has the discipline of nursing developed to the stage where nurses do "think nursing?" *Journal of Advanced Nursing, 10*, 31-37.

Phillips, S. J. (1988). *Clinical judgment of students in professional nursing programs: An inductive approach.* Unpublished doctoral dissertation, Case Western Reserve University, Cleveland, OH.

Powell, J. H. (1989). The reflective practitioner in nursing. *Journal of Advanced Nursing, 14*, 824-832.

Schmieding, N. J. (1970). The relationship of nursing to the process of chronicity. *Nursing Outlook, 18*(2), 58-62.

Schmieding, N. J. (1983). *A description and analysis of the directive process used by directors of nursing, supervisors, and head nurses in problematic situations based on Orlando's theory of nursing experience.* Unpublished doctoral dissertation, Boston University. (University Microfilms No. 83-19936)

Schmieding, N. J. (1984). Putting Orlando's theory into practice. *American Journal of Nursing, 84*(6), 759-761.

Schmieding, N. J. (1987). Analyzing managerial responses in face-to-face contacts. *Journal of Advanced Nursing, 12*(3), 357-365.

Schmieding, N. J. (1987). Face-to-face contacts: Exploring their meaning. *Nursing Management, 12*(11), 82-86.

Schmieding, N. J. (1990). The analysis of the patient's immediate experience through the use of Orlando's theory. In *Proceedings of the first and second Rosemary Ellis scholars' retreat* (pp. 155-158). Cleveland, OH: Case Western Reserve University, Frances Payne Bolton School of Nursing.

Schmieding, N. J. (1990). Foreword. In I. J. Orlando, *The dynamic nurse-patient relationship: Function, process and principle* (pp. xvii-xix). New York: National League for Nursing.

Schmieding, N. J. (1990). An integrative nursing theoretical framework. *Journal of Advanced Nursing, 15*(4), 463-467.

Schmieding, N. J. (1993). Empowerment through context, structure, and process. *Journal of Professional Nursing, 9*(4), 239-245.

620   FOUNDATIONS OF NURSING THEORY

Schmieding, N. J. (1993). Successful superior-subordinate relationships require mutual management. *Health Care Supervisor, 11*(4), 52-63.

Silva, M. C. (1979). Effects of orientation information on spouses' anxieties and attitudes toward hospitalization and surgery. *Research in Nursing and Health, 2,* 127-136.

Skipper, J. K., Jr., Leonard, R. C., & Rhymes, J. (1968). Child hospitalization and social interaction: An experimental study of mothers' feelings of stress, adaptation and satisfaction. *Medical Care, 6*(6), 496-506.

Wallston, K. A., Cohen, B. D., Wallston, B. S., Smith, R. A., & DeVellis, B. M. (1978). Increasing nurses' person-centeredness. *Nursing Research, 27*(3), 156-159.

Wiedenbach, E. (1958). *Family-centered maternity nursing.* New York: G. P. Putnam.

Williamson, Y. M. (1978). Methodologic dilemmas in tapping the concept of patient needs. *Nursing Research, 27*(3), 172-177.

Wooldridge, P. J., Leonard, R. C., & Skipper, J. K., Jr. (1978). *Methods of clinical experimentation to improve patient care.* St. Louis: C. V. Mosby.

Author Index

Subject Index

About the Editors

Chris Metzger McQuiston, PhD, RN, CFNP, received an ADN from Sinclair Community College in 1973, a BSN from the University of Cincinnati in 1975, an MSN from the Medical College of Virginia/ Virginia Commonwealth University in 1981, and recently completed a PhD in nursing at Wayne State University in Detroit in 1993. She has published and been funded in the area of sexually transmitted diseases and was an NIH predoctoral fellow while at Wayne. She is particularly interested in power in relationships as it relates to condom use and the prevention of sexually transmitted disease and self-care agency. Both her clinical practice and research are theory driven. She is also interested in theoretical substruction and Orem's Self-Care Deficit Theory of Nursing. She has taught and maintained a clinical practice as a family nurse practitioner for 13 years and recently began teaching in the FNP Primary Care program at the University of North Carolina at Chapel Hill. She is a member of the American Academy of Nurse Practitioners, the American Nurses' Association, and the Lamda Chapter of Sigma Theta Tau.

Adele A. Webb, PhD, RN, received her BSN from the University of Akron in 1983, her MS in nursing from Ohio State University in 1985, and the PhD in nursing from Wayne State University in 1989. She is an Associate Professor at the University of Akron College of Nursing where she is Chair of the Child and Adolescent track of the graduate program. She is also Director of Nursing Research at Akron General Medical Center and maintains a theory-based clinical practice in the emergency room at Children's Hospital Medical Center of Akron. In 1994, she completed a clinical fellowship at the National Pediatric HIV Resource Center in Newark, New Jersey. Since earning her PhD, she has taught nursing theory in the graduate program and has been published and funded in her clinical focus. Her areas of research include ethics, AIDS, and theory-based practice using Roy and Nightingale's models.

About the Authors

Sheila McGuire Bunting, PhD, RN, has spent many years in nursing practice, education, and administration and is Assistant Professor of Community Health Nursing at the University of Tennessee in Memphis. She received her PhD in nursing from Wayne State University. Earlier nursing degrees were received from St. Ambrose College in Davenport, Iowa, the University of Illinois, and Northern Illinois University. Topics of her publications and presentations include feminist and ethical theories and their relationships to and influences on nursing. Her research pursuits have involved, in addition to nursing ethics, the specific needs and strategies of individuals with HIV and, most recently, the stories of women with children who are living with AIDS. Her dissertation research, funded by the National Institutes of Health, Lambda Chapter of Sigma Theta Tau, and the Michigan Commission of Health and Education, was a grounded theory study of persons with AIDS and their caregivers.

Cheryl Forchuk, PhD, MSN, RN, has a joint appointment as a Nurse Scientist with the Research Institute at Victoria Hospital and Associate Professor with the University of Western Ontario in London, Ontario, Canada. She received her BS in nursing and BA in psychology from the University of Windsor, her MSN with a clinical specialty in mental health nursing from the University of Toronto, and her PhD from the College of Nursing at Wayne State University in Detroit. She has published on many topics, including denial, health promotion, sexuality, and Peplau's interpersonal theory of nursing. Her current research includes exploring the orientation phase of the nurse-client relationship.

Donna L. Hartweg is an Associate Professor in and Director of the School of Nursing at Illinois Wesleyan University in Bloomington, where she has taught in the Orem guided curriculum for over 10 years. She has presented at national and international conferences on Self-Care Deficit Theory of nursing and is author and coauthor of several self-care articles. Her most recent work is on Health Promotion Self-Care within Orem's general theory of nursing, published in the *Journal of Advanced Nursing*. Her current research is on the health promotion self-care practices of healthy middle-aged women. Throughout her doctoral studies in the College of Nursing at Wayne State University in Detroit, she was active in the Orem Research Group.

Madeleine M. Leininger, PhD, PhD Nsc, LHD, DS, RN, CTN, FAAN, is Professor of Nursing and Anthropology in the Colleges of Nursing and Liberal Arts at Wayne State University in Detroit. She is an internationally known educator, author, theorist, administrator, re-searcher, consultant, and a frequently sought after public speaker. Her areas of expertise are transcultural nursing, comparative human care, qualitative research methods, cultural care theory, culture of nursing and health fields, anthropology, nursing, and the future of nursing. She established transcultural nursing as a formal field of study and practice and started the Transcultural Nursing Society in 1974 and the International Association of Human Care (formerly the National Research Care Conference) in 1978. She served as dean, professor of nursing, and director of the centers of nursing and health research at the University of Utah and Wayne State University. Author or editor of 25 books, she has also authored 200 articles, chapters, and films. Extensive field research has been done in Western and non-Western cultures. In the early 1960s, she was the first transcultural nurse to do an ethnographic and ethnonursing study with the Gadsup of the Eastern Highlands of New Guinea. Since then, ethnonursing and ethno-care studies have been conducted with a number of cultures ranging from Appalachia to Africa to the Philippines. She was an early leader in the development and use of qualitative research methods.

Louette R. Johnson Lutjens, PhD, RN, is Associate Professor of Nursing at Grand Valley State University in Allendale, Michigan. She received her doctorate in nursing in 1990 from Wayne State University in Detroit. Her research interests include nursing administrative issues related to nursing diagnosis, interventions, and aggregate patient outcomes and theory development and testing.

Joanne Marchione is a scholar of theories related to health and human caring. For more than a decade she has explored theory development and application with students from nursing and other disciplines. She has also mentored and advised faculty on the application of theory and praxis research. Her B.A. was received from Francis Payne Bolton School of Nursing at Case Western University, and her graduate degrees are in education and anthropology with an emphasis on nursing science. Over the years she has focused on a multicultural approach to the health of families and children. She has studied at many universities in the United States, Europe, and Canada in a continued effort to improve her teaching relative to higher education, theories, cultural diversity, health, child and family health, and nursing. She received certification from the University of Washington to teach parent-child interpersonal and environmental assessment skills. She has studied child health, family health, and comparative health systems and has presented her findings to local, national, and international professional assemblies. Currently, she is studying children in homeless family situations.

Nancy O'Connor, MSN, RNC, is Assistant Professor of Nursing at Oakland University in Rochester, Michigan, and is also certified by the American Nurses' Association as an Adult Nurse Practitioner. She is currently a doctoral student in nursing at Wayne State University in Detroit, Michigan. Her research interests include the nurse-patient relationship, primary care nursing practice, and nursing education for advanced clinical practice.

Karen S. Reed is an Associate Professor in the College of Nursing at the University of Akron, Ohio. Her association with Betty Neuman began in 1979 at Ohio University, where Dr. Neuman first encouraged her to explore the idea of family as a client system. That work was published in the 1982 edition of *The Neuman Systems Model*. She has spent the past 12 years continuing to incorporate family constructs within the Neuman model and was a contributor to the 1989 edition of Neuman's book. She has presented the family-focused material at several national and international conferences on nursing theory and family nursing. Her most recent work has focused on developing a family assessment model based on the Neuman systems model (NFAM). Her current research interests focus on testing the family assessment model and the impact of perinatal loss on families. Recent publications include an article on miscarriages in *Image*, an article on the development of NFAM in *Nursing Science Quarterly*, and two book chapters on family and psychiatric disorders in children in the pediatric textbook *Child Health Nursing*.

Cheryl L. Reynolds, PhD, MS, RN, served as a hospital corpswoman in the U.S. Navy and the U.S. Naval Reserve and was awarded a special commendation with her honorable discharge. She received her BSN from Northern Michigan University in Marquette and her MS from Arizona State University in Tempe. She has been a professor of nursing for the past 10 years at Northern Michigan University where she teaches both graduate and undergraduate students, has been instrumental in the development and delivery of the Adult Health Clinical Nurse Specialist program, and has received numerous awards and honors for her scholarship. Her area of special expertise is research and theory development related to health promotion phenomena. During her doctoral studies in nursing at Wayne State University in Detroit, she studied the health promotion beliefs of the Ojibwe people.

Norma Jean Schmieding, EdD, RN, is Professor of Nursing at the University of Rhode Island College of Nursing. She is a diploma graduate of Lincoln General Hospital School of Nursing in Lincoln, Nebraska, and has a BS from Nebraska Wesleyan University, also in Lincoln. Her master's degree in nursing administration was obtained at Boston University, where she also received her doctorate in 1983. Her career has been divided between nursing service and nursing education. In the early 1970s, as Director of Nursing Service at Boston City Hospital she implemented Orlando's theory. She is an expert on Orlando's theory and has used it extensively in nursing service and research. Her publications include those on theoretical and concept analyses, research, and application to nursing service.

Louise C. Selanders, EdD, RN, is Assistant Professor of Nursing at Michigan State University in East Lansing. She completed her doctorate in educational leadership at Western Michigan University in Kalamazoo. Her research interests include nursing history, sociological issues in nursing education, and nursing administration.

Christina L. Sieloff, RN, MSN, CNA, received her BSN in 1970 from Wayne State University's College of Nursing in Detroit, Michigan. In 1977, she returned to Wayne State for her MSN (major: Nursing Administration; minor: Psychiatric/Mental Health Nursing with Children and Adolescents) and is now a doctoral student in nursing there. Certified by the American Nurses' Association as a Nurse Administrator, she is Clinical Director of an inpatient adult psychiatric unit at Oakland General Hospital in Madison Heights, Michigan. A member of the Detroit District of the Michigan Nurses' Association, American Nurses' Association, she is active at the district, state, and national levels. She is also a member of Sigma Theta Tau and the Wayne State University Alumni Association and has written several publications that focus on psychiatric nursing and nursing administration.